Rosemary Gladstar's
FAMILY HERBAL

Rosemary Gladstar's

FAMILYHERBAL

A Guide to Living Life
with Energy, Health, and Vitality

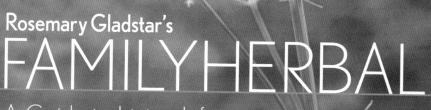

STOREY
BOOKS

North Adams, Massachusetts

The mission of Storey Publishing is to serve our customers by publishing practical information that encourages personal independence in harmony with the environment.

This publication is intended to provide educational information for the reader on the covered subject. It is not intended to take the place of personalized medical counseling, diagnosis, and treatment from a trained health professional.

Edited by Nancy W. Ringer
Cover and text design by Wendy Palitz
Book layout by Susan Bernier and Erin Lincourt
Photograph credits given on page 399
Indexed by Susan Olason, Indexes & Knowledge Maps

Printed in China by Regent Publishing
10 9 8 7 6 5 4 3 2 1

Library of Congress Cataloging-in-Publication Data

Gladstar, Rosemary.
[Family Herbal]
Rosemary Gladstar's family herbal: a guide to living life with energy, health, and vitality.
p. cm.
Includes index.
ISBN 1-58017-425-6 (alk. paper)
1. Herbs—Therapeutic use. 2. Health. I. Title: Family herbal.
RM666.H33 G528 2001
615'.321—dc21
                                          2001032783

Contents

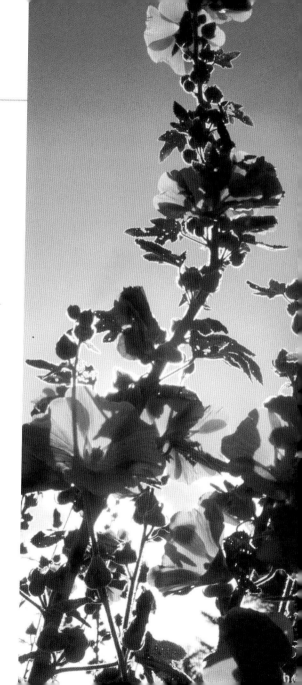

Dedication

There is a circle, green hands enfolded, lives entwined, of fellow herbalists. I've held each of their hands and laughed and prayed with them, these old friends who influenced my earliest teachings. Their thoughts are embedded in my heart and flow into the words of this book. At a time when herbalism wasn't popular or faddish, we "followed our bliss," our green passion. Now practically elders, ever more impassioned by the green world, we face a new millennium, wondering not what the world has in store for herbalism but what the herbs have in store for us.

With all my heart, this book is dedicated to my family of fellow herbalists. You have guided, nourished, and fed me on this journey into the green. You are the sparks that light my way. May the circle ever grow and the weeds be plentiful.

And in sweet memory of Gail Ulrich; she walked the beauty way.

Acknowledgments

A book is never born alone but is the collective vision and hard work of many. First, I must thank my partner and dearest friend, Robert Chartier, for his unending support, kindness, and passion for the earth. He makes my life more joyful. Great credit must be given to my editor, Nancy Ringer, whose patience and gentlest prodding are the only reasons this book ever made it past the first rough draft. She was a wonder in every way. I also wish to thank Deborah Balmuth of Storey Books for her integrity and vision, as well as the entire Storey staff — what delightful people! I felt nourished and supported in every way.

Thanks also flow readily to Rocio Alarcon, Svevo Brooks, Stephen Buhner, Cascade Anderson Geller, Christopher Hobbs, Tieraona Low Dog, Paul Strauss, and David Winston; their teachings continue to inspire me and are woven into the leafy fabric of my own lessons. My gratitude is great.

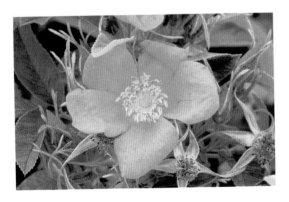

Foreword by James A. Duke, Ph.D.

Rosemary, the herb of remembrance, and the memorable Rosemary Gladstar have much in common. Both are stimulating, ethereal, and volatile, beautifully enhancing any setting they chance to alight in. Inspirational, effervescent, innervating . . . enlightening to both the mood and the intellect . . . challenging, whether with aromatic vapors or ephemeral ideas . . . these characteristics are the essence of R(r)osemary.

Photosynthesis, the manufacture of useful things from simple ingredients in the presence of sunshine, blesses our planet with oxygen, green foods, and green medicines; it embraces and purifies the soil, rescues the atmosphere from pollutants, and provides communion and peace. Through photosynthesis, plants draw on the sun's power to prepare the chemicals necessary for life on earth. Anyone who sees Rosemary Gladstar in her green gardens, caressed by spring, summer, and autumn light, wonders whether she, too, might draw her unending energy from the sun. It's no wonder that she is the driving force behind the herbalist movement. She may not have chlorophyll, but she certainly has green charisma, green passion, green wisdom, and green spirit.

It is not only Rosemary's enthusiastic and authoritative lectures, teachings, and writings that I praise, but her unflagging dedication to green causes, such as United Plant Savers, which vigorously promotes the salvation of endangered medicinal plants in North America. Having brought so much to the herbalist movement, Rosemary now brings us this great and useful book, *Rosemary Gladstar's Family Herbal.* A delightful guide to a green lifestyle, it will certainly help you and your loved ones live healthier, happier, more joyful lives. As Rosemary writes, "Everyday radiant well-being, in mind, body, and soul, is a function of everyday self-care. It's a prescription for life. It's a part of what you do, what you take into your body, and what you feed your mind. Radiant well-being is . . . finding your joy in life. Exploring your passions. . . . Whatever you choose to do, do it well, and do it joyously." The information, advice, recipes, and stories that Rosemary — the gladdest of herbalism's superstars — provides in this treasury will help and inspire you and your family to achieve radiant well-being and enjoy a well-lived life.

To your health! Think green!

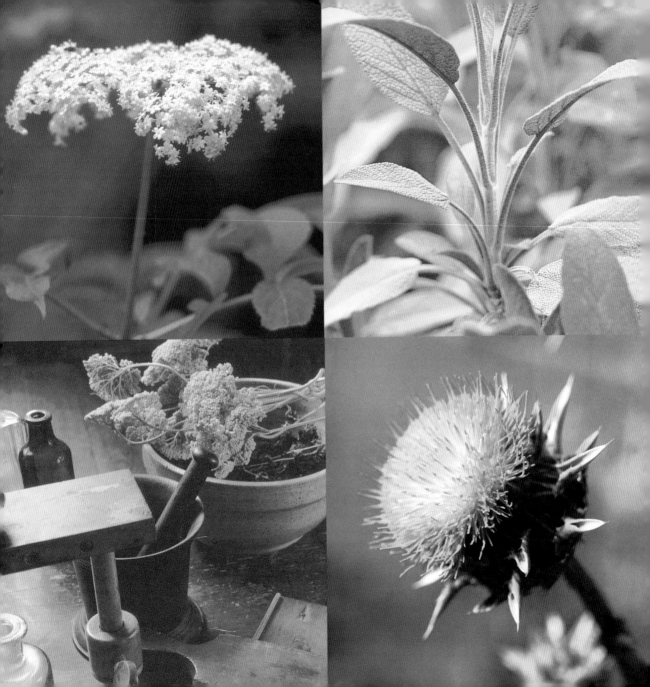

1 Eco-Logical Herbalism

This book began, at the urging of my friends, as a project to collect my various writings and teachings that span the past 30 years into one volume that could serve as a practical home guide to herbal health care. I must admit, I was reluctant at first to take on the project. I couldn't imagine what I might possibly add to the rich treasury of herbal medicine that hasn't already been written — and, in many cases, written quite well. But months later, as I finished up the pages of what has turned out to be a rather hefty volume, I realized that the teachings shared here have a vitally important purpose. They are not necessarily new, astounding, or complex, but they serve as a firm reminder of the roots of herbalism: Our heartfelt connection to the plants. I wanted to create a guide to sustainable herbal medicine for the entire family. My hope is that this book will be used and cherished, the pages dog-eared and the cover crackled with time, and, just as important, that it will bring to the forefront of our consciousness the idea that our health is integrally linked to that of the world around us. Then I will know the book is truly worth not only my time — and yours — but also, perhaps, the lives of the trees that were used to make it.

ancient medicine for modern times

At a time when herbalism is being overrun with the "-tions" of modern culture — that is, standardization, legalization, certification, and other such bureaucratic challenges — I wish simply to remind each of you who pick up this book that herbs have been used by humans as food and as medicine for hundreds of thousands of years, far back into the recesses of time. We have evolved thanks to the generosity of our green neighbors, our lives dependent on them for oxygen, food, medicine, clothing, and spiritual insight. If there's even the smallest shred of truth in the adage "You are what you eat," our bodies are enmeshed with theirs. Plant life has been the basis of our food chain for the past several thousand years. Before we took those first upright awkward steps,

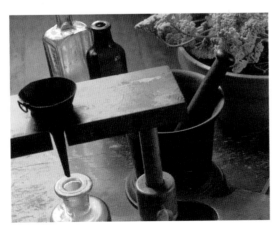

teetered, then realized we could run, hunt, and kill, we were gatherers, our sole source of nutrients coming from the plants, the green biomass that grows from the heart of the earth. Plants were our first and greatest medicine. In fact, the World Health Organization estimates that more than 80 percent of the world's population still uses herbal medicine as a primary system of healing. In this day and age of modern miracle medicine, we're sometimes encouraged to believe that herbalism is merely myths and old wives' tales. If herbs weren't effective medicine, wouldn't a species intelligent enough to put a man on the moon have discarded them a long time ago? In fact, it is in part because plant medicine has been so effective, despite raging plagues, disease, famine, and warfare, that humans have not only survived but multiplied beyond reason.

The terminology of plant medicine changes through the ages, different systems evolve depending on climate and costume, and various plants rise and fall in popularity, but the core truth remains the same: Herbalism is an effective, natural, and inexpensive system of healing readily available to every human who chooses to use it. We have eons of human experience to prove it.

Modern science often validates through meticulous study what our ancestors instinctively knew about the medicinal power of plants. This research has the potential to provide another window into the world of plants. Unfortunately, however, the information provided by science can be misleading because it is often based on studies of a single plant constituent or dosages that are far more concentrated than nature ever intended to provide. Though it's interesting to speculate how herbs work on the body, we're not much closer than we were a few centuries ago to understanding what makes a plant work. The myriad constituents each plant contains only partially explain its complex actions on the human body. When you consider how many thousands of plants there are, each with its own unique chemical blueprint, you begin to understand the daunting nature of this approach. What's been proved by centuries of empirical evidence is not easily proved by science. The plants pay no attention to our modern predicament. These most ancient of beings simply go on living and growing, thriving and multiplying, providing the substances of our life: food, shelter, medicine, oxygen, and beauty.

honoring the plants

Long before we had electronic databases or comprehensive scientific tomes filled with information about herbs, humans knew and understood the healing power of plants. I am convinced that this knowing came from an intrinsic sense of relationship with the plants, not simply a trial-and-error process, as we often postulate. Imagine, if you would, our ancestors, suffering from burning

There are innumerable **great minds and souls** who, by their words, deeds, and writings, contributed to the rich body of herbal knowledge that has been passed down to us. Most of the herbalists who were instrumental in creating and recording this collective system of healing will never receive recognition, yet we carry the **seeds of their knowledge** each time we use plants as medicine. So when someone asks me if a particular formula or recipe is my own, I have to smile. What I know about herbs is shared information, passed down to me sometimes from people I know well and often from people who lived hundreds of years before me. It is our collective treasury, **our birthright,** and it is meant to be freely shared.

getting perspective on safety

Many reports have surfaced recently about the dangers of herbal medicine. Even perfectly benign plants such as chamomile and peppermint are finding themselves on the "herbal blacklist." Are we just now discovering the dangers of herbs? No — but we are now able to ingest herbs in tremendously potent forms. In the past, herbs were most often taken as teas, tinctures, and syrups. But herbal capsules, which make it easy for us to swallow as much herb as we wish, and standardized preparations, which contain extracts of herbal constituents that are far more concentrated than nature ever intended, have not been available until recently.

Few herbs are actually toxic, but just about any herb may occasionally stimulate an idiosyncratic reaction in an individual. Strawberries, for example, are sweet nectar to some and noxious to others. This doesn't make the berry toxic; it's just a poor choice for that particular individual.

Don't be scared off from herbal medicine by a few dramatic news stories. Use your head. Herbs are powerful medicine, but they don't always have the same effect on everyone. Take the time to get to know the herbs and how they affect you; you'll reap the benefits of energy, health, and vitality for years to come.

fevers, congestive croup, or bloody wounds, trying, by trial and error, to figure out which plant worked best for the situation. There are hundreds of thousands of plants on this earth and thousands that grow in any given area. It would have taken eons longer than we've been on this planet to document the information that we know about the medicinal uses of plants. Did we simply experiment until we got it right? No. Trial and error played a part in our understanding, but most of what we know about plant medicines came through and from the plants themselves.

Plants have an innate ability to communicate with people. Although I believe that almost anybody can learn to listen to the plants, there are certain people — the green witches, herbalists, healers, botanists, keepers of the green — who lend an ear more readily. In traditional cultures, herb gatherers asked permission from the plant before harvesting it for medicine. This was considered essential for learning and retaining the healing power of the plant, and it was also a gesture of respect. Sometimes when I'm trying to find an appropriate remedy, I ask the plants themselves for help, and I get a feeling about which plant is right. This isn't a special gift; many people have it, but most forget how to use it. As you become more familiar with working with plants and using herbal remedies, this skill begins to mature. It won't replace book learning, but it will guide your understanding of plant medicine.

nurturing herbal wisdom in today's world

In the past, in cultures around the world, children who had a special gift with plants were recognized early. These children underwent a lengthy, rigorous apprenticeship with the local herbalist, community healer, or shaman. They became the healers of their communities, and so the tradition was carried down through the ages.

Today we still have children who are "plant sensitives," who seem to carry a gene of "green blood" in them. You recognize them at family gatherings, on playgrounds, and in schools: girls and boys absorbed in grass and weeds, lost in play for hours in the garden, enchanted by the pollen-covered insects and butterflies lazing on the launching pads of freshly opened blossoms. They play games with the flowers and woodland plants, speak of gnomes and fairies in the wild, and seem to have a special rapport with all of nature. They must be called and called and called again when it's time for them to come inside. Watch for these children. In the old days, they were the "keepers of the green," and they were recognized as future wise ones and healers.

Though herbology is generally recognized and honored as our oldest system of healing, much of the art of herbalism is at risk today. It suffers from lack of understanding, bureaucratic tangles, economic pressure, environmental destruction, and loss of connection with the earth. Our future healers are pulled away from their calling by television, concrete, and the carefully supervised, filled-to-the-minute schedules that today's children live by. We must take our children to the wild, introduce them to the plants, and teach them of their connection to the earth. In instilling in our children a respect for plant medicine, we not only care for their tender bodies but help pass along the seeds

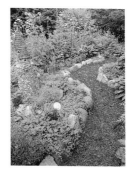

of a tradition that is as old as human life itself. We teach them to respect and care for the planet, for you cannot have a relationship with the plants without entering fully into a relationship with Gaia, the living earth.

replanting the fields

Not only the art of herbalism but also the plants themselves are threatened. A gypsy at heart and by blood, I've traveled a fair amount in my life. I have seen many places of botanical beauty and have sat at the feet of many wise practitioners of plant medicine. However, I've also observed a trend that frightens me: Almost everywhere I've traveled, even in places where herbal traditions are alive and well, native plant populations are in dire straits. China, for example, long regarded for its

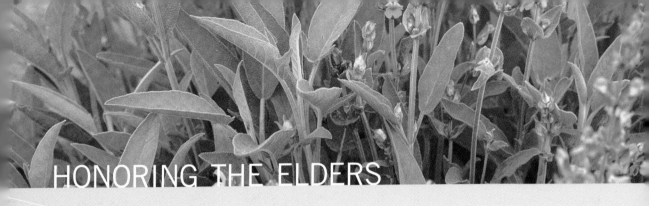

HONORING THE ELDERS

Sambucus nigra, **the elder tree,** is often planted in the center of the herb garden and is said to be the guardian of the garden, the keeper of the green. The other plants in the garden look to it for protection, wisdom, and strength. So it is with the elders of our herbal community.

As a teenager, my stepdaughter Melanie said to me, "Herbalists are like fine wine, aren't they? They become more valuable as they age." Though I had never looked at it quite in that light, she was right. In the herbal community, elders are still considered the wisdom keepers, and their knowledge of the plants and teachings are sought after. At conferences and events they are guests of honor, and younger herbalists travel great distances to meet and study with them. Why is this?

Aside from the fact that these individuals are often great characters, wonderfully entertaining and full of stories, they have lived rich and meaningful lives, and their experiences reach in and touch us, giving our own lives meaning. It is the elders who have kept the teachings of herbalism alive through generations of time, the wise ones who taught the children how to find the plants, how to speak with them, and how to make medicine from them. This lineage, though weakened, still lives on, and our hearts hunger for this connection to our traditions.

Often, we find in our herbal elders a passion for and a commitment to their vision and life that is extraordinary. They light the way for us. Though many of the elders I have known and loved have passed on, their teachings live on in those whose lives they've touched. And, likewise, the teachings of the green will live on through us.

enduring herbal tradition, is almost entirely devoid of its most important wild medicinal plants, their populations having been almost completely annihilated by wildcrafters. India, with two million acres of herbs under cultivation, is the world's largest producer of medicinal plants, but its wild native plant populations are sparse and scarce. In modern Greece, one is hard-pressed to find the fields of wild herbs or the great majestic forests that Homer described so poetically in the *Iliad*. Everywhere you look, the wild kingdom of plants is under siege, and failing fast.

When I return home to my own Vermont woodlands, I marvel anew at the great expanse of wilderness that stretches before me. I've come to fully appreciate the wealth of biodiversity that remains in this young, eager land and the degree to which it is changing before our very eyes. As elsewhere in the world, habitat loss, overpopulation, poor logging practices, and poor wildcrafting practices are diminishing plant populations in North America. Sudden surges in popularity for a particular plant — consider the 1990s St.-John's-wort craze — can cause irreparable harm to that plant's population status, if not monitored carefully. Perhaps the fact that herbal medicine became widely unpopular and even illegal to practice in the United States from the 1940s through the late 1980s (in fact, herbal medicine is still technically illegal to practice, despite its popularity) was the saving grace for our native wild plant populations. Forced underground, the plants and the tradition that grew from them set deep roots and flourished quietly.

The Price of Popularity

Habitat loss is, without a doubt, the greatest threat to plants. But what effect is the sudden resurgence of interest in herbal medicine having on our dwindling plant resources? The herbal industry reached the $5 billion mark at the turn of the millennium and is growing rapidly. Large drug companies have entered the herbal marketplace with their usual "profit at any cost" attitude. Hundreds of small and midsize herbal-product companies have sprung up across North America in the past few years, and herb shops can be found in almost every community. Where do all the plants needed for this vast amount of industry originate? Until very recently, large-scale cultivation of medicinal herbs in the United

"Frances Thompson, the English poet, once wrote that **one could not pluck a flower without troubling a star.** If we cannot pluck a flower without troubling a star, what then if we lose a species?"

— **Loren Isrealson**
Board member, United Plant Savers

States was rare. Almost all of the resources used in making botanical medicine came either from third-world countries, which generally have less than ideal growing agricultural practices, or from our wildlands.

But our wildlands are in stress. In 1998, a 20-year, 16-organization, worldwide study was released. It reported that approximately 12.5 percent, or 34,000 of the world's plant species, were threatened, and that in the United States, 29 percent of the nation's 16,000 species were in imminent danger of extinction. Until recently, little attention has been paid to the destruction of plant species except in the tropical rain forest. As Steven Foster, well-known author and plant photographer, commented, "Plants, unlike animals, are not warm, cute, or fuzzy and, therefore, don't catch the public's attention so readily." Yet without plants, we can't survive. And who would want to? Imagine a world devoid of plants — barren, cold, lifeless.

"Never doubt that a small group of thoughtful, **committed citizens can change the world**; indeed, it is the only thing that ever has."

—Margaret Mead

Shortly after moving to my wilderness home in the Green Mountains of Vermont, I began to realize that many of the oldest plants of the eastern deciduous forests, including many important medicinal plants, had either completely disappeared or were in short supply. One spring as I was hiking, stepping over the wake-robins and adder's-tongues of early spring, feeling a certain despair, an abiding loss at the disappearance of these sweet earth medicines, I heard a voice ascending from the forest around me. It was plain and directive and said rather simply, "Plant us. Bring us back to our communities." Having listened to plants all my life, I had no doubt about what I heard and what I was being asked to do. That fall, I ordered several pounds of endangered plants — American ginseng, goldenseal, black cohosh, and bloodroot — and reintroduced them to my woodlands. I planted them back into the native landscape where once — before logging, before sheep farming, before haying and mowing, before the stone walls of the early New England farmers — these plants had thrived in abundant communities. To be honest, I really didn't know what I was doing, and many of these early plantings fared poorly. Soil conditions, pH factors, the changing overstory, and the quality of the rootstock I ordered were all factors I hardly thought to consider. I was acting from pure enthusiasm and ignorance, an impractical combination, but it lit a fire in my heart and fueled me onward.

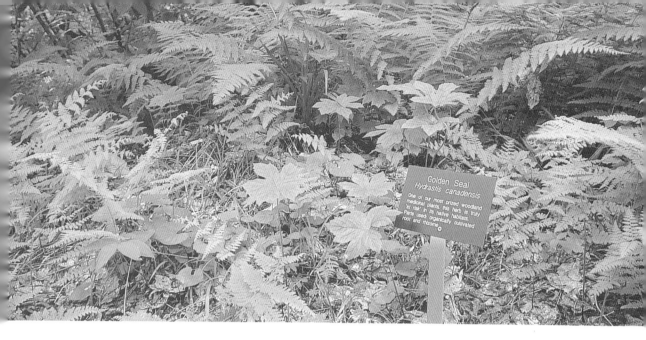

Those early plantings were the beginning of a project that has since reshaped my life's work and become a driving passion. Having spent the greater part of my life studying medicinal plants, working as a community herbalist, wildcrafting, making herbal products, and educating others about the ancient and marvelous system of herbal medicine, I suddenly found myself thrust into new territory: the intricate network of wild plant communities. How did these healing plants grow in their native landscape? How did the plant communities fare when important members of the medicinal clan disappeared from their ecosystem? These powerful plants are as valued for the well-being of the earth and the wild plant communities as they are for the two-leggeds, the humans who have been dependent on them for thousands of years. What happens when a plant community becomes unbalanced? When a medicine is removed from the community? Are the ever-diminishing numbers of these powerful medicine plants one of the reasons there are so many more diseases attacking both our native plant and human populations?

United Plant Savers

Out of a deep concern for what I felt was happening to our wild plant communities, I began talking with fellow herbalists, and I found that many of them had similar concerns. Feeling a growing need, a small group of dedicated individuals met at the International Herb

Symposium held at Wheaton College, near Boston, in 1994 to discuss native medicinal plant conservation and what we could do to become a voice for the plants. We became the United Plant Savers (UpS). Dedicated to the conservation and cultivation of North American medicinal plants and the habitat they thrive in, UpS has grown to be the major voice for medicinal plant conservation in the United States.

"The beauty and genius of a work of art
May be reconceived,
Though its first material expression
 be destroyed;
A vanished harmony may yet again
Inspire the composer;
But, when the last individual of a
 race of living beings
Breathes no more,
Another heaven and another earth
 must pass
Before such a one can be again."

— A sign at the Belize City Zoo
for Endangered Species

Formed in the spirit of hope by people who love and know plants, our organization reflects the great diversity of American herbalism. Our membership includes herbalists, doctors, nurses, naturopaths, botanists, organic farmers, business owners, wildcrafters, seed savers, manufacturers, and plant lovers from all walks of life.

United Plant Savers has initiated a number of projects, including plant giveaways in which more than 50,000 goldenseal roots and several thousand other at-risk plants have been distributed to members to plant on their land. Our most complex task to date was defining and developing the medicinal plant At Risk List and the accompanying To Watch List (see page 400), which have become guiding sources for the herbal industry, herbalists, and those who use herbal products. We encourage people to act as stewards of existing wild medicinal plants by spreading seed within the habitat and by weeding out nonnative species. We also encourage gardeners to propagate at-risk medicinal plants in their backyards, gardens, farms, and privately owned lands, and to monitor their status from season to season. A few years ago, UpS purchased a 370-acre farm in southeastern Ohio. This beautiful piece of earth holds a rich repository of medicinal herbs, many of which are on the UpS At Risk List. A teaching center, farm, and outdoor research "lab," this site is being set up as a model of a sustainable botanical sanctuary.

Of great importance, UpS encourages people who love and use plants to become responsible consumers: Know where the plants you are using come from. Know if they're listed on the UpS At Risk List or are considered rare or endangered in your region. Buy organically cultivated herbs when possible, supporting the survival not only of the wild plant communities but also of another endangered species, the American farmer.

herbalism for the future

Herbal medicine is truly a wonderful system of medicine. Used joyously and judiciously, herbs are capable of bringing incredible health, energy, and vitality into our lives. But, in turn, if we choose to use plants as our medicine, we then become accountable for the wild gardens, for their health and upkeep. We undertake a partnership with the plants, giving back what we receive — health, nourishment, beauty, and protection.

We have reached a time in history when not to respect and replenish the cocreative relationship we have with the resources we use on this small and beautiful planet would be disastrous. We are at a critical point in our planetary evolution. With this book, I invite you to take part in creating a vibrant, radiant world that supports all beings, great and small, in balance and in health. I invite you to join in the effort to help seed the future with eco-logical herbalism.

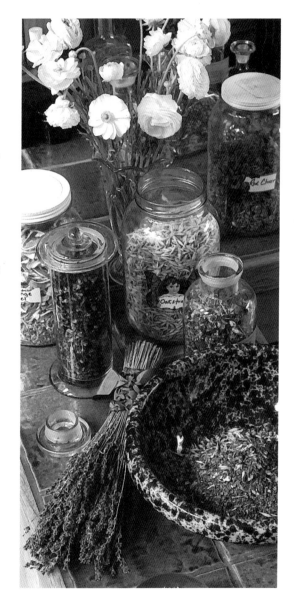

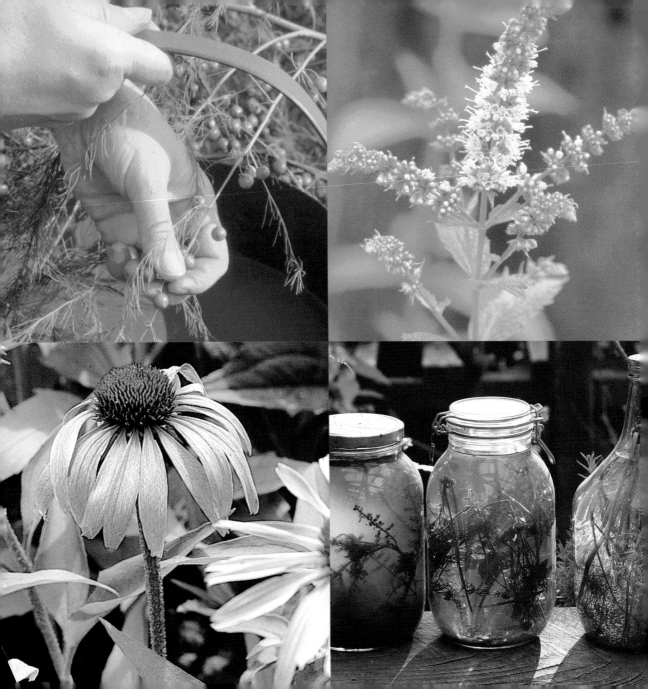

2 A Prescription for Life

There is no great secret to good health. Despite the bombardment of advertising from the health and beauty industries that offers an instant pill or cure-all for the woes and illnesses of life, good health is, in truth, the practice of living healthfully every day. If we become susceptible to illness, lack vitality, or feel unfocused or lethargic, it's generally due not to any mysterious illness but, rather, to lack of exercise, lack of sleep, poor dietary practices, and too little quality time with friends and family.

You can't get energy, health, and vitality from a pill, or even from a cup of herbal tea. Everyday radiant well-being, in mind, body, and soul, is a function of everyday self-care. It's a prescription for life. It's a part of what you do, what you take into your body, and what you feed your mind. Radiant well-being is not taking a pill for this pain, a dose of X for that problem, a quick fix to get rid of the lethargy you're dragging around with you. Radiant well-being is, instead, finding your joy in life. Exploring your passions. Getting up from your chair and moving your body. Wiggling. Eating good food. Playing hard and resting well. Putting your mind to work. Laughing.

Whatever you choose to do, do it well, and do it joyously. There is no greater benefactor to well-being than the satisfaction of a well-lived life.

living healthy

Achieving radiant health and vitality doesn't have to be difficult, nor does it require "medical" intervention. Your body is designed to run at optimal levels, and given the opportunity, it will. All it needs is a little care from you, including exercise, good food, and enough sleep. By putting into practice the simple guidelines that follow, you can reinvigorate your body, your mind, and your life.

"We need the tonic of the wilderness," said Henry David Thoreau. The ocean, the mountains, the deserts, a wooded grove — all contain the **"magic"** needed to restore pure radiant energy to a stressed soul. Mother Earth in all of her infinite compassion and strength has remarkable powers to restore vitality. **Wash yourself in the pure water** of the streams, put your bare feet on the good earth, fall asleep in the arms of an ancient tree. There is good medicine to be found in nature. It is long lasting and heals the soul.

For even more ideas on the practices of healthy living, consult my favorite little book on the topic: *The Art of Good Living*, written by naturopathic doctor Svevo Brooks.

Exercise Is Essential

Humans need to exercise. We were not meant to sit at desks all day, not moving our bodies. Fatigue and ill health are often the result of oxygen-deficient cells. Vigorous physical work is accompanied by an increase in breathing and heartbeat, which causes a rapid exchange of oxygen on a cellular level. The entire body is revitalized and uplifted via the cells.

Mental work, in which so many people are involved today, is far more fatiguing than physical work. The brain requires a greater rejuvenation time than the body, and mental work definitely does not increase oxygen levels in the body. For good health, exercise daily. Any type of exercise will do, depending on your individual needs.

Some people respond best to mind-quieting yoga practices, while others are able to "let off steam" in aerobic activities. It's important to realize that the body needs movement every day, and you need to find the kind of activity that works best for you. I might also suggest that you not forgo "life exercise" in favor of a gym regimen. Be sure to get out and hike, bike, ski, and play games, and let your body and spirit interact with the life around you. For me, there's something far more physically satisfying in stacking a cord of wood than in pedaling a stationary bike.

Maintain a Balanced Diet

Diet is another of those simple, marvelously effective keys to health and vitality. It's not always necessary or even beneficial to follow strict dietary disciplines. Rather, follow the laws of healthy eating: Eat food as close to nature as possible, eat what's in season, prepare it simply, chew slowly, and give thanks. Your diet is perfect when it is really enhancing who you are — your skin looks good, your hair looks good, and you just glow wonderfully. It is a simple thing for us to be aware of. If I'm feeling a little sluggish, I know that I've had too many cookies or that I'm not drinking enough water; whatever the case may be, the message is very clear: My body is telling me that I'm not eating well.

We've all heard that old saying, wise in its simplicity, "You are what you eat." Perhaps it's just as true that you are what you don't eat. What we do and don't eat, a healthy daily dose of exercise, good sleeping habits, and a positive perspective on life are the golden keys to a high-quality, productive life.

Whole foods contain all the nutrients your body needs to properly assimilate and use the food. While high-quality therapeutic supplements are fine for remedying problems, they do not provide the whole spectrum of nutrients,

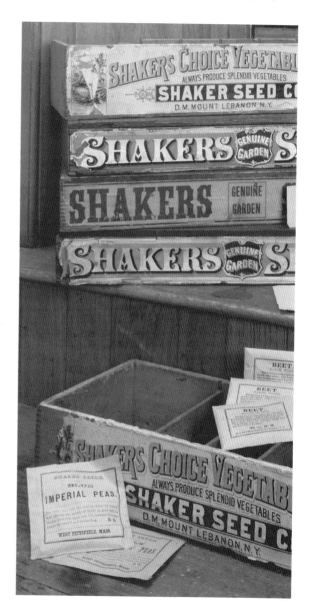

and they certainly don't provide them in a manner that our bodies have been evolving with for many centuries. Supplements are excellent at times, but I think we have fooled ourselves into thinking they are natural foods; they are not. They are most often made in chemical labs; they are not at all like the food that nature designed for us to eat. It's not that I don't use or recommend vitamins; I just use them as I would use drugs: for serious health issues.

There is an ongoing debate among nutritionists concerning our supposed inability to obtain all the nutrients we need from food. This is a sad argument at best. Organic agriculture based on sustainable, renewable practices replenishes both the earth and our bodies and provides wholesome, high-quality food rich in the total spectrum of nutrients. If we insist on eating demineralized processed food, then, yes, the chances of getting all the necessary nutrients are highly questionable. If one further argues that organic food is priced beyond the average person, check out the price of vitamin and mineral supplements. What we save on supplementing our diet with these pills can buy a lot of organic food. But everyone, even those with the smallest garden space, can grow an organic vegetable garden. In fact, in addition to providing high-quality food and the satisfaction of restoring the earth, gardening is one of the best therapies available for stress and anxiety.

yin/yang: the theory of opposites

Throughout this book, I use the terms *yang* and *yin,* which refer to certain complementary energetics inherent in all life forms. *Yin* and *yang* make up an ancient Chinese philosophy of opposites.

Generally speaking, *yang* refers to an expansive energy. Qualities associated with yang include warm, dry, male, sun, day, fire, light, heaven. Yang energy moves up and outward, expanding into the world. It is the creative or firm principle.

Yin refers to a contractive or inward force. Qualities associated with yin are cool, moon, night, water, cold, dampness, darkness, female, earth. Yin energy moves downward and inward. It is the receptive or yielding principle.

Men and women, food, movement, art — all of life can be represented to varying degrees by the principles of yin and yang. A healthy, harmonious life is created by continuously striving for a balance between yin and yang, the contractive and the expansive.

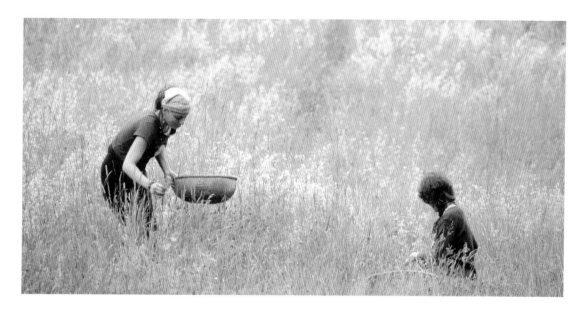

Get the Rest and Relaxation Your Body Needs

Just as important as exercise are appropriate amounts of rest and relaxation. So often in our lives, as we're buried under the stress of unbalanced living, we forget to care lovingly for ourselves. Some of the most basic human needs, such as a loving and supportive environment, good nutrition, exercise, rest, and relaxation, are sacrificed. We look for instant cures and remedies in the drugs that are available today and dig ourselves further into the pits of our despair. But remedies are more often found in basic lifestyle changes; these are the true "medicines" that create balance and harmony.

Chemicals such as seratonin are produced only during particular times of sleep and are vitally necessary for mental function. Sleep is needed not so much to rest our bodies as to rest our minds. The body needs little more than two hours of sleep per day to function, but parts of the brain need seven to eight hours to be fully recharged and rested. There are simple but highly effective methods that ensure that one gets more rest in times of stress. Above all, remember to avoid staying up late at night, and learn to say no to extra activities, especially those in the late evening. Though they may be fun and entertaining, many of those extra activities require the very energy needed to refuel and restore a depleted nervous system. Whenever something seems really important or necessary to do, ask yourself how much energy it will require. Remind yourself that what is most important in your life at this time is feeling really good, rested, and vital. I think often of the biblical story of Joseph and the coffers of grain he stored as insurance against famine. To me, this story is a reminder of the access we have to plentiful energy. But for that energy to be everlasting, we must not use it all up. We must also replenish the energy we borrow from the coffers by sleeping, eating well, exercising, and striving to live lives of harmony and balance.

what are we talking about?

Homeostasis: A maintained state of health where all checks and balances among interdependent elements of mind, body, and spirit are functioning harmoniously (as defined in *From Earth to Herbalist*, by Gregory Tilford)

Longevity: A long duration of individual life

Vitality: Capacity to live and develop; physical or mental vigor; power of enduring

Well-being: The state of being happy, healthy, or prosperous

You also may wish to review the suggestions for relieving insomnia (see page 61) for tips and natural therapies that can help ensure that you get deep, restful sleep every night.

Eliminate Undue Stress

If we are to believe what our centenarians tell us, the key precept for good health and long life is simple: Eliminate chronic stress.

There are many different kinds of stress. A passionate kiss is stressful; it excites your being. The excitement of going on a journey is stressful. For me, getting up and giving lectures creates a lot of stress. I always say that I'm an introvert living in an extrovert's body. Speaking in public still makes me nervous. But sometimes stress is useful. It can help you work more efficiently, act more quickly, and take on challenges you might otherwise turn away from.

However, a little stress goes a long way. Many of us, in our hectic and harried lives, face undue or overwhelming stress almost every minute of the day. If your body is not in an excellent state of health — which chronic stress can severely compromise — stress leads to anxiety, emotional imbalance, and physical illness.

If you find that you are having trouble handling stressful situations or that you feel "burned out" from chronic stress, see chapter 4 for suggestions on strengthening and revitalizing your nervous system.

Use Herbs Every Day for Health and Vitality

Don't wait until you're sick to use herbs. The best way to cure illness is not to become ill, and there is a wonderful variety of longevity, nutritive, and tonic herbs that can and should be used daily to enhance wellness.

Nutritive herbs to make a regular part of your diet include horsetail, passionflower, cleavers, chickweed, red clover, and lemon balm.

Tonic herbs feed, tone, rehabilitate, and strengthen particular body systems. Tonics for particular systems are listed in the chart at right.

Longevity herbs are not life extenders; what they will do is increase quality of life, so that you feel better and better as you grow older. I consider our very common weeds to be America's most vital healing plants. They are powerful and abundant, and the more you try to run over them and dig them out, the happier they are. When I teach classes on longevity, I stress many of these plants, such as dandelion, nettle, burdock, and oats, not only because they offer chemical benefits but also because they embody a tremendous determination to survive. We tend to love the exotica, those very shy, very beautiful plants. They have special energy, certainly. But it is the weeds, those vulgar plants that grow everywhere, challenging us, that espouse true vitality and a passion for life. These are the longevity herbs. When their hardy spirits come into you, they feed you and make you stronger.

REVITALIZING HERBS AND SUPPLEMENTS

This is a quick look at the herbs and supplements that are used to maintain the health and vitality of various parts of the body. Use these herbs on a regular basis for best effect.

Body Part or System	Herb or Supplement
Blood	Burdock, dandelion
Bones	Nettle, oats
Brain	Ginkgo, gotu kola
Eyes	Bilberry, lutein
Heart (cardiovascular system)	Cayenne, garlic, hawthorn
Kidneys	Dandelion leaf, nettle
Liver	Burdock root, dandelion root
Muscles	Fo-ti, glucosamine sulfate
Nerves	Ginseng, nettle, oats
Nervous system (endurance and stamina)	Fo-ti, American ginseng, Siberian ginseng
Spirit	Flower essences, kava-kava

superfoods for well-being

Superfoods are whole foods that are naturally concentrated with important nutrients. They are nature's original vitamin and mineral supplements and may actually be the precursor of the supplement industry. Although vitamin and mineral supplement have their place and are useful therapeutic agents, superfoods provide whole-spectrum nutrients as only nature can. Most supplements, while useful in the same manner that drugs can be valuable, are generally made from unnatural substances — contrary to what the labels may claim.

> "These primitive organisms [algae] were among the first life forms. In spirulina, we find **three and one-half billion years of life** on this planet encoded in nucleic acids (RNA/DNA). At the same time, algae supplies that fresh burst of primal essence that manifested when life was in its birthing stages."
>
> — **Paul Pitchford,**
> ***Healing with Whole Foods***

Spirulina: The Protein Powerhouse

Spirulina is a blue-green algae that grows on freshwater ponds. Respected in many cultures for centuries as an excellent source of nutrition, it found its way into the U.S. diet just a decade or two ago, and only in a limited manner. Its use is primarily restricted to those who shop in natural foods stores. Too bad, as it could benefit so many!

Spirulina is 55 to 70 percent protein by weight. It is considered the greatest plant source of usable protein and is rich in B vitamins and gammalinolenic acid (GLA). It is second only to dried whole eggs as a protein source. People often complain about the flavor of spirulina, but let me assure you, it is far better than that of dried eggs!

Spirulina is available in tablet and powder form. I recommend the powder for quality and economy, but most people find the "green" taste and appearance overpowering and opt for the tablets. A recommended amount is 6 to 10 tablets or 2 tablespoons of the powder daily. If you use the powder, mix it into a blender drink or sprinkle it onto stir-fries and salads.

Though people sometimes balk at the high price of spirulina, it is quite economical when purchased in bulk. My favorite way to take spirulina is in a drink available through Empowered Herbals (see Resources). It can be purchased in bulk from Frontier Herbs or Trinity Herbs at very reasonable prices (see Resources).

Seaweed: The Mineral Supplement

There are a number of seaweeds available, harvested off the many coastlines around the world. Though they have several nutritional factors in common, they vary greatly in flavor and texture. If you try one and don't like it, don't dismiss them all.

Seaweeds are our richest plant source of minerals, providing 10 to 20 times the minerals of land-based plants. In fact, they contain a wider range and broader spectrum of minerals necessary for human metabolism than any other known organism. They have been used for thousands of years to promote longevity, prevent disease, and impart health to those wise enough to use them.

The many types of seaweed lend themselves to a variety of dishes. My favorites include hiziki, arame, kelp, and dulse. Eat seaweed several times a week in salads, soups, Asian dishes, and salad dressings. Some seaweeds, such as dulse, are nice to snack on by themselves.

Bee Pollen: The Energizer

The tiny grains of bee pollen, a combined miracle of flowers and bees, provide some of nature's finest nutrition. A wonderfully uplifting food, bee pollen captures the essence of flowers and the energy of bees and transforms that energy into food for our human nervous system.

Bee pollen is a concentrated form of nearly all known nutrients and provides a powerhouse of energy for the nervous system. It is a complete

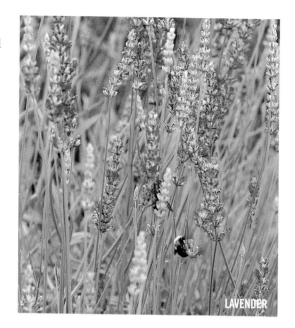

LAVENDER

protein, containing all 22 amino acids, and has a higher concentration of the eight amino acids essential to human health (those not produced in our bodies) than most other forms of protein. In addition, bee pollen contains high levels of 27 minerals, enzymes, and coenzymes; vitamins B_1, B_2, and B_6; niacin, pantothenic acid, and folic acid; vitamin C; and the fat-soluble vitamins A and E.

Use only small amounts of bee pollen, out of respect for the energy that the bees put into collecting these golden grains. And never waste a kernel; it takes the bees hundreds of visits to flowers to produce even a small pinch of pollen.

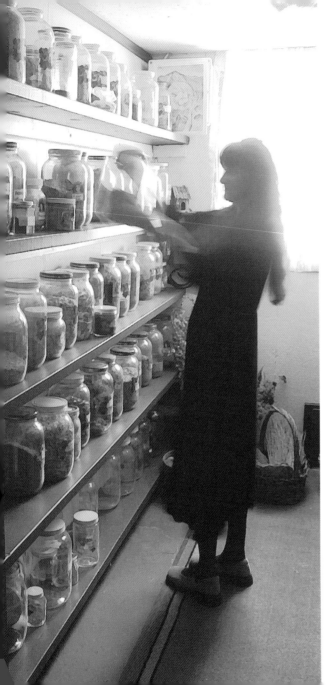

I recommend that you eat no more than 1 to 2 teaspoons a day — each teaspoon contains 4.8 billion grains of pollen! For the best-quality pollen, use it fresh, not in tablet form. Always eat it raw, sprinkled over salads or yogurt, by itself, or in blender drinks.

Some people suffer allergic reactions to bee pollen; others claim it helps clear their allergies. The first time you try some, take just a few grains to test for allergic reactions.

Flaxseed: The Heart Healer

Much has been written in the past few years about flaxseed and flaxseed oil, especially since the rise in the incidence of heart disease and other degenerative illnesses.

Flaxseed is one of the richest sources of omega-3 fatty acids, which are important for keeping the arteries clean, the heart functioning, and the immune system in good health.

One tablespoon of the oil daily is sufficient. Be certain to buy only cold-pressed oil and store it in the refrigerator. Two to four tablespoons of the ground seeds (they are easily ground in a spice and seed mill or coffee grinder) added to your daily meals not only helps prevent heart disease and improve your immune health but will add a beautiful glow to your skin and hair. The mucilaginous quality of the seeds aids in digestion and makes them mildly laxative. Flaxseed oil goes rancid quickly, so store seeds in the refrigerator and grind only a few days' supply at a time.

Shiitake Mushrooms: Immune-System Defenders

The shiitake mushroom is a staple of the traditional Japanese diet and has long been used in Asia to enhance the body's resistance to infection and disease. This mushroom is not only exotically delicious but also easy to grow. You can grow a mushroom log in your basement or under your kitchen sink.

Shiitakes contain lentinan, a polysaccharide complex that has been shown to possess significant immune-enhancing properties. It also stimulates the production of interferon, macrophages, and lymphocytes, infection-fighting agents that

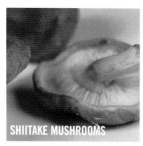

SHIITAKE MUSHROOMS

form the first line of defense against viral infections and other illnesses. The shiitake also has antitumor properties and is useful in the treatment of ovarian cysts and tumors and as part of a nutritional therapy for people with cancer. In addition, it lowers blood cholesterol and is good for the heart.

Include shiitake mushrooms in your meals as a food for well-being several times a week. Shiitakes are best fresh but are fine dried as well. They can be expensive and, unfortunately, what's available in the supermarket is often not of the best quality. Try your hand at growing them, join a shiitake mushroom club (they'll deliver the highest-quality mushrooms at the best prices directly to your doorstep), or buy good-quality dried ones.

Nutritional Yeast: A Superior Supplement

Nutritional yeast, commonly referred to as brewer's yeast (it is *not* baker's yeast), is a superior source of protein and includes all of the essential amino acids. It is 50 percent protein and is one of the best sources of the entire B-vitamin complex, excluding B_{12}. Nutritional yeast is also an excellent source of many minerals and trace elements, including selenium, chromium, iron, potassium, and phosphorus, and it is extraordinarily rich in nucleic acids, including RNA factors.

Yeast comes in powder, flakes, and tablets. The powder is the most potent, the flakes dissolve more easily and often taste the best, and the tablets are the least effective and most costly. Cooking yeast will destroy some of the B vitamins and nutrients, so it is best to eat it in its raw state. There are numerous creative ways to enjoy this potent, vitamin-laden substance. Mix it with juices and blender drinks; sprinkle it on vegetables, salads, soups, casseroles, and popcorn.

When I began using nutritional yeast 25 years ago, there was only one kind available — the by-product of beer breweries — and it was bitter. But I have always appreciated its high nutritional content and found ways to enjoy it in tomato juice, with cottage cheese, and in soups and salads. Today, many of the flavors of the nutritional yeast are actually enjoyable. To help your taste buds adjust to the flavor, start by taking small amounts of nutritional yeast (1 teaspoon twice a day) and work up to 1 to 2 tablespoons per day.

If you are depleted in B vitamins, large amounts of nutritional yeast may at first cause gas and bloating; experiment with small amounts until you find the portion that works best for you. It's often recommended that people who suffer

yeast and beer?

Many people shy away from eating nutritional yeast because of the flavor. Originally a by-product of the beer-making industry, this microscopic plant organism, *Saccharomyces cerevisiae,* was grown in vats containing grain, malt, and hops. The yeast took on the characteristic bitter flavor of the hops. Most yeast on the market today, however, does not come from breweries. It is grown on various media, including molasses, sugar beets, whey, and wood sugar, for the purpose of being sold as a nutritional supplement, and the flavor has greatly improved.

from yeast infections *(Candida albicans)* should not eat yeast or fermented foods, as they may agitate the infection. I have not found this to be the case, but it is the current popular opinion and I will respectfully pass it on.

B Vitamins: The Emotional Balancers

The B-vitamin complex comprises 11 essential vitamins. All are dependent on one another and are essential for mental health, a well-balanced nervous system, and well-functioning metabolism. Symptoms of mental distress or disorders such as irritability, nervousness, panic attacks, excess fear, depression, or suicidal tendencies often indicate a B-vitamin deficiency.

Though each B vitamin has a specific role in the physiology of the body and the psychology of the mind, they are synergistic with one another. An excess of one of the B vitamins for a long period of time will, sooner or later, result in a deficiency of the others. B vitamins are most effective taken as a complex.

Vitamin B_5 is the most important of the B vitamins for relieving stress. Vitamin B_6, together with vitamin C, helps form the brain chemical serotonin, which promotes calm moods and deep sleep. (Another important factor for normal serotonin levels is enough sleep. People who are sleep deprived often suffer from low serotonin levels, resulting in anxiety, stress, and mental distress.)

Some of the highest concentrations of B vitamins are found in the superfoods nutritional yeast, spirulina, and bee pollen. B vitamins are also found in high concentrations in dark-green leafy vegetables, whole grains, whole wheat, brown rice, oatmeal, yogurt, kefir, wheat germ, blackstrap molasses, dried beans, and some nuts and seeds.

Herbs high in B vitamins include:

- Dandelion greens
- Nettle
- Parsley
- Seaweed
- Sesame seeds
- Wild oats

Antioxidants: The Anti-Agers

Antioxidants are chemicals produced by the body to keep free radicals — atoms or groups of atoms with one or more unpaired electrons — in check. They accomplish this by circulating throughout the system and neutralizing any unpaired electrons they come upon, thereby rendering them inactive. However, if the body is unable to produce enough antioxidants to meet the demands caused by excess stress factors, free radicals continue to multiply, opening the door to imbalance and illness.

Supplements and foods rich in antioxidants support the body's inherent ability to produce antioxidants and have a marked healthful effect

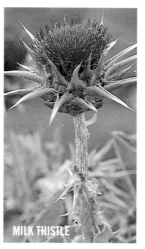

MILK THISTLE

on the body, especially the immune system. All the antioxidants you need should come from your regular diet; they are found in good, healthful foods such as fresh fruits and vegetables and teas made from antioxidant-rich herbs. But if you have been ill or are under tremendous stress, you may want to consider taking antioxidant supplements.

Herbs rich in antioxidants include bilberry, cayenne, garlic, ginkgo, hawthorn, milk thistle, and green and black tea. Vitamin E has long been recognized as a potent antioxidant, as have vitamin C and beta-carotene.

I always tell women, if you love your husband, start feeding him hawthorn berries when he turns 40. Hawthorn berries not only are very rich in antioxidants but also protect the heart; they've been proved to reduce angina attacks as well as to lower blood pressure and serum cholesterol levels. You don't have to persuade him to take a tincture, either; you can simply spread hawthorn jam and jelly on his morning toast. Hawthorn is also good for women, of course, but it's particularly excellent for men because of its effects on the heart.

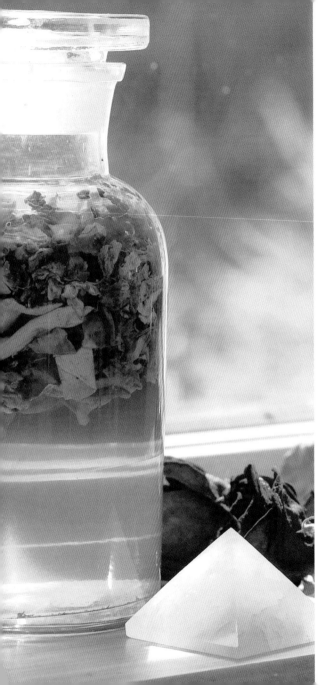

building enduring energy and stamina

Are you tired all the time? Have difficulty starting your day? Can't get out of bed? Before investing in expensive vitamins and minerals or energy supplements, before taking herbs, even, try this simple prescription: For the next 2 weeks, get at least 6 to 8 solid hours of uninterrupted sleep. If sleeping soundly is difficult for you due to stress or anxiety, you may wish to use a combination of valerian and hops tincture just before bed to ensure a sound sleep. Skullcap can also help you turn your brain off at night. You may just find that the reason behind your exhaustion and mental depression is lack of sleep and not enough dream time, and that the magical elixir is just a healthy dose of ZZZs. It's simple enough to try, costs nothing, and is certainly worth the effort.

Most people in our culture are content with quick bursts of energy that often leave them feeling more strained and depleted. When younger, the body has remarkable abilities to call on its energy sources at any given moment. There is little thought of replenishing or restoring the energy used. However, as we grow older, those bursts of quick energy begin to take their toll, and our internal energy reserves often seem drained. People become "addicted" to substances and activities that give them a quick pick-me-up, and often depend on stimulants to get them out of bed and going in the morning. Not good, especially if longevity and radiant well-being are what you strive for.

We don't have to drain those energy reserves if we remember to restore and replenish the resources we use (sounds like an environmental lesson, doesn't it?). The steps are simple, but challenging for most people to follow.

Step 1: Cut Back on Stimulants

Eliminate or cut back on your daily need for stimulants, especially coffee. Coffee is high in a variety of alkaloids that are very taxing to the system. Caffeine, in particular, has a very negative impact on the adrenal glands if used over a period of time. Symptoms of adrenal exhaustion are almost identical to what some women consider the symptoms of menopause: depression, anxiety, insomnia or the need to sleep all the time, and extreme fatigue. Usually, what women are experiencing is not brought on by menopause but by adrenal exhaustion from too many high-powered stimulants and too much stress.

battling free radicals

In my youth, a free radical was something that many of us strove to be. I have to admit, at first I suspected that these unpaired electrons were a metaphor for my generation. And they may well be.

A free radical is a molecule with an unpaired electron. These molecules are formed as part of the body's normal metabolic process and perform a number of important activities that promote well-being. They help keep inflammation in check, fight bacteria, and help regulate normal activity of the blood vessels and organs by keeping the smooth muscles in tone.

Daily exposure to stress and irritants, however, stimulates the body to produce excess free radicals. The stress factors that produce this overabundance of free radicals are wide-ranging, from pollution and cigarette smoke to poor dietary choices and electromagnetic fields. The unpaired electrons begin a frantic search for a partner and often will attach themselves to electrons that are already paired, eroding their cell membranes and altering genetic material by oxidation.

More than 60 age-related conditions are generally attributed to excess free radicals roaming the system.

An occasional cup of coffee can be a wonderfully uplifting and stimulating experience. Daily consumption, especially after you reach the midlife years, can have a very detrimental effect on overall energy and vitality and will drain, not restore, your energy reserves.

Step 2: Build Energy with Herbs

Take those herbs daily that have a reputation for restoring and replenishing energy. There are many excellent herbal energy tonics, including burdock, dandelion, fo-ti, ginkgo, gotu kola,

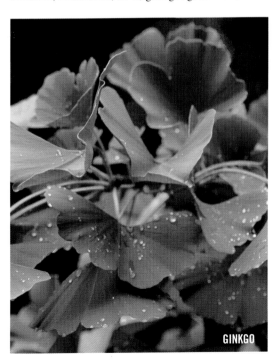

GINKGO

licorice, lycium berries, nettle, oats, and Siberian ginseng. All will build and restore energy if used over a period of time.

Step 3: Strengthen Your Nervous System

Focus on supporting and strengthening the nervous system. Often we feel worn out or mentally exhausted simply because our nerves are overtaxed. By using herbs that strengthen and nourish the nervous system, such as nettle, oats, and Siberian ginseng, we begin to experience a sense of calm and relaxation. It is when we reside in the center of calmness that tremendous energy is available. It is in this center that our chi, or life force, is stored.

See chapter 3 for more information on strengthening and supporting the nervous system.

improving your mental acuity

Because of the ravaging effects of Alzheimer's disease, there is often fear among the elderly every time they forget something. Children forget, too, to put their clothes on, where they left their jackets and shoes, and what time bedtime is — even though it's been the same time every night for several years. Teenagers are notorious for forgetting everything they don't want to remember.

I've noticed that as we grow older, there is a resistance to remembering certain details and facts, a selective memory process, and I wonder if this isn't a natural process meant to draw us into ourselves, away from the mundane, into the inner journey of knowing. Perhaps our inner clock is telling us it's time to forget those details that seem so important to the world but that are hardly worth thinking about, and to get on with the more important quests of life.

In any event, no matter what you choose to contemplate, it is important to have a mind that's sharp and clear. The one thing that clears the mind like magic is peace and calm. Even the most confused states of mind are relieved by a few days near a quiet lake, a hike in the great outdoors, a walk on the beach, or a journey into an old-growth forest. If these are not feasible, meditation and yoga provide a similar calming and peaceful experience.

Herbs That Feed the Brain

For long-term mental acuity, the following herbs are extremely beneficial and should be used on a regular basis by those who find themselves frequently in "brain fog."

Ashwagandha. This herb contains alkaloids and steroidal lactones that relax the central nervous system, as well as concentrations of several key amino acids that bolster the brain's natural supplies. Ashwagandha has a long reputation for clearing the mind, calming the nervous system, and promoting deep sleep.

"We have about **2,000 thought processes** occurring every minute. Just about all — 99.9 percent — are from yesterday or the day before. Your brain may be on overload."

— Ayurvedic physician
Virender Sodhi, M.D.

Ginkgo. One of the best substances to take for brain function is ginkgo. It has been used for several thousand years and has been subjected to much testing in modern times. Most people will notice a marked improvement, but it must be taken over an extended period of time (at least 4 to 6 weeks) to be effective. Ginkgo increases cerebral blood flow, is a powerful antioxidant, and increases short- and long-term memory. Recent studies confirm that it does slow cognitive decline in patients with early-onset Alzheimer's.

Ginseng. All varieties of ginseng are longtime brain rejuvenators that increase cognitive function. They are especially useful for brain fatigue, when one just can't think anymore. Ginseng is restorative and tonic in action.

Gotu kola. This is the most noted herb in Ayurvedic medicine, the ancient healing art of

India, for brain function. It is also used extensively in China for memory and mental acuity. It is used specifically for brains that are stressed by deadlines and intense intellectual activity.

These herbal brain nutrients must be used over a period of several weeks or months to be effective. I generally suggest taking herbs on a rotational basis of 5 days on, 2 days off, repeated for up to 3 months. Rest for 3 to 4 weeks, then repeat the cycle again. Here are the usual adult dosages:

Capsules: 3 capsules two times daily

Tincture/Extract: ½ to 1 teaspoon two or three times daily

Tea: 1 cup three times daily

standardized ginkgo

You'll often find standardized ginkgo products on the market. They are very effective for Alzheimer's disease and I would recommend them as well as tea and whole-plant tincture. However, for most other problems, it is not necessary to use ginkgo in standardized preparations to be effective. Instead, use products made from the whole leaves of the ginkgo plant.

"Smart Drugs"

Along with the herbs used for improving cognitive powers, there are a host of trendy "smart drugs," both synthetic and natural, sweeping the country. Substances such as acetyl-L-carnitine (transports fatty acids into the energy-generating mitochondria in cells), DMAE (crucial to the production of acetylcholine, a major brain neurotransmitter), DHA (a polyunsaturated omega-3 fatty acid crucial for communication between neurons), and phosphatidyl serine and phosphatidyl choline (important for the flexibility of brain-cell membranes) can be found in every health food store and are hot market items.

Though some of these brain nutrients look promising, little is known about them or their long-term effects on the brain. Accolades are high, coming mainly from the companies that market the products, but research to substantiate their claims is lacking. These "brain nutrients" may be useful for corrective procedures such as "brain fog," depression (check with your doctor first), early-onset Alzheimer's, or mental exhaustion; but for long-term brain maintenance and memory function, I would certainly recommend trying first those herbs that have been tested and used for hundreds of years. (For more information on brain nutrients and smart drugs, see Ward Dean's *Smart Drugs and Nutrients, Smart Drugs II* by Ward Dean, John Margenthaler, and Steven Fowkes, and *Brain Longevity* by Dharma Singh Khalsa.)

recipes for longevity and radiant well-being

Age is not an illness, so it's not necessary to take these herbal formulas in the rather orthodox form of medicinal capsules or tinctures. The herbs in these recipes are not "prescribed" as medicine but meant to be used daily as food in soups, teas, elixirs, condiments, and whatever other creative way strikes your fancy. This is a great opportunity to have fun and enjoy "making medicine."

Herbs are not always the best medicine for crisis situations, but when used regularly over time, they reduce the incidence of those crisis situations. The true direction of herbalism is to create excellent health and energy through the *daily use* of herbs and natural tonics. This theory of healing is one that our ancestors knew well, and that we must make every effort to re-create. Bringing medicinal herbs into the kitchen is a good way to get started.

If you study medicinal herbalism through culinary history, you'll notice that kitchen herbs tend to aid the digestion of the dishes in which they are used. For example, horseradish is used to make tartar sauce, a common accompaniment to German food, which tends to be heavy, oily, and meaty. And horseradish absolutely stimulates digestion. Sweet basil is another good example. Tomatoes and basil are natural partners, used for making sauces, pizza, salads, and more. Tomatoes

A CAUTION ON USING IMPORTED HERBS

When using herbs imported from overseas, particularly from China and India, it is important, and sobering, to remember that many of these plants are treated with sulfates and other harsh chemicals, both during cultivation and while in transport. Do not be merely content for a company to tell you its imported herbs are untreated. Rather, ask what the company's policy regarding chemical exposure is, and what its wildcrafting standards are. Find out how they treat the farmers who grow for them. In this way, we all help one another become responsible.

contain a high percentage of acids, and chemically basil aids the body's digestion of acids. The more basil you ingest, the lesser the effects tomato's acids have on your body, which can range from indigestion to exacerbating the symptoms of arthritis.

Coming to medicinal herbalism through cooking is really a fascinating approach, and it sums up where the real art of herbal healing is — in daily life, through what we put into our bodies and into our minds.

7-HERB LONG-LIFE SOUP

A highly nourishing and restorative blend, 7-Herb Long-Life Soup is an excellent broth to serve someone who is sick or recovering from illness. This is a wonderful recipe that can incorporate any number of tonic or adaptogenic herbs. Use fresh herbs whenever possible, but if they're unavailable, chopped dried roots will do. This soup also may be made in a chicken broth base.

Extra-virgin olive oil

2 onions, sliced or chopped

2 or 3 cloves of garlic, chopped

3 quarts water

8 large shiitake mushrooms (fresh or dried), chopped

4 ounces fresh burdock root (or 2 ounces dried), thinly sliced

4 ounces fresh dandelion root (or 2 ounces dried), thinly sliced

2 ounces lycium berries

1 ounce astragalus, thinly sliced

1 ounce fo-ti (ho shou wu), cut and sifted

1 tablespoon fresh grated ginger root

1 ounce ginseng root (any variety)

Miso paste of choice

1. In a large pot, heat just enough olive oil to coat the bottom of the pan. Add the onions and garlic and sauté until tender and golden.

2. Add the water and bring to a boil.

3. Add the mushrooms and herbs, turn down the heat, and simmer over low heat for several hours.

4. When the roots are tender, turn off the heat and strain out the herbs. (I often leave the herbs in, especially if most of them are fresh.) Add miso paste to taste. Do not boil the miso, as it destroys its valuable enzymes. Add other seasonings and chopped vegetables as desired.

pickled nettles, anyone?

One of my favorite ways to prepare fresh nettles is to pickle them. Served with toast, feta, and olives, pickled nettles are a rare treat. Pick the fresh tender tops of the plant. Place them raw in a quart pickling jar. Fill the jar to the top with vinegar, being sure that no nettles surface above the vinegar. A few garlic cloves and whole cayenne peppers are nice additions. Cap tightly, and let sit for 8 to 12 weeks.

NETTLE SPANAKOPITA

You can play with the filling in this recipe — leave out the rice, leave out the eggs, leave out everything but the herbs, for that matter — but this is the blend I love the best. It is rich, aromatic, and mouthwatering.

Ready-made phyllo dough is sold in the frozen foods section of most grocery stores. It must be completely defrosted and at room temperature.

Be careful while handling "mother nettle," who will sting right up to the time she's cooked.

> 2 cups water
> 1 cup brown rice
> 3 quarts fresh nettle tops
> Extra-virgin olive oil
> 3 large onions, chopped
> 1 full head of garlic, chopped
> Basil, marjoram, oregano, and thyme
> 1 cup ricotta cheese
> ½ cup grated provolone or Cheddar cheese
> 2 eggs
> ½ cup butter
> 1 package phyllo dough at room temperature
> ½ pound feta cheese, crumbled

1. Preheat the oven to 350°F. Bring the water to a boil, add the rice, cover, and simmer over low heat for 45 minutes, or until done. While the rice is cooking, steam the nettle tops for about 20 minutes, or until completely steamed through.

2. In a skillet, heat just a few drops of olive oil. Sauté the onions and garlic until translucent. Add basil, marjoram, oregano, and thyme to taste.

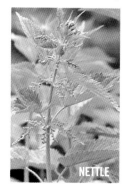
NETTLE

3. For the filling, combine the rice, nettles, and onions and garlic in a large bowl. Add the cheeses and eggs; stir well.

4. Melt the butter in a small saucepan. Place the phyllo under a damp towel to prevent it from drying out, and work quickly. If exposed to the air too long, the phyllo will become dry, brittle, and unworkable.

5. Butter the bottom and sides of a 9- by 13-inch baking dish. Place a layer of phyllo on the bottom of the dish and brush lightly with the butter, using a pastry brush. Add another layer of phyllo and butter lightly. Repeat this process until you have used half the package of phyllo.

6. Pour the filling over the phyllo and sprinkle the feta on top. Place a layer of phyllo over the filling and butter lightly. Repeat until you have used all the phyllo or until you get tired of layering and buttering. Cut into diamond-shaped pieces before baking.

7. Bake for about 1 hour, or until lightly browned. Serve with a fresh wild herb salad or Greek nettle marinade, French bread, and hearty red wine.

SEAWEED SALAD

It is sometimes challenging for people to learn to cook with seaweed. The following recipe is an interesting combination of flavors and creates a marvelous dish. The hundreds of people I have served it to have loved seaweed prepared this way.

Though you can use any variety of seaweed in this dish, my favorite is hiziki (sometimes spelled hijike) or arame. These are both delicious, mild-flavored seaweeds. Wash the seaweed thoroughly and chop it into bite-sized pieces. If using dried seaweed, you will need to reconstitute it by soaking it in cold water for approximately ½ hour.

Olive or sesame oil
2 onions, chopped
1 to 4 cloves of garlic, chopped
1 tablespoon grated fresh ginger
2 cups carrots, thinly sliced
¼ cup water
1 cup seaweed (more or less, to taste)
2 cups cooked brown rice
½ cup tamari (soy sauce)
¼ cup honey
2 or 3 tablespoons toasted sesame oil
Cayenne

1. In a saucepan, heat just enough olive or sesame oil to coat the bottom of the pan. Add the onions and sauté until they are golden brown. Add the garlic and ginger. Cook a few minutes longer. Add the carrots and water. Cover the pan and let steam over very low heat for 8 to 10 minutes, or until the carrots are soft.

2. Drain the seaweed, add it to the pan, and cook a few minutes longer. Add the rice and stir well.

3. In a separate saucepan, warm together the tamari, honey, sesame oil, and cayenne to taste. Adjust the flavors and pour over the rice-and-seaweed mixture. It will taste sweet, hot, and spicy. This dish is traditionally served cold, but it is delicious hot as well.

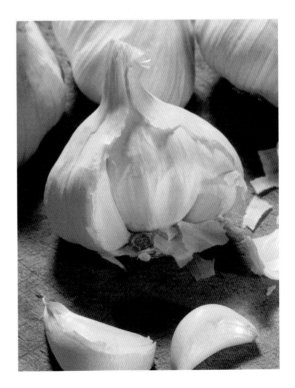

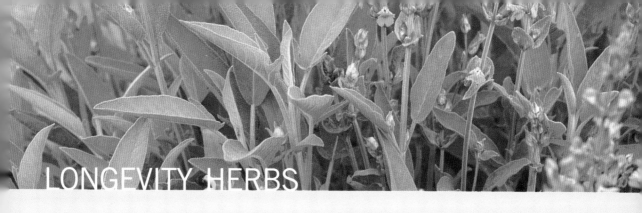

LONGEVITY HERBS

When we think of herbs for longevity, plants from China and India come most quickly to mind. Both countries have a renowned history of traditional herbal medicine that dates back thousands of years. Herbs known to restore energy and promote well-being were among their most highly prized medicines. These herbs were used on a regular basis to build and maintain radiant health.

Though we have far fewer stories to tell of longevity herbs of the North American herbal tradition, it is not, as people often suppose, that they didn't abound. Native peoples of the North and South American continents developed a highly sophisticated and earth-oriented herbal system. We had shamans and healers who had direct communications with the spirits of the plants, knew how to evoke the plants' medicine power, healed with energy, could shapeshift into other entities, and knew which plants were best used to commune with the spirits. These traditions evolved orally, passed down from generation to generation within each culture.

When these cultures were destroyed, shortly after Columbus landed on the shores of America, nearly all of the traditions of these earth-centered herbalists, with their vast body of information on herbs and healing, were lost. Teachers of these old ways are hard to find and eagerly sought, and the herbs from the North American continent are among the most popular and sought-after botanicals in the world.

In Europe, before the Inquisition claimed the lives of more than nine million healers and herbalists, there had evolved another earth-centered herbal tradition. It, too, was largely an oral tradition passed down from generation to generation. Much of the magic of this earth-centered practice was destroyed in the great fires fueled by the bones of our ancestors that burned in the night skies for more than 300 years. The last witch-hunt ended a mere 100 years ago, with the hangings in Marblehead, Massachusetts.

There were books written at that time and earlier that hold remnants of this western European herbal tradition. Much of our Western system of herbalism is based on these writings. But a great deal of the magic and the knowledge that had been passed down was lost during the burning times of the Middle Ages.

This quick and admittedly lopsided look at history is mentioned not as a distraction but as a possible explanation of why herbs such as ashwagandha, fo-ti, ginkgo, ginseng, lycium berries, and others popular in China and East India are generally mentioned in discussions about longevity, while the equally tremendous bounty of tonic and longevity herbs found on the North American continent and throughout western Europe are largely ignored. Did the people of these lands not care about longevity and radiant well-being? I find that doubtful. Were the secrets buried or burned with the cultures that kept them? A much more likely answer.

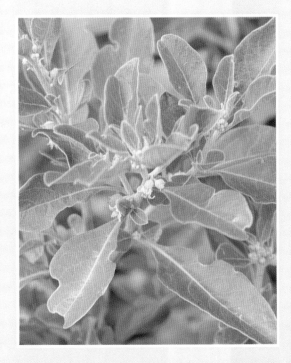

ZOOM BALLS

Zoom Balls combine the energetics of nourishing herbs with high-powered stimulants to provide a balanced form of energy. This recipe makes 60 large, superdelicious Zoom Balls.

> 3 cups tahini (drain excess oil from the top)
> 1 cup cashew or almond butter
> 2 cups honey (more or less to taste)
> 5 ounces guarana powder
> 2 ounces kola nut powder
> 2 ounces Siberian ginseng powder
> 1 tablespoon cardamom powder
> 1 ounce Asian ginseng powder
> ½ ounce nutmeg and/or mace
> 2 ounces bee pollen
> 2 vials royal jelly
> 1 package carob or bittersweet chocolate chips
> 8 ounces unsweetened shredded coconut,
>   lightly toasted
> 1 cup finely chopped almonds
> Unsweetened cocoa powder
> 2 pounds bittersweet dipping chocolate (optional)

1. Mix the tahini, nut butter, and honey until smooth. Combine the herbal powders, bee pollen, and royal jelly and add to the tahini mix.

2. Add the carob or chocolate chips, coconut, and almonds and mix in well (this usually requires mixing with your hands). Mix in enough cocoa powder to bring the dough to the desired thickness.

3. Roll the dough into small balls. If you want to coat the balls with chocolate, chill them in the refrigerator for easier dipping. You can also spread the mixture onto a baking sheet, chill, and cut into squares.

4. Melt the dipping chocolate in a double boiler. Dip the balls one at a time into the melted chocolate, and place them on wax paper to cool.

5. Store the balls in baking tins in a cool place. They will last a few weeks. Have a ball!

FIRE CIDER ZEST

A warming, energizing concoction, Fire Cider Zest is designed to light your fires. It can be added to salad dressings, used to flavor steamed veggies, and sprinkled on steamed grains.

> ½ cup chopped ginseng root, fresh or dried
> ¼ cup freshly grated ginger root
> ¼ cup freshly grated horseradish
> ⅛ cup chopped garlic
> Cayenne to taste
> Apple cider vinegar
> Honey

1. Place the herbs in a glass jar. Pour in enough vinegar to cover the herbs by an inch or two, then seal tightly. Let sit for 4 weeks.

2. Strain the herbs from the vinegar. Sweeten with honey to taste.

LONGEVITY TONIC

I've found that you can formulate delicious herbal pastes by blending finely powdered herbs with honey and fruit concentrate or rose water. These pastes can be spread on toast, licked from the spoon, or added to boiling water for instant tea. Stored in the refrigerator, the paste will last for several weeks.

You can prepare any number of formulas this way. Even bitter, unpleasant-tasting herbs can usually be "hidden" if you blend them with warming spices and enough fruit concentrate and honey!

2 parts fo-ti powder
1 part ashwagandha powder
1 part astragalus powder
1 part cardamom powder
1 part cinnamon powder
1 part licorice root powder
1 part Siberian ginseng powder
½ part echinacea powder
¼ part ginger powder
Honey
Fruit concentrate

Mix all the herbs together in a bowl. Add enough honey and fruit concentrate to make a paste. Pure rose water can be added for an exotic flavor. Be sure that the paste isn't too dry. It will dry out a bit in the refrigerator, even when tightly closed. If it becomes too dry, moisten with a little more fruit concentrate and honey mixture.

LONGEVITY CHAI

A robust, spicy herbal blend originating in India, Nepal, and Tibet, chai comes in literally thousands of varieties. The following chai blend is especially formulated for longevity. Serve it hot or chilled with frothy steamed milk. You can easily make frothy milk at home with an inexpensive kitchen device that looks like a French coffee press, or whip it in a blender.

5 tablespoons black tea leaves
6 slices fresh ginger root, grated
3 tablespoons cinnamon chips (or 1 stick
broken into small pieces)
1 tablespoon sliced fo-ti
1 tablespoon sliced ginseng root
1 tablespoon sliced licorice root
2 teaspoons cardamom, crushed
6 black peppercorns
4 whole cloves
6 cups water
Honey
Frothy milk (can be soy or rice milk)
Nutmeg or cinnamon

1. Gently warm the herbs and water in a covered saucepan for 10 to 15 minutes. Do not boil.
2. Strain the mixture into a warmed teapot and add honey to taste. Pour the chai into a large cup, add a generous heap of frothy milk, and sprinkle with nutmeg or cinnamon.

LONG-LIFE ELIXIR

This is an herbal tonic that builds strength and vitality. Although it can be used by both sexes, it is predominately a yang (masculine) type of tonic and was formulated especially for men.

This recipe invites your creativity; in fact, it begs for it. You can use different herbs, different proportions, and different flavoring agents. Truthfully, I've never followed the exact recipe twice myself, though each batch is similar. For each quart of tincture, use two nice-sized, good-quality ginseng roots, or whatever you can afford. This strong herbal tonic will taste like a rich liqueur and is excellent for you. Serve it in a fine little goblet and sip it as an aperitif.

> 2 parts damiana leaf
> 2 parts fo-ti
> 2 parts ginger root
> 2 parts licorice
> 2 parts sassafras root bark
> 1 part astragalus
> 1 part Chinese star anise
> ¼ part saw palmetto berries
> Asian ginseng roots (2 per quart of elixir)
> Brandy
> Black cherry concentrate (available at
>   most health food stores)

1. Place the herbs in a widemouthed glass jar and cover with a good-quality brandy. Seal with a tight-fitting lid and let sit for 6 to 8 weeks; the longer, the better.

2. Strain. Discard the herbs and reserve the liquid. To each cup of liquid, add ½ cup of black cherry concentrate. Be sure this is a fruit concentrate, not a fruit juice, and do not add more than ½ cup per cup of tincture. Shake well; rebottle. I often put the whole ginseng roots back into the tincture, but they also can be sliced first. A standard daily dose is about ⅛ cup.

astragalus and energy

Astragalus is one of the most popular tonic herbs in China and is often called the "young people's ginseng," as it is specifically indicated as an energizer for younger people. It is described in Chinese medicine as affecting the "outer" energy, while ginseng affects the "inner" energy. It is one of the most important herbs used in Chinese Fu Zheng therapy, a system of herbalism that treats disease by enhancing the system and normalizing the chi, or central energy of the body.

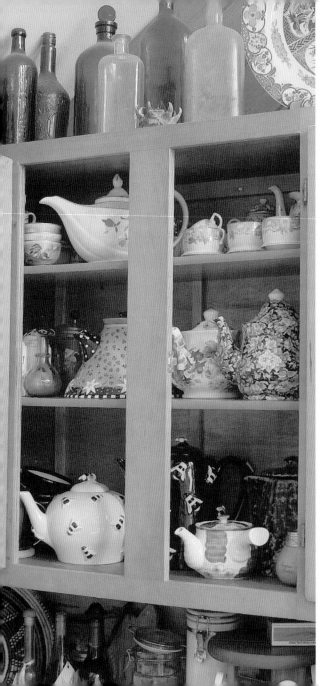

BRAIN TONIC TINCTURE

This is my favorite brain tonic formula, and the first tincture I teach my students to make. Hundreds of people have attested to its effectiveness. However, it must be used consistently for at least 6 to 8 weeks.

Don't expect to wake up one morning feeling like Einstein. But you may remember where you put that shopping list. You know the tonic is really working when you remember everything on the list — or you no longer need a list.

2 parts ginkgo leaf
2 parts gotu kola
1 part peppermint
½ part rosemary
½ part sage
Brandy or vodka (80 proof)

1. Place the herbs in a widemouthed jar and cover with brandy or vodka. Seal the jar with a tight-fitting lid and place it in a warm, shaded area for 6 to 8 weeks. Shake the bottle every few days to prevent the herbs from settling on the bottom.

2. Strain and rebottle the alcohol. The recommended dosage is ½ to 1 teaspoon of tincture diluted in ¼ cup warm water, juice, or tea three times daily for 2 to 3 months.

LONGEVITY LIQUEUR

This wonderful liqueur is a perfect way to enjoy the benefits of damiana and ginseng. Be creative; other herbs, such as astragalus and fo-ti, can be added. This stuff is dangerously lip-smacking good — and daringly easy to prepare. Prepare it ahead of time and serve it at the beginning of a hot date.

> 1 ounce dried damiana leaves
> 1 ounce fresh ginseng (a dried root will also do)
> 2 cups vodka or brandy
> 1½ cups springwater
> 1 cup honey
> Vanilla extract
> Rose water

1. Soak the damiana leaves and ginseng root in the vodka or brandy for 5 days. Strain; reserve the liquid. Return the ginseng leaves to the alcohol.

2. Soak the alcohol-drenched leaves in the springwater for 3 days. Strain; reserve the liquid.

3. Over low heat, gently warm the water extract and dissolve the honey in it. Combine both of the extracts (water and alcohol) and stir well. Pour into a clean bottle and add a dash of vanilla and a touch of rose water for flavor. Let it mellow for 1 month or longer; it gets smoother with age.

ginseng honey

I often preserve my herbs in honey. Occasionally, when I use fresh ginseng roots, which have a high moisture content, the honey ferments and I end up with ginseng–honey mead. If you don't want mead (it's rather strong tasting), partially dry your roots before using them.

Of course, you can mix other herbs with your Ginseng Honey. Try ashwagandha, astragalus, fo-ti, and any combination of spices, such as cardamom, cinnamon, and ginger (one of my favorite blends).

All you need to make this tasty spread is:

• Ginseng roots
• Honey

Slice the roots like carrots and place them in a widemouthed jar. If the roots are dried, you may have to soak them in water before slicing them. Pour in enough warmed honey to cover the roots and let sit for 2 to 3 weeks. The honey will take on the qualities of the ginseng and can be used in tea and in cooking.

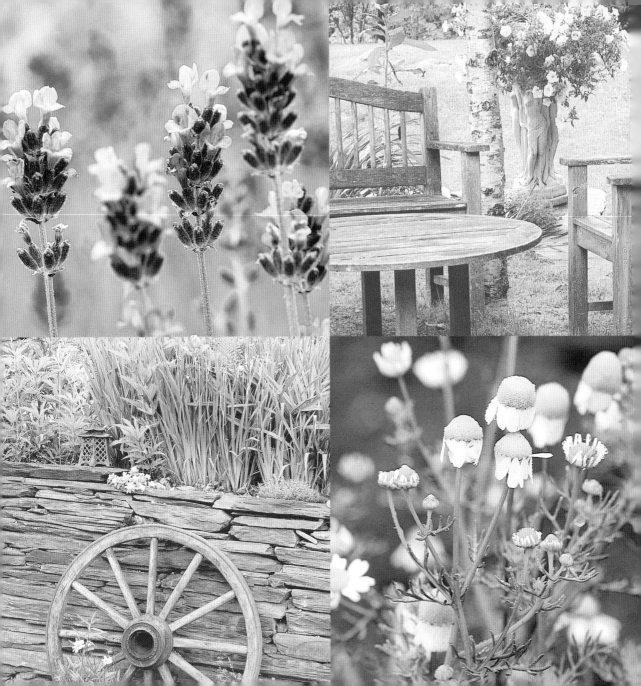

3 Taming Stress and Anxiety

The mind–body connection is fraught with controversy and mystery. How do physical experiences affect the mind, and how do mental experiences influence the body? No one yet knows for sure, but we do know that a link between the mind and the body exists.

Until recently, the majority of Western scientists were unwilling to recognize the connection between these two seemingly independent forces. But today, in the face of a host of modern depression-related disorders, people everywhere are turning to the natural world to heal themselves from the inside out.

Whatever your philosophy of life, the nervous system is your only means of connecting and interacting with your world. If you treat your nervous system like the sensitive instrument it is, it will play back the finest music to enrich your being. Keep it tuned and healthy, feed it well, and protect it from overuse and exploitation, and your reward will be a life of exquisite quality. Through even the most stressful events, you will feel centered and empowered. Abuse the nervous system, however, and the music turns to a cacophony of sound, the colors fade and run, the joy and zest for life drain away into indifference.

This chapter contains remedies for common nervous system ailments, as well as — perhaps more importantly — advice for strengthening and supporting the nervous system. That part of you that can't be measured or quantified, that part that understands these words and makes rich associations from them, that part that can transcend all physical boundaries through the creative thought process — it is encompassed within the nervous system. The nervous system is your instrument of creation. You alone get to decide what kind of music you wish to play, what dance you wish to dance.

understanding the nervous system

The nervous system is our link to our environment. It has three basic functions: to receive, to interpret, and to respond. Within the limited paradigm of modern Western science, this involves only our physical being and the physical world in which we live. We have our five basic senses to experience our external environment, and countless internal sensory neurons to monitor our internal environment. Then there are the some 12 billion cells that constitute our brain, the central computer or main station of the mind.

"**Stress can be** anything from the lash of a whip to a passionate kiss."

—**Hans Selye**
(1979 cofounder of the
Canadian Institute of Stress)

That alone would make the nervous system the most important system of our body. It is what provides integration and coordination to our lives. It allows us to see, feel, touch, act, and react. Without this basic physical nervous system response, there could be no life. To the degree that it is impaired, the quality, tone, color, and richness of life are diminished.

But the nervous system serves in a far greater capacity than just that of the physical quarterback of our body. It is that place where life itself, conscious self-awareness, attaches to the physical vehicle and converts the "puppet" into the "puppeteer." It is the interface where we can dream, think abstractly, create, and receive intuitive impressions. It is our primary connection to Universal Consciousness, or the divine in all of us.

The Final Frontier?

Western scientific culture and experimental techniques have shed great light on the workings of the human entity and the disease processes that affect it; however, there are many frontiers in medicine that continue to baffle the most ardent of researchers. As we discover more answers, we are confronted with even more difficult questions.

The continuing exploration of the biological sciences provides us with the gross understanding of the human body and how it interacts with its environment. This progress has carried us to the exploration of ever more subtle areas of human metabolism. In these more elusive areas, the psychologist, the physicist, the microbiologist, the physiologist, the biochemist, and others must combine their thinking to push back the boundaries of our understanding. The foremost physicists of the world are now adding the mystics and metaphysicians to their think tanks because particle physics has revealed that, no matter how much you dissect and reduce something, you cannot understand the whole by learning only about its tangible physical parts.

Interpreting the Signals

This, in part, is why the nervous system is such an exciting aspect of humankind. We cannot understand consciousness or the interpretation of impulses by dissecting a brain. We cannot understand how logical, rational thought occurs or, even more baffling, how creative ideas spontaneously form in our minds.

We know which autonomic nerves control which involuntary body functions, what the

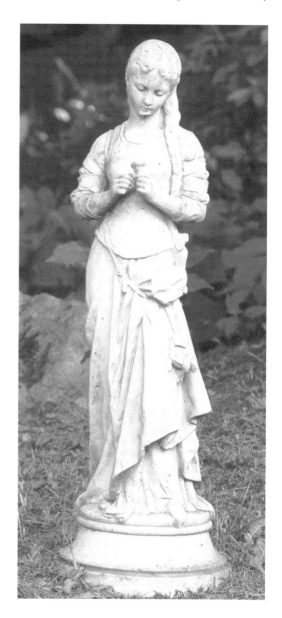

neurochemical transmitters and their target sites are, and what part of the brain controls these processes. But can anyone pinpoint the location of the original awareness that understands the need to send the message in the first place? And how does this awareness transmit its desires or needs to the physical brain so the impulses can be sent?

We don't even really know what pain is, or why similar impulses can be interpreted as either pain or ecstasy. What hypotheses do we possess to define and explain emotions and feelings, where they originate, and what effects they have on our systems?

Why does the heart keep beating and the breath continue to flow without our "conscious" intervention? And what causes them to eventually stop, likewise without our apparent conscious intervention?

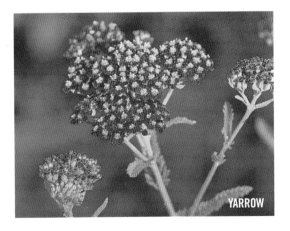
YARROW

Asking the Right Questions

As much as we have learned about the nervous system, we are only scratching the surface. There comes a point where deductive and inductive reasoning and dissection arrive at an impasse. Without including the idea of a higher consciousness or higher order of the universe in their theoretical constructs, right-brain scientists are completely stymied in answering what many of us consider the real questions about life: how it works and what its purpose may be.

With these thoughts in mind, it is important (perhaps with the nervous system more so than with any other system of the body) to address health and lack thereof from a perspective that considers more than physical symptoms and treatments. Allopathic medicine, however appropriate for certain circumstances, treats nervous system disease primarily with drugs that interfere with or block the system's transmission and interpretation of impulses, or by surgical removal of unhealthy tissue. Considering how limited our knowledge in this field is, the irreversible nature of surgery should always make it a last resort, after every other option has been explored.

treating the nervous system

The proprioceptive side of the nerves, the sensory receptors that respond to stimuli, provides feedback to the brain and consciousness about vital body information. If we are suffering pain or distress, it is a warning of imbalance or danger to us. These warnings are only the symptoms, not the originating causes. If the smoke detector in your house goes off, the solution isn't to "deaden" it with a hammer. Wouldn't you be better advised to look for a fire somewhere?

To continue the analogy, it is often appropriate to shut off the alarm and stop the noise while searching for the source of the smoke. Allopathic medication often functions beautifully to alleviate acute pain. Unfortunately, for many, when the immediate pain subsides we forget to continue to "search for the fire."

Will Herbs Work?

The approach presented in this book is to provide tried-and-true ways to strengthen and build a healthy nervous system using natural therapies. Holistic treatments can be used in conjunction with conventional allopathic treatments to promote healing at all levels of life: physical, emotional, mental, and spiritual. In the great circle of holistic healing, all systems are part of the whole and should be used when appropriate.

The healthier the nervous system is, the better equipped it is to provide sensory input and motor response that facilitate optimum quality in our lives. Herbs and natural therapies play a vital role in the health and well-being of the nervous system. Not only are herbs

The wise words of an ancient physician, spoken in 1200 B.C., still apply: "First the word, then the plant, lastly the knife."

important both nutritionally and medicinally, but they also form a direct link with intuition and higher intelligence.

Far more than just "green matter," herbs have an inherent ability to channel life energy and to connect with those places in us that are "disconnected" and in need of healing. Herbs contain chemicals that have no apparent function for the life processes of the plant. However, these very chemicals have a direct and positive influence on the human body. Is some divine plan at work here? Perhaps it is true that humankind's oldest system of medicine offers a form of healing that transcends the physical and connects us directly with a higher consciousness.

There are numerous physical ways that herbs benefit the nervous system. Because they serve as a source of energy and vitality for the entire body, herbs benefit the whole body while caring for the nervous system. Drinking a warm cup of chamomile tea after a long day at work is certainly a simple and rewarding way to relax the entire body. Immersing oneself in a warming, soothing bath in times of stress can be quite sustaining. Using herbs over an extended period of time for chronic stress problems can have long-term benefits. There are many excellent herbs and herbal formulas to use for relieving stress, anxiety, and mental tension.

Though herbs are not as effective as orthodox medicine in dealing with acute pain, they can help relieve and soothe the pain through toning and nourishing the affected areas. Using herbs on a routine basis is a wonderful way to maintain a healthy, strong nervous system. In this way, herbs serve as preventive "medicine" — truly the best medicine of all.

the herbal home medicine chest

There are a number of remarkable herbs that reduce stress and anxiety and directly benefit the nervous system. These herbs are generally referred to as herbal nervines. Unlike conventional medicines for nervous system disorders, which either deaden or nullify nerve response, nervine herbs are often toning and/or adaptogenic (helping the body adapt to stress) in action and have nutritive benefits for the nervous system. They reconnect the nerve channels in the body, gently stimulating or "reawakening" them, strengthening the nervous system so that it can better respond to pain. In

essence, herbal nervine therapy increases our ability to cope with the stress of daily life.

The following categories are helpful in defining the action of herbs on the nervous system. There is great overlap among these categories, but grouping the herbs gives some definition of how and what they are doing in the body. Most herbal nervines do not manipulate life energy but, rather, work in harmony with it. Those herbs strong enough to change energy patterns through manipulation are often the plant substances synthesized by drug companies, and most are not legally available without prescription.

Nerve Tonics

Herbs that feed, tone, rehabilitate, and strengthen the nervous system are called nerve tonics. These herbs strengthen or fortify the nerve tissue directly and are generally high in calcium, magnesium, B vitamins, and protein. Though very effective, most are mild in action and can be taken over a long period of time. Herbs from this category are included in every formula for nervous system disorders.

Examples of nerve-tonic herbs are oatstraw, skullcap, wood betony, chamomile, valerian, hops, and lemon balm.

Nerve Sedatives

These herbs directly relax the nervous system and help reduce pain, ease tension, and encourage

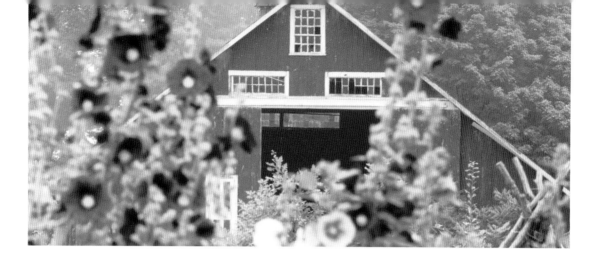

sleep. Unlike allopathic drugs, they accomplish this not by deadening nerve endings but, rather, by a gentle action that soothes and nourishes the peripheral nerves and muscle tissue.

Nerve sedatives include California poppy, passionflower, St.-John's-wort, catnip, valerian, lemon balm, hops, lobelia, skullcap, and cramp bark. Also included with the nerve sedatives are the antispasmodic herbs that help relieve muscle spasms and cramping.

Nervine Demulcents

These herbs are soothing and healing to irritated and inflamed nerve endings. The demulcent herbs have a gel-like consistency that coats and protects the nerve endings. Their actions are general and not specific to the nervous system, but they are included in almost all nervine formulas for their soothing, healing qualities and nutritional benefits.

Slippery elm bark, oats, barley, flaxseed, and marsh mallow root are all good examples of nervine demulcents.

Nervine Stimulants

It is not often that stimulants, as we usually think of them, are recommended for nervous system disorders. When you are stressed, depressed, and worn out, the last thing you need is to have your system roused with caffeine-rich foods, sugar, or drugs — all common "remedies" for the blues. Instead, mild herbs that gently and surely nourish and spark the system are appropriate; they activate the nerve endings by increasing circulation, providing nutrients, and increasing vitality and zest. They neither provoke the system nor agitate it.

Try lemon balm, peppermint, ginkgo, gotu kola, spearmint, wintergreen, cayenne, ginger, bee pollen, eleutherococcus, ginseng, spirulina, rosemary, and sage if you need a stimulant.

herbal formulas for strengthening the nervous system

The following herbal formulas are among my favorites for the nervous system. Some of them are calming or pain relieving. Others supply a spark to gently energize. But all of the herbs included here provide nutrients that help strengthen and support this marvelous system.

As with most forms of natural healing, consistency is the key to health and well-being. Herbs and natural remedies will not always alleviate pain and nervous stress as quickly as allopathic drugs that are designed to quickly and effectively deaden our senses. Natural therapies will, when used over an extended period of time, rebuild the nerve connections and create a lasting flow of vibrant energy. Most natural therapies for nervous system disorders are based on nutrition, herbs, exercise, and a reevaluation of lifestyle.

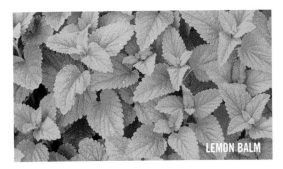

LEMON BALM

VALERIAN TEA BLEND

A hearty, relaxing tea, Valerian Tea Blend is one of the better-tasting valerian formulas.

> ½ part licorice root
> 2 parts lemon balm
> 1 part valerian root

Following the instructions on page 381, decoct the licorice root for 15 minutes. Turn off the heat and add the lemon balm and valerian root. Infuse for 45 minutes. Strain; drink as much and as often as needed.

NERVE TONIC FORMULA #1

Drink this general rejuvenator for the nervous system daily for 2 to 3 months. Feel the stress just slip away.

> 3 parts lemon balm
> 1 part chamomile
> 1 part oats
> ½ part chrysanthemum flowers
> ½ part rose petals
> ¼ part lavender flowers
> Stevia to taste (optional)

Combine the herbs. Prepare as an infusion, following the instructions on page 380. Drink 1 cup three or four times daily.

NERVE TONIC FORMULA #2

This is a very energizing and revitalizing root blend.

- **2 parts dandelion root**
- **2 parts Siberian ginseng**
- **1 part astragalus**
- **1 part burdock root**
- **1 part cinnamon**
- **1 part licorice root**
- **½ part cardamom seeds**
- **½ part ginger**
- **½ part ginseng root, sliced**

Combine the herbs. Prepare as a decoction, following the instructions on page 381. Drink 1 cup three times a day.

HIGH-CALCIUM TEA

This calcium-rich tea is soothing and calming to the nerves. It is most effective when used over a 3- to 4-month period.

- **1 part horsetail (shave grass)**
- **1 part nettle**
- **1 part oats and oatstraw**

Combine the herbs. Prepare as an infusion, following the instructions on page 380. Drink 3 to 4 cups daily.

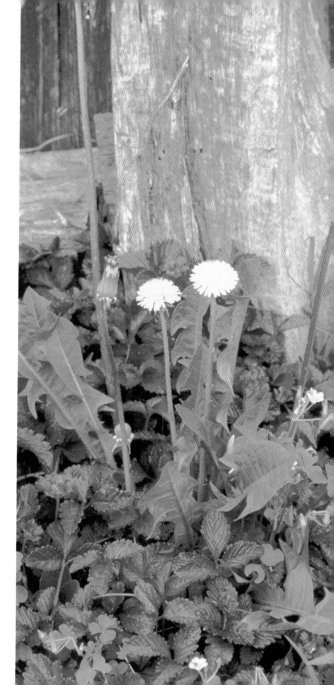

flower essences: nature's most radiant remedies

Flower essences were "discovered" and made popular by the great master of healing, Dr. Edward Bach. A prominent physician in England during the early 20th century, Bach became dissatisfied with the conventional healing modalities of modern medicine and returned to the fields of his childhood. There he discovered the healing power inherent in flowers. Devising a remarkably simple, safe, and effective system of healing from the flowers, he treated all manner of illness by addressing the emotions behind the problems. The system is brilliant in its simplicity and humbling in its effectiveness. Though many may find it hard to believe that flower essences have medicinal power, there are thousands of recorded cases of their effectiveness in treating physical ailments.

Since Dr. Bach's death in the early '50s, many people have chosen to carry on his work and have developed thousands of flower essences for all manner of disorders. But, always and foremost, the flowers address the spirit of the illness, the underlying cause, the emotional being.

Because I am most familiar with Dr. Bach's remedies, I continue to use them. However, I am convinced that those essences made from North American plants have a special affinity for people who live on this continent. No matter which flower essences you choose, be sure that they are ethically prepared. Flower essences are energetic medicines working on the powerful yet subtle vibrational levels of healing; how the medicines are prepared is of the utmost importance.

Flower essences are available in natural foods stores across the country. In fact, you can find flower essences in most countries of the world, a testament to their effectiveness. They are liquid extracts that can be used with any other system of healing or medication with no harmful side effects. You simply place a drop or two of the

woodland essence: a cut above

My good friends Kate Gilday and Don Babineau of Woodland Essence have been making essences from endangered plants. By gently bending the blossoms into springwater or sprinkling water over the flowers, they are able to capture the medicinal properties without injury to the plants. These exquisite remedies are already proving to be invaluable in treating rare and unusual illnesses. (See Resources for the address of Woodland Essence.)

selected essence under the tongue several times a day. Flower essences are tasteless and odorless. They are absorbed instantly into the system and begin their healing work seconds after they're ingested.

For trauma, anxiety, stress, and other nervous system disorders, there are a number of flower essences that are particularly valuable. The chart below offers guidelines for using some of the more common flower remedies.

A GUIDE TO FLOWER ESSENCES FOR STRESS AND ANXIETY

Flower Essence	Use
Aspen	Indicated for fear of the unknown, vague anxiety and apprehension, hidden fears, and nightmares.
Gorse	Used for feelings of discouragement, hopelessness, and resignation.
Hornbean	Indicated for fatigue, weariness, or when daily life is seen as an overwhelming burden.
Impatiens	Recommended for impatience, irritation, tension, and intolerance.
Mimulus	Used for known fears of everyday life and shyness.
Mustard	Indicated for melancholy, gloom, despair, and general depression without obvious cause.
Olive	Excellent for complete exhaustion after a long struggle.
Rescue Remedy (also called Five-Flower Remedy)	The most famous of all the flower essences, this combination of five flowers is especially suited for trauma and stressful situations.
Rock Rose	Suggested for deep fear, terror, panic attacks, fear of death or annihilation.
Star of Bethlehem	Used for shock or trauma, either recent or from a past experience; also indicated for the need for comfort and reassurance from the spiritual world.
Vervain	Recommended for nervous exhaustion from overstriving.
White Chestnut	Indicated for a worrisome, chattering mind.
Wild Rose	Indicated for resignation, lack of hope, or lingering illness.

how to maintain mental equilibrium

We all yearn to feel balanced, in harmony, at peace with our environment. Often we are distracted by the chaotic nature of the world we live in and then expect a "quick ride" back to our place of center, of calm. This can be difficult. Thankfully, there are ways to be fully present and involved in the chaos of the world but still remain calm, centered, and at peace with our inner environment.

I have found that even in the busiest of lifestyles it is easy to maintain that sense of center we long for, but it requires basic common-sense practices and a maintenance program to sustain that feeling. Knowing what the connection is between our nervous system and our environment is helpful; knowing what foods feed and build our nervous system is also helpful. Equally important is being conscious of what creates for us as individuals that feeling of calm in the eye of the hurricane.

Lots of natural therapies support nervous system health and vitality. Combined with herbs, diet, and whole food supplements, these simple practices will help guide you to that perfect place

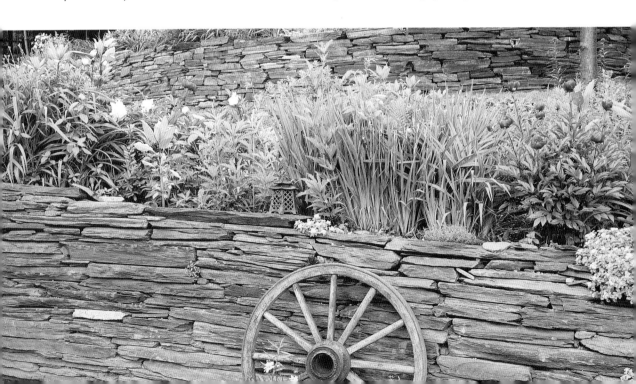

of calm. They are especially useful when combined with other therapies for nervous system disorders.

Eat Foods That Support the Nervous System

Dietary imbalances and unhealthy eating patterns contribute to many of the problems of nervous system disorders, especially those associated with stress and anxiety. Likewise, a well-balanced diet will support and build a healthy nervous system.

A diet specific to nervous system health should emphasize alkalizing foods such as fresh sprouts, high-quality protein, whole grains, green leafy vegetables, root vegetables, cultured milk products (such as yogurt, kefir, and buttermilk), lemons and grapefruit, and seeds and nuts.

Also include the energizing and mentally balancing superfoods described in chapter 2: spirulina, bee pollen, and nutritional yeast.

Add Calcium to Your Diet

Calcium is well known for its role in building strong bones and teeth, and it is also essential for healthy nerve function. Proper amounts of blood calcium prevent nervousness, irritability, muscle spasms, muscle cramping, hyperactivity, and insomnia. Fortunately, calcium is abundant in our diets and is found in easily digestible forms in seaweed, yogurt and other cultured milk products, and most dark-green leafy vegetables such as spinach, chard, broccoli, turnip greens, kale, beet greens, and parsley. It is also found in high amounts in almonds and sesame seeds. Though milk is touted as a good source of calcium, it is, in fact, sorely lacking in the amounts and type needed by our bodies.

Seaweeds are particularly high in calcium. A major food source in many parts of the world, seaweed is often neglected as a high-calcium food in American diets. For comparison, 3½ ounces of cow's milk contain 118 mg of calcium. The same amount of hizike (a mild-flavored seaweed) contains 1,400 mg. Kelp contains 1,093 mg, and wakame, 1,300 mg.

Along with eating foods high in calcium, you may wish to add a calcium supplement to your diet during times of high stress or anxiety, or when working on nervous system disorders. Look for supplements that are biochelated for easier assimilation. Also consider drinking High-Calcium Tea (see the recipe on page 51) daily.

Many herbs are excellent sources of high-quality calcium. These include:

- Amaranth
- Chickweed
- Dandelion greens
- Horsetail
- Mustard greens
- Nettle
- Oats
- Watercress

Avoid Foods That Stress the Nervous System

The dietary suggestions given in this chapter, basic though they are, are guaranteed to enhance the health of your nervous system. But if you are to achieve optimum health, there are certain foods that you must avoid. Rather than repeating the obvious (most people are aware that these foods are potential troublemakers), I'm listing them here with a gentle reminder that, ultimately, they really are not worth the trouble they cause.

Chocolate

Called "the food of the gods" in the languages of the people who discovered and first used it, chocolate was and is a "holy" food. Like most substances held sacred, it was not intended to be consumed often, certainly not every day. Chocolate originally was not served with sugar. In fact, it may have been considered an abomination to sweeten chocolate. It was most often mixed with other bitter herbs and spiced with a bit of hot pepper to make a delicious, spicy beverage. The original formula is, by my standards, a far more interesting and delicious drink.

Coffee and Other Caffeine-Rich Foods

Stimulants are contraindicated in most cases involving imbalances of the nervous system. Foods high in caffeine especially are to be avoided. Not only do they overstimulate an already tired system, but they further agitate the adrenal glands, contributing to adrenal exhaustion, fatigue, and depression. Adrenal exhaustion is the root cause of many of the problems associated with the nervous system and plays a big part in depression and anxiety disorders.

Prescribed in therapeutic dosages, coffee and other caffeine-rich foods have been successfully used to ward off migraines (if taken at the early signs). They also serve as excellent "emergency energy" for situations such as late-night driving. Of course, caffeine addiction and withdrawal symptoms are a prime source of agitation for the nervous system. There are basically two methods recommended to withdraw from this most common of all addictions: going cold turkey or undertaking a gradual, steady withdrawal.

Processed, Refined Foods

The foods that fall into this category fill huge grocery stores and occupy most of the space on people's kitchen shelves. In a short period of history, we have digressed from an almost totally natural diet dependent on the earth's simple riches — foods that have evolved over centuries for compatibility with our genetic makeup — to a diet replete with food colorings, pesticides, synthetic hormones, and, most recently, genetically engineered foods. This chemical bath we subject our bodies to daily has taken its toll. For a complete discussion on the effects of this change in the eating patterns of our species, I direct you to two excellent books: *Nourishing Traditions* by Sally Fallon and *Healing with Whole Foods* by Paul Pitchford. If you believe that diet doesn't affect your health, follow the guidelines that Andrew Weil sets forth in *8 Weeks to Optimum Health.* If you do not feel better after eight weeks on his suggested regime, then you are one of those very rare individuals whom food doesn't affect.

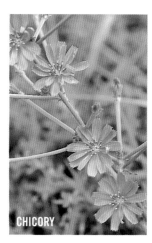

CHICORY

Sugars and Sweets

Sugar in all its many forms provides quick, high-powered energy to the body. The problem is that the energy is used quickly, often leaving you feeling more tired than ever. The huge sugar consumption of Americans — more than 126 pounds per person per year — may be more directly linked to the abnormally high percentage of depression, anxiety, and personality disorders experienced in the United States than we have previously thought.

Aside from providing short-term energy, sugar further depletes the nervous system by forcing the body to use up precious calcium in its digestive process. The nervous system is dependent on high levels of blood calcium in order to function at its maximum potential. Sugar competes for this calcium. It's no wonder you feel agitated, annoyed, or depressed after a sugar binge has worn off! The calcium levels drop as the sugar is digested, leaving nerve endings — and therefore you — irritated.

Alcohol

When you're suffering from a nervous system disorder, even small amounts of alcohol can be disorienting. Alcohol is often sought as a crutch during times of stress and depression, but it actually further depresses the system, worsening instead of improving the situation. It is a highly addictive substance for some people; oddly, those who need it the least are the ones most avidly addicted to it. Alcoholism — as with addictions of any kind — is challenging at best, and devastating at worst. It's difficult to escape its grip without personal loss and an ironclad will.

Alcohol, like sugar, demands calcium in its digestive process, thus leaching the nervous system of valuable nutrients. When suffering from nervous system imbalances, it is best to avoid alcohol altogether, or to drink only moderate amounts. If there is a tendency toward alcohol sensitivity, depression, anxiety, or panic attacks, avoid alcohol as if your life depended on it. It may. Don't use alcohol-based tinctures. Instead, use tinctures made from glycerin or vinegar, or take your herbs in capsules and tea instead.

Reenergize with Herbal Bathing

For many people, stress focuses in their heads. It gets stuck, so to speak, in the mental plane. This is perhaps why stress so often results in headaches and mental disorders. Though hot herbal baths feel great anytime, they are especially recommended for headaches and mental stress. They are deeply relaxing, easy to prepare, and an excellent remedy for head tension.

Taking a bath does take more time than swallowing an aspirin, but the results will be deeply satisfying and long lasting.

A warm footbath is one of my favorite ways to relax after a long day or when I'm feeling anxious or stressed. All of the 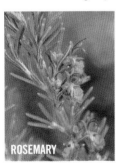 nerves in the entire body pass through the feet and the hands, making them a map of our inner being. And footbaths encourage good circulation, dilating the blood vessels in the feet and drawing blood downward, away from your head, often alleviating throbbing stress headaches. In fact, soaking your feet in a warm bath while resting with a cold pack on your head will often stop a migraine in its tracks.

ROSEMARY

HERBAL FOOTBATH

This is a soothing, aromatic formula, but you may, of course, use any combination of relaxing herbs you have at hand. Mustard powder, ginger, sage, and rosemary are all good herbs for footbaths. Oatmeal is excellent, also, and will do in a pinch.

> **2 parts lavender**
> **1 part hops**
> **1 part sage**
> **½ part rosemary**
> **A few drops of lavender essential oil (optional)**

1. Place the herbs in a large pot and fill with water. Cover tightly and bring to a low simmer. Simmer over low heat for 5 to 10 minutes. Pour into a large basin and adjust the temperature with cold water. It is important to keep the footbath water very hot. It should be hot enough to be almost uncomfortable but without burning the feet.

2. Make yourself comfortable in the softest, coziest chair you have. Slowly immerse your feet in the water. Cover the basin with a thick towel to keep the heat in. It helps to have a friend massage your feet, head, and shoulders. Refill the basin with hot herbal tea as it cools. Play quiet, relaxing music in the background or listen to the silence. While bathing your feet, sip a cup of chamomile or feverfew–lavender tea.

Get Regular Massages

Massage is among my favorite ways to relieve stress. Much of the psychological tension of the nervous system is held in the physical body. A well-trained massage practitioner not only has the ability to work out the aches and pains of present tension but also is able to train the body to release tension as it builds.

Many people consider massage an unaffordable luxury, but in times of nervous stress and life upheavals, it is often the *best* use of your time and money. There are many systems of massage, from gentle Swedish-style massage to deep tissue work. As with most therapies, you may have to experiment and research the various systems before deciding which form works best for you.

Massage helps not only with the physical symptoms of muscle stress but also with our internal programming — the stress held deep in the inner recesses of the body. Painful memories can become reasons for stress and physical pain as much as actual injury. Often trauma, fear, panic attacks, and severe depression respond to the touch of a skilled bodyworker.

A couple of years ago, I was in a fairly bad car accident. Although the three of us in the car were basically unharmed, the car rolled several times. The only injury was to my shoulder, but at the time it seemed hardly worth mentioning. We declined a ride in the ambulance to the local hospital, took a little Rescue Remedy, and decided a

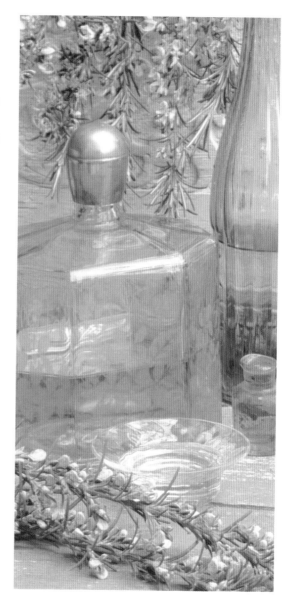

soak at a local hot tub was the remedy needed to wash away our aches and fears.

Several weeks later, my shoulder began aching severely, as much from the stress of the accident, I think, as from the injury to the muscle. I tried stretching, resting, moving, and holding it, and finally called my favorite masseurs, Matthais and Andrea Reisen. Bodyworkers for many years, these two expert therapists specialize in cranial sacral

When I was going through the upheaval of divorce several years ago, I took up running. I always ran on the same woodland path, as the **familiarity** of it gave me some reassurance. Along with the physical benefits of running, I began to notice how much quieter my mind felt after the run. But the **greatest benefit** was making all those friends en route. I would pass the same plants, the same grand trees. I would stop each day and talk to a huge old yellow birch, telling it my troubles and how I was doing that day. Exercise helped, but **Nature, my running partner,** helped even more.

massage, a form of bodywork that moves energy through the body and helps unlock old memories and patterns experienced as blockages. After three sessions of cranial sacral work, my shoulder no longer held on to the trauma and was able to release whatever residual pain remained.

Exercise!

Physical exercise is one of the best methods we have available to release the stress and tension of our minds and our bodies. Like massage therapy and bathing, exercise helps transform the disorders and tension of the mind into physical matter, and the physical body is better able to release it as energy into the universe.

Exercise ensures a good flow of blood to all parts of the body. It helps move us out of our heads, where so much of our stress is stuck. Exercise is a valuable part of any therapy for nervous system disorders. When you find yourself facing life changes or upheavals, or are under stress, be absolutely sure you increase your exercise accordingly.

There are so many forms of exercise available today, from outdoor sports to TV aerobics, from yoga and gentle stretching to weight lifting at the local gym. There are suitable exercise programs for every body type, age, and condition. Your responsibility is to find the type most suitable for you and to make the time in your life to enjoy the changes that begin to happen as you take care of yourself.

Treasure Your Sleep

During periods of extreme tension or nervous system disorders, some people find that they don't sleep well. If they fall asleep, it is restless and disturbed. For others, the reverse is true; they fall into periods of deep sleep and never seem to wake up fully. Both problems stem from a similar nervous system imbalance and both can be corrected with proper nutrition and natural herbal remedies. The proper amounts of rest and relaxation are extremely important for nervous system health and balance.

One out of three Americans suffers from insomnia at some time. Purportedly caused by stress, anxiety, depression, and physiological disorders, insomnia aggravates and is aggravated by nervous system disorders. Though the body needs only a couple of hours of rest to recharge its battery, the brain and nervous system suffer without the necessary 6 to 8 hours of sleep a night.

If you suffer from insomnia, these steps will help remedy the problem. But remember that insomnia is only a symptom of an imbalance. It is important to look at the greater picture and correct the cause.

Step 1. Beginning 4 hours before bedtime, take valerian–skullcap tincture, ¼ teaspoon every hour. Also, take a calcium–magnesium supplement or drink a cup of High-Calcium Tea (see the recipe on page 51).

Step 2. About 20 minutes before bedtime, take either a warm lavender oil bath or an invigorating

developing awareness

Temporary insomnia can be used as a tool to develop psychic awareness. Those unusual waking hours are an excellent time to write in your journal, pray, and do "inner" work that is difficult to find time for during the day. If insomnia persists, however, it will wear down the psyche, as rest is essential to the health of the nervous system.

walk outdoors. If you're walking on grass, walk barefoot for a time to connect with the earth.

Step 3. Right before bedtime, drink a warm cup of milk (or soy, almond, or rice milk) with cinnamon and honey added. These alternative milks, unlike cow's milk, do not have high amounts of tryptophan, but they are tasty and soothing. Set the valerian–skullcap tincture by your bedside. Then slip into bed.

Step 4. If you do wake up, which you may, do not try to force yourself back to sleep. That is an exhausting process and seldom works. Instead, take ½ to 1 teaspoon of the valerian–skullcap tincture. Read a boring book or draw a hot herbal bath and soak for 30 minutes or so. Sip a strong nervine tea while you're soaking.

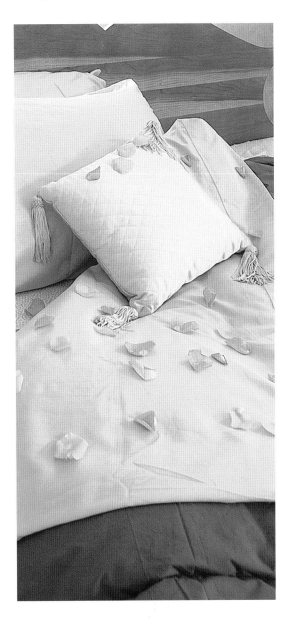

If you are experiencing a long-term period of insomnia, follow the suggestions in this chapter for building the nervous system. Include massage, hand baths and footbaths, lavender oil baths, and daily exercise. Make a sleep pillow for your bed, and begin taking the Nerve Formula for Insomnia (see the recipe at right) as a regular pre-bedtime supplement.

SLEEP PILLOW

One of my favorite ways to use hops is to sew them into a small pouch that gets tucked inside a bed pillow. These sleep or dream pillows, as they're called, have been used for hundreds of years to aid in inducing deep, restful sleep. In this recipe, the lavender oil enhances the herbs' relaxing effects and adds a lovely scent. For vivid dreams, add 1 part of mugwort to the blend.

> 1 part dried chamomile
> 1 part dried hops
> 1 part dried lavender
> 1 part dried roses
> 1 or 2 drops lavender essential oil

Mix the herbs. Stuff a small pillow or pouch with the herb mixture. Sleep with it tucked into your pillowcase.

NERVE FORMULA FOR INSOMNIA

This blend is extremely effective if taken in frequent doses just before bedtime. The hops make it quite bitter; for palatability, you may wish to tincture the formula, in which case increase the amounts of hops and valerian.

> **3 parts chamomile**
> **1 part oats**
> **1 part passionflower**
> **1 part valerian**
> **½ part hops**

Combine the herbs and prepare as an infusion, following the instructions on page 380. Take small, frequent doses beginning about 3 hours before bedtime.

reducing anxiety and panic attacks

At one time or another we've all felt overcome by anxiety at the thought of something fearful, either real or imagined. Talking in front of a group of people, a first date, a car coming head-on at you — these are all reasons for anxiety. Occasional apprehension is normal and sometimes the sanest response to a situation; frequent feelings of anxiety are not. The physical symptoms include accelerated heartbeat, rapid breathing, restlessness, and difficulty concentrating. Anxiety almost always precedes panic attacks. Living in a constant state of apprehension is a sign of major nervous system stress and should be attended to immediately.

Extreme, uncontrollable fear, often agoraphobic in nature, characterizes panic attacks. The fear frequently stems from unknown causes. Panic attacks may be a sane reaction to life in an insane world, the body's attempt to sound a loud, clear alarm. Unfortunately, panic attacks often do more harm than good to the person experiencing them, eroding self-confidence, leaving him or her shaken, scared, and fearing another attack.

Panic attacks tend to be preceded by periods of stress, insomnia, or poor dietary habits. It is essential when addressing a panic attack to seek out the reason behind it and work from there, correcting the underlying problem.

What You Can Do About It

To relieve chronic anxiety and prevent panic attacks, it's imperative that you follow strict dietary guidelines for nervous system health. Avoid all foods that irritate the nervous system, especially stimulants. Concentrate on nervine tonics and sedatives such as California poppy, hops, kava-kava, lemon balm, oat tops, and valerian. Drink 3 to 4 cups of relaxing teas every day. If you are feeling particularly apprehensive, take valerian tincture every hour until the anxiety subsides.

Flower essences are excellent for relieving anxiety. If you are prone to feelings of overwhelming anxiety, carry an appropriate flower essence (see page 53 for suggestions) with you at all times. Use it at the first sign of anxiety. For panic attacks, use Rescue Remedy.

High noise levels often amplify feelings of fear and uncertainty. Do your best to surround yourself with calm. Taking warm baths, playing soothing music, and staying quiet are often the best remedies for the overanxious individual.

Watch for symptoms of anxiety in children and treat them with the same remedies and therapies as you would adults; simply adjust the formulas accordingly (see page 168).

MELISSA TEA BLEND

Melissa, or lemon balm, is a wonderfully relaxing yet gently stimulating herb. It increases energy in the system by helping release energy blocks and stress.

> 3 parts lemon balm
> 1 part borage flowers and leaves, if available
> 1 part chamomile
> 1 part lemon verbena
> 1 part St.-John's-wort

Combine the herbs; prepare as an infusion, following the directions on page 380. Drink as often and as much as needed.

CALIFORNIA POPPY BLEND

This is a very soothing nervine tea, perfect for infants and children to help soothe the cares of the day.

> 1 part California poppy flowers and/or seeds
> 1 part chamomile
> 1 part oats, milky green tops
> ½ part marsh mallow root

Combine the herbs; prepare as an infusion, following the directions on page 380. This is a very gentle formula, so drink as much and as often as needed.

CHAMOMILE TISANE

A relaxing, tasty evening drink, Chamomile Tisane gently soothes irritated nerve endings and eases away the day's tension.

> 4 parts chamomile blossoms
> 3 parts rose hips
> 2 parts lemon balm
> 1 part borage flowers and leaves, if available

Combine the herbs; prepare as an infusion, following the directions on page 380. Drink as much and as often as needed.

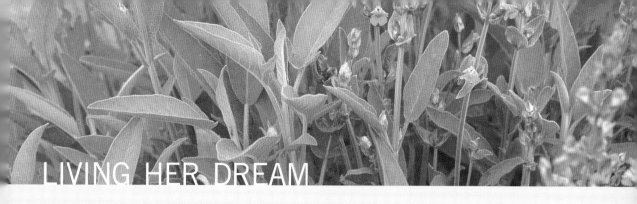

LIVING HER DREAM

Tasha Tudor may be simply one of the most inspiring people I have ever met. A world-renowned illustrator and author, Tasha not only is an artist but lives her life as a work of art. I believe that Tasha was born into the wrong century, so she went back to a time in history that suited her better, the late 18th century. She has created around her a world that is uniquely her own, and it is so filled with magic and delight that it enchants all who have the great good fortune to be invited into it.

I was still new to New England, having lived there only a couple of years, when I received a large box in the mail. Inside was a basket filled with all manner of dried herbs and flowers and a short note from Tasha invit-ing me to tea. Of course I was delighted. We were well into winter, the world covered in a thick layer of snow, when I drove to her home in southern Vermont for that first visit. I remember feeling that I had entered fully into another time. Here was a most enchanting elder with the spryness of a child. We had tea served in cups that were her grandmother's or her great-grandmother's, shared next to the warm friendliness of the fire. After tea, we wound our way through the great old house to the greenhouse, to the goat barn, to the dovecote, and back into the house, without ever having to step foot outdoors. The green-house is what I recall best; in the middle of winter, in the whiteness of snow, it was alive with green and the sweet breathing of plants.

If Tasha is passionate about anything — and she is passionate about many things — it's gardening. The gardens surrounding her country home are, I feel, the most beautiful in New England. The work of over thirty years of tilling, planning, and planting, they reflect the hard work and vision of this inspiring woman. I dream of being lost in those gardens, and when I emerge, I, too, would hope to be found in another time and place.

This elderly woman still gathers her own firewood, grows flax in her fields, weaves and dyes the flax into fabric, and makes her own clothing. She keeps a small herd of goats and milks them daily, and her goat cheese and ice cream are the best I've ever tasted. Though she would never say so, in my definition Tasha is a skilled herbalist. We've shared many a lively afternoon in her kitchen making all sorts of herbal products.

I love Tasha's spirit, her generosity, her strength, her creative power, her will, and her wonderful unconventionality. Though Tasha has been featured in many books, magazines, and television programs, her spirit is a hundred times brighter than the pictures they paint of her. I've often heard her quote Thoreau: "If one advances confidently in the direction of his dreams, and endeavors to live the life which he has imagined, he will meet with a success unexpected in common hours." She is living her dream, and she is an inspiration to others who want to live theirs.

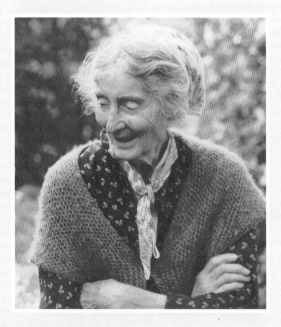

overcoming depression

Depression is characterized by extreme sadness, a sense of hopelessness and despair. It is caused by a variety of "lack factors," including lack of sleep, lack of nutrients, lack of light, and lack of love. Adrenal exhaustion, cold and damp conditions in the body, and hormonal and chemical imbalances can also contribute to depression.

· Depression is marked by varying degrees of either insomnia or hypersomnia, appetite irregularities (including excessive weight gain or loss), loss of energy accompanied by a sense of fatigue, diminished ability to think clearly, and general loss of interest in life. Though there are many and complex reasons for depression, herbs and proper nutrition can help all types. In fact, along with supportive counseling, nutritional support with a strong emphasis on biogenic amines (also known as monoamines) is becoming one of the most effective ways to treat depression.

The biogenic amine hypothesis links biochemical derangements such as depression with imbalances of amino acids in the delicate ecology of our system. Amino acids are essential to the healthy formation of neurotransmitters, complex compounds that form communication links between the nerve cells. Many practitioners are including biogenic amines with other holistic therapies to successfully treat depression. Results are promising. For a more in-depth discussion of biogenic amine therapy for the treatment of depression, see the *Encyclopedia of Natural Medicine* by Drs. Michael T. Murray and Joseph E. Pizzorno.

Sometimes depression is simply caused by a series of very sad, life-challenging or -threatening events. Like that smoke detector, depression is the symptom, not the cause, and is an indicator that things are awry. Fortunately, there are many treatments that can help alleviate depression.

healing through reading

A wonderful book to read during times of depression is Thomas Moore's *Care of the Soul: A Guide to Cultivating Depth and Sacredness in Everyday Life.* I have found Moore's words to be incredibly uplifting. Though the book is certainly not about depression, it is in essence a guide to living soulfully in a troubled world — and this is soul food for a troubled spirit. But don't limit yourself to just one book; read any kind of literature that lifts your spirits and soothes your soul.

Embrace Life and Love

The best thing we can do for ourselves during times of depression is to embrace ourselves, like a loving parent to a favorite child. Create love in your life, whether of people, of books, or even of gardening, hiking, or sailing. It is essential to connect with nature during times of great depression. Find every reason you can to love yourself and everyone else. Generally, people who love others are loved by others.

I suspect that depression is a sort of wake-up call, a sign that we're alive and well and attempting to respond sanely to an insane situation. I've found that the times I've been most depressed have been when I was not listening to some deep, biological, sacred song within me. A more simple way to explain this may be to say that when you know you have to do something, stop resisting and just do it. Follow your heart; it is the pathway to the soul.

Supplement with St.-John's-Wort

Probably the most promising herb for depression is St.-John's-wort. Though marketed as if it were a recent discovery, St.-John's-wort has been used for centuries for depression, anxiety, and nerve damage. It's interesting that the American public woke up and discovered St.-John's-wort at the same time that the most popular antidepressant drugs were being consumed like candy. At least the herb is an effective alternative for those choosing to manage their nervous stress differently.

St.-John's-wort works best for people with mild depression, though it can be used for clinical cases as part of an overall program supported by diet, counseling, and exercise. Take ½ teaspoon of the tincture three or four times daily or 2 capsules three times daily. Many people recommend extracts standardized to 0.3 percent hypericin, but I have found that the whole-plant extract works

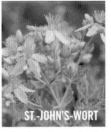

ST.-JOHN'S-WORT

just as well when it is prepared properly. St.-John's-wort definitely has that ability to brighten one's day, but it doesn't have an immediate effect; use it for 3 to 4 weeks before deciding whether it works for you.

Build and Strengthen the Nervous System

To break out of a state of depression, you must strengthen the nervous system so that it can serve as the marvelous receptor and distributor of energy that it is meant to be. Review Superfoods for Well-Being (page 20). Emphasize a diet that is high in calcium and B vitamins. Drink 3 cups daily of High-Calcium Tea (page 51), Nerve Tonic Formula #1 or #2 (pages 50 and 51), or Nerve Formula for Depression (at right).

Concentrate on the herbs that are indicated for depression and sadness, such as lavender, lemon balm, oats, and St.-John's-wort. St.-John's-wort has gained such fame as an antidepressant that it has eclipsed other important nervine herbs. Oats (leafy tops, stalks, and oatmeal) are an incredible herb for depression and anxiety. They slowly and surely build the myelin sheath of the nerves, reducing stress and irritability. Passionflower is another herb indicated for nerve stress; it strengthens and tones the entire nervous system. Combine it with lemon balm, oats, and St.-John's-wort for an excellent antidepressant tea. Valerian can help regulate sleep, while ashwagandha, astragalus, ginseng, and licorice help energize the system on a cellular level.

Take evening baths of lavender and lemon balm. If you have a garden, collect roses and borage flowers and add them to the bath. Herbal bathing can be soothing to a weary soul. You might even consider installing an outdoor tub in your garden. It's a bit hard to remain depressed for long while soaking in a flower-strewn tub surrounded by plants in the garden. However short, this respite from the cares of the world is welcome relief.

NERVE FORMULA FOR DEPRESSION

2 parts chamomile
1 part borage flowers, if available
1 part lemon balm
½ part lavender flowers
½ part roses

Mix the herbs. Make an infusion following the directions on page 380. Drink 1 cup three times a day.

Implement an Overall Health Care Program

Depression, though often associated with loss and emotions, may be more closely related to chemical imbalances in our body that are helped by herbs, supplements, rest, diet, and exercise. The proper diet makes a big difference; during times of depression and anxiety, find a holistic health care practitioner who can help you create a nutritional supplement program to support you through the critical stages of the illness.

Exercise is an important component of any program for depression. Find a routine that you can stick to. Though gym exercise is fine, nothing lifts the spirits more than interacting with nature: walking, hiking, bike riding, canoeing. Take your cares to Mother Earth and the great healing spirit of nature.

Make massage a part of your daily routine. Sometimes, treating yourself from the outside in helps heal the source of the problem.

Use Flower Essences

Flower essences are strongly indicated for depression and go straight to the issues, even when you're uncertain what they are. Find a flower essence practitioner in your area and make an appointment for a consultation, or use one of the excellent books that guide you, step by step, through the process of selecting a flower essence. See page 53 for a list of flower essences most often recommended for nervous system disorders.

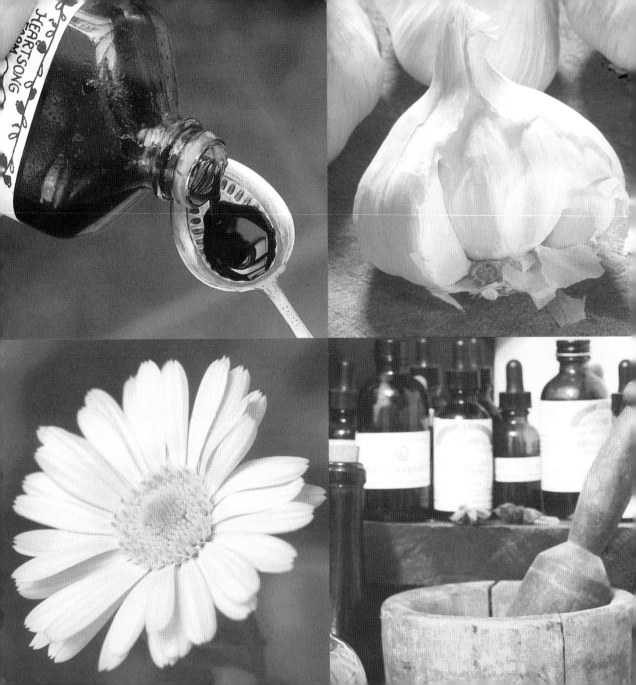

4 Home Remedies for Everyday Ailments

In the past, injuries and illnesses were treated either by a family member or by the community healer or herbalist. Choosing among the vast selection of health care traditions, techniques, and modalities readily available today, however, can be challenging. When you or someone in your family is ill or injured, what is the most responsible and wise course of action? Should you visit the hospital? Call a holistic health care practitioner for advice? Wait and see if the ailment responds to treatment at home? Each situation is different, of course. In one, antibiotics and a hospital visit may be advisable; in another, herbal remedies and home treatments may be the most responsible approach to take. But how do you decide?

My philosophy is this: If your grandmother would have treated the problem at home, you probably can, too. This is a sweeping statement, I know, and of course there are many exceptions to it. But herbs have truly amazing healing powers to offer us, if we know how to take advantage of them. Though they can be, and are, effectively used for complex and sometimes even life-threatening health situations, herbs truly shine as a home health care system. When you study and connect with the plants, you can rely on them, and yourself, for most of the ailments that you and your family will experience.

herbalism versus allopathic medicine

Herbalism and Western allopathic medicine often seem at odds with each other. But they are, in fact, complementary and work extremely well together, increasing the possibilities for achieving and maintaining well-being. Though some of the strongest herbs should not be used in combination with allopathic drugs, most herbs do not interfere with the actions of the drugs and can be used to support or enhance allopathic treatments.

While allopathic drugs actively kill bacteria and viruses, herbal medicines build and restore the system. Allopathic medication generally has a specific agenda; herbs, through a complex biochemical process, take the whole person into consideration and replenish the entire body. When taken correctly, herbs do not upset the body's innate sense of harmony, so there are few or no side effects. In fact, using herbal therapies as a complement to chemical drugs often helps eliminate or lessen the drugs' side effects.

Unlike allopathic medicine, herbalism is a supreme preventive medicine. Herbs build and strengthen the body's natural immunity and defense mechanisms. They nourish the deep inner ecology of our systems on a cellular level. Our bodies recognize and make good use of the medicine of plants simply because we have been evolving with them on this planet for several million years, breathing the air they make for us at every moment, eating the food they provide for us, and drinking in the beauty they create around us.

COMBINING HERBS AND DRUGS

If you are taking any form of prescription medicine, speak with a health care practitioner (ideally one who is well versed in natural therapies) before augmenting with herbs. Some herbs are quite powerful and can cause adverse reactions when combined with prescription drugs.

When to Use Herbs

Each situation requiring medical attention is different. But here are some guidelines for recognizing when herbal treatments can be better than allopathic treatments.

As preventive medicine. Herbs are inimitable for building and strengthening the body's natural immunity and defense mechanisms. They are also powerful adaptogens, increasing the body's ability to adapt to the ever-changing environment and increased stresses of life. Our bodies are familiar with herbs, recognize them, and efficiently use them. Used every day, herbs prevent ailments from occurring.

In most nonemergency medical situations. Everyday problems such as bruises, inflammation, sprains, cuts, wounds, colds, low-grade fevers, and burns respond well to herbal remedies. Herbs can also be an effective first-aid treatment for emergency situations when medical help is unavailable or on its way.

As therapeutic agents. If you choose to undergo more radical forms of treatment for serious illnesses such as cancer, AIDS, and other autoimmune disorders, herbs serve as excellent secondary therapeutic agents, supporting and replenishing the life energy. Herbs and allopathic medicine work compatibly in these critical situations and can be used to complement and enhance each other.

When to Seek Help

I have offered here what I have found to be the most effective natural remedies for the most common maladies that affect humankind. Most illnesses, imbalances, and injuries respond well to nourishment, rest, and these gentle natural treatments. If your body does not respond in an appropriate manner or does not respond quickly enough for the situation, consult a medical practitioner, ideally one who is interested in and knowledgeable about holistic treatments. And, of course, in a crisis or life-threatening situation, get yourself to a hospital or emergency clinic as quickly as possible.

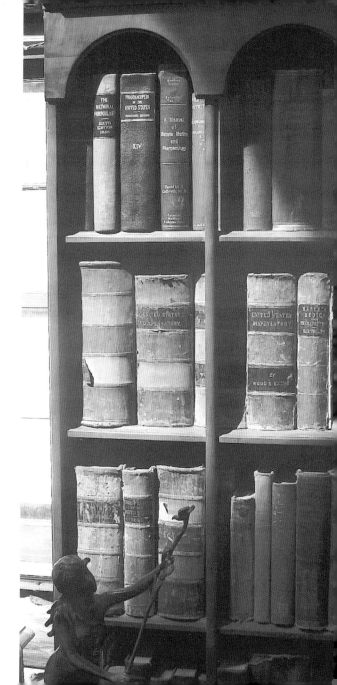

athlete's foot

Athlete's foot is a fungal infection of the feet. Often itchy, it can spread to the hands. In dealing with athlete's foot, it is important to keep your feet dry, to keep your socks clean, and to go shoeless or wear sandals as much as possible to air your feet.

Several treatments are available for this common infection. Try sprinkling tea tree essential oil directly on the area that is infected. Soak your feet several nights a week in a hot footbath with chaparral and tea tree essential oil added to the water. Or try one of the following recipes.

ANTIFUNGAL POWDER

This is an effective powder that is also simple to make. Use only organically grown goldenseal; if you can't find it, eliminate it from the recipe.

½ cup white cosmetic-grade clay
   or arrowroot powder
1 tablespoon powdered chaparral
1 tablespoon powdered black walnut hulls
1 teaspoon powdered organically grown goldenseal
1 teaspoon tea tree essential oil

Combine the powders. Add the tea tree essential oil and mix well. Let the mixture dry; store in a shaker bottle in a cool, dry location. Apply to your feet once or twice daily.

ANTIFUNGAL SALVE

This salve was created for athlete's foot and works especially well for dry, chapped areas, lesions, and cracks. I have used this salve successfully for other fungal infections, as well as for mange on animals. If you can't find organically grown goldenseal, just omit it from this formula.

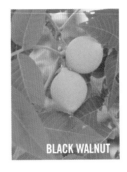

BLACK WALNUT

2 parts chaparral
2 parts black walnut hulls
1 part organically grown
   goldenseal
1 part myrrh
1 part echinacea
A few drops of tea tree
   essential oil

Follow the instructions for making a salve on page 384. Apply twice daily, once in the morning and again in the evening.

burns

Burns can be caused by fire, sunlight, or chemicals. First- and second-degree burns can generally be treated effectively at home, but you must be certain to keep the area clean to avoid infection. If infection should occur, seek medical advice. Always seek medical attention for third-degree burns.

To treat a burn, first cool the area, thus "putting out the fire." Immerse the area in ice water or apply a diluted apple cider vinegar compress to the damaged area for at least 30 minutes. Next, choose one or more of the following treatments:

- Apply a cooling disinfectant poultice made of 2 or 3 drops of peppermint essential oil added to ¼ cup of honey.
- Apply aloe vera gel, which is cooling, disinfectant, and healing, to the burn.
- Take valerian tincture to help alleviate pain (see page 379 for dosage guidelines).
- For burns on the roof of the mouth from hot foods, make a pill ball (see the instructions on page 386) with slippery elm and honey to heal the burn and lessen the pain.
- Apply St.-John's-wort salve (see the recipe at right), which is helpful for healing any kind of damaged nerve endings.

ST.-JOHN'S-WORT SALVE

St.-John's-wort salve or oil applied topically is especially helpful for healing burns. This particular salve is also an excellent all-purpose treatment for rashes, cuts, and wounds. I first crafted this recipe back in 1974 and found it so effective that I have been making it ever since.

> **1 part calendula flower**
> **1 part comfrey leaf**
> **1 part St.-John's-wort (leaf and flower)**

Follow the instructions on page 384 for making a salve. Apply to the affected area two or three times daily.

the versatile aloe

The fresh gel from the aloe vera plant is easy to extract. Choose a large succulent leaf and slice it carefully off the mother aplant. (The plant will ooze a gel-like substance from the location of the cut, which will heal itself within a few hours.) Slice along the edge of the leaf lengthwise (cutting only as far as you need to for one application of gel). Scoop out the gel from the interior of the leaf, scraping the skin clean. This gel can be applied directly to any burn, wound, or rash. If you don't use the entire leaf, wrap the remainder in plastic wrap and store it in the refrigerator. It will keep for several months.

Note: Never use aloe vera gel on a staph infection. It will seal in the bacteria, creating a perfect petri environment for the staph to multiply.

colds and flus

Colds and flus are infections of the upper respiratory tract, often involving the throat, eyes, nose, and head. Bed rest is always recommended to treat these illnesses, but not always feasible. There are many other readily available, inexpensive treatments.

To recover from a cold or flu, eat lightly, avoiding all dairy products and anything else that will cause more mucus in the system, such as sugar and orange juice. Foods should be simple and warming. Hot broth was made for colds; drink it throughout the day. Add medicinal herbs such as astragalus and echinacea to the soup. And, of course, eat onions and garlic, nature's best remedies for colds and flus. Traditional curry blends are a mix of medicinal herbs, including turmeric and cayenne, which stimulate and activate the immune system. Sauté onion slices and whole cloves of garlic with lots of curry powder.

cold kicker

Make your own echinacea tincture (see page 384 for instructions) before the cold season starts. In order for echinacea to ward off a cold, you must take ½ teaspoon of it every 30 minutes at the first sign of infection. If you already have a cold, take 1 teaspoon of the tincture every 2 hours.

It tastes divine and clears the sinuses while effectively fighting the cold or flu virus.

Drink several cups a day of yarrow, peppermint, and elder tea (an old Gypsy formula) or hot ginger tea made from freshly grated ginger with honey and lemon. For an extra punch, I often sprinkle a bit of cayenne into the ginger tea. Both of these remedies will help you sweat out the cold.

HAIR-RAISING CIDER

This is another of my favorite remedies that is effective, easy to make, tasty, but not for the weak of heart. Make a batch before the cold season starts.

> 1 quart vinegar
> 1 onion, chopped
> 1 head of garlic, peeled and chopped
> ¼ cup grated fresh horseradish
> 2 tablespoons powdered turmeric
> Cayenne
> 1 cup honey (more or less to taste)

1. Combine the vinegar, horseradish, onion, garlic, turmeric, and a pinch or two of cayenne. Cover and let sit in a warm place for 3 to 4 weeks.

2. Strain the mixture, add the honey, and rebottle. Refrigerate. Take 1 to 2 tablespoons at the first sign of a cold and continue throughout the day (approximately every 2 to 3 hours) until the symptoms subside.

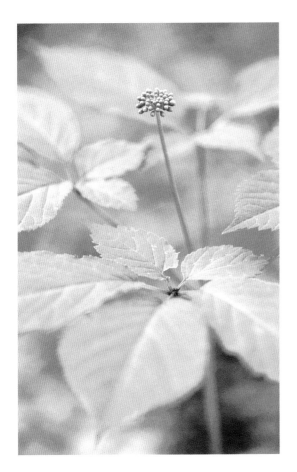

Conjunctivitis often occurs in people whose immune systems are compromised. Use echinacea tincture to boost natural immunity. Administer ½ to 1 teaspoon every hour, decreasing the dosage as the symptoms subside.

For severe itching and irritation, make a tea of equal amounts of chamomile, lavender, and lemon balm; drink several cups a day. Augment the relaxing and pain-relieving properties of the tea with 1 teaspoon of valerian tincture several times daily.

HERBAL EYEWASH

Use this eyewash to treat conjunctivitis without antibiotics. Be sure to strain the liquid well; you don't want any herb particles to get into the water. If you prefer, mix the herbs into a paste with a small amount of warm water, then spread the paste on a piece of gauze and apply as a poultice over the eyes.

   1 tablespoon powdered comfrey root
   1 teaspoon powdered organically grown goldenseal
   1 cup boiling water

1. Combine the herbs and the water. Strain through two or three layers of muslin or a fine coffee filter. Allow the liquid to cool to room temperature.
2. Using an eyecup or an eyedropper, wash the eyes several times a day with the eyewash. Apply daily until symptoms subside, usually within 4 or 5 days.

conjunctivitis

A highly contagious inflammation of the eye, conjunctivitis causes the eye to become red, swollen, and itchy. The tendency is to rub the itchy eye and then, unthinkingly, rub the other eye, thus infecting both eyes.

constipation

Herbs are the best treatment for infrequent or difficult bowel movement. I do not recommend allopathic medicine for constipation; it is designed not to correct the situation but to remedy the symptoms. If constipation is chronic, consult a holistic health care practitioner.

If you don't have a regular bowel movement at least once a day, you suffer from constipation. You must make every effort to eliminate dietary factors that may be contributing to the problem; cheese, pasta, and bread are just a few of the foods that frequently cause constipation. For many people, stress and tension are the major causes of constipation; exercise is always helpful in these cases. Constipation can also be caused by dehydration; drink 6 to 8 cups of pure water daily.

A good daily remedy is a mixture of 1 tablespoon each of ground psyllium seeds and ground flaxseed. Add the ground seeds to cereal, salads, or other foods. You must drink several cups of water daily when using these seeds.

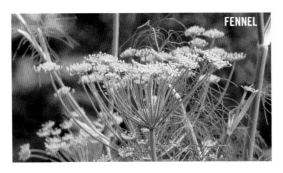

FENNEL

YELLOW DOCK CONSTIPATION REMEDY

I've found yellow dock to be excellent for constipation, and it doesn't create any dependency issues.

> 2 parts yellow dock root
> 1 part dandelion root
> 1 part licorice root

Combine the herbs. Prepare as a decoction, following the instructions on page 381. Drink 3 cups a day.

EMERGENCY CONSTIPATION REMEDY

On occasion, when you need a good formula to get things going, try this one. Don't use it regularly, though, as senna and cascara are quite powerful and can create dependencies when used too often.

> 4 parts fennel seed
> 3 parts licorice root
> 2 parts yellow dock root
> 1 part cascara sagrada
> 1 part psyllium seed
> 1 part senna

Combine the herbs and prepare as a decoction, following the instructions on page 381. Drink 1 to 2 cups to start, and increase the dosage if needed.

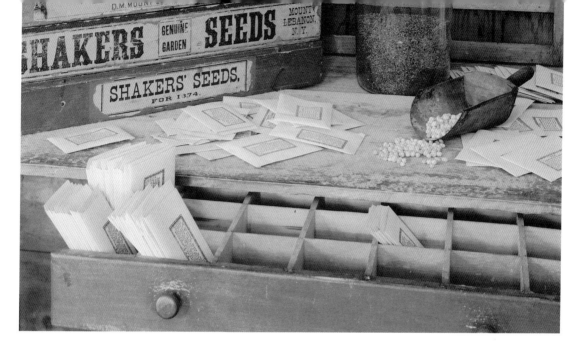

cuts and wounds

Lesions, open wounds, and surface cuts are often, though not always, accompanied by bleeding and pain. Large or deep wounds will need medical attention, but you can treat minor cuts at home.

Wash all cuts and wounds with an antiseptic solution consisting of witch hazel and tea tree essential oil (use 6 to 8 drops of tea tree essential oil for every cup of witch hazel extract). If necessary, disinfect the area with Kloss's Liniment (see the recipe on the following page).

To stop bleeding, apply a poultice or compress until the wound stops bleeding. Shepherd's purse and yarrow are excellent for this purpose, as are, believe it or not, clean cobwebs. Simply apply the cobwebs as you would a poultice, having been sure to first remove any resident spiders.

If the wound contains a splinter, soak the area in water and Epsom salts, or apply a thick pack of clay (green or red) directly to the spot. Change once or twice during the day until you are able to easily remove the splinter. Then disinfect the area with Kloss's Liniment or a similar remedy.

When the wound has been properly cleaned and the area disinfected, apply St.-John's-wort salve (see the recipe on page 75). Wrap the wound in a gauze bandage or cotton flannel cloth to keep it clean. If the cut is painful, drink lemon balm, valerian, and chamomile tea or tincture to help soothe the nerves.

KLOSS'S LINIMENT

This is a very old, very strong recipe, and it's one of the finest disinfectant remedies you'll ever have on hand. First concocted by that famous old herbalist Dr. Jethro Kloss, this liniment is useful for reducing inflammation of the muscles, cleansing wounds, and soothing insect bites.

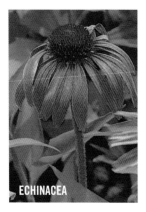
ECHINACEA

If you can't find goldenseal that has been organically cultivated, substitute chaparral or Oregon grape root.

1 ounce echinacea powder

1 ounce organically grown goldenseal powder

1 ounce myrrh powder

¼ ounce cayenne powder

1 pint rubbing alcohol

1. Place the powders in a jar and cover with rubbing alcohol (a food-grade alcohol can be used, but rubbing alcohol seems to work best), leaving a good 2-inch margin above the herbs. Cover with a tight-fitting lid. Place the mixture in a warm location and let it sit for 4 weeks.

2. Strain and rebottle. Label the bottle clearly FOR EXTERNAL USE ONLY.

GOLDENSEAL SALVE

This salve is excellent when an astringent, disinfectant action is needed. It also serves as an emollient. If organically grown goldenseal is not available, substitute chaparral.

1 part organically grown goldenseal

1 part myrrh gum

Follow the instructions on page 384 for making a salve.

diarrhea

One of the most common ailments, diarrhea is characterized by loose, watery bowel movements. This problem can be caused by factors such as infection, unbalanced diet, and even stress. While everyone experiences diarrhea from time to time, if you have chronic diarrhea, you should consult a medical practitioner.

Effective natural remedies for diarrhea include:

• **Blackberry root tincture.** Blackberry root tincture is my favorite remedy for diarrhea. At the first sign of diarrhea, take ½ teaspoon every 30 minutes until symptoms subside. You may have to make your own, because it's seldom found in herb shops; follow the directions for making tinctures on page 384.

• **Astringent herbs.** If blackberry root is not available, any strong astringent such as white oak bark, witch hazel bark (not the extract sold in pharmacies), or raspberry leaf will do. Black tea also works in a pinch.

- **Mucilaginous herbs.** Use a tincture of mucilaginous herbs such as marsh mallow, licorice, and slippery elm to soothe the irritated bowels. Make a tea using 2 parts blackberry root and 1 part licorice root to augment the tincture. Drink 3 to 4 cups daily. If the diarrhea is persistent, add chaparral or organically cultivated goldenseal to the tea. You can also mix slippery elm with oatmeal porridge for a soothing, non-irritating, edible remedy.

It is essential to drink sufficient quantities of water when experiencing diarrhea; it is very easy to become dehydrated and exacerbate the illness as a result. Be especially mindful of this with small children, and ensure that their liquid intake is sufficient (several cups of water a day in addition to their medicinal tea).

earaches

Earaches are infections of the inner or outer ear signified by pain, redness, and sometimes itchiness around the outer ear. If the pain becomes severe or is prolonged, consult a medical practitioner, ideally one who is well versed in natural therapies.

Generally, earaches are accompanied by colds and flus. Treat the related symptoms (see page 76) and eliminate foods that may be congesting

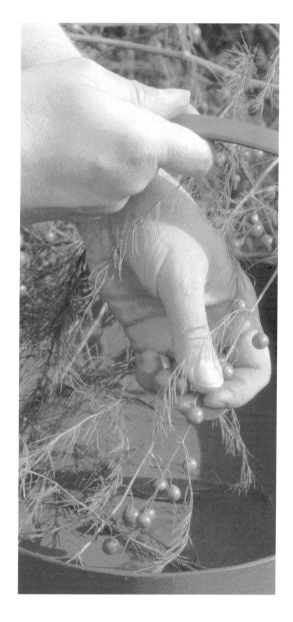

to the eardrums. Dairy, sugar, and citrus products (with the exception of lemons and grapefruit) are the primary culprits. Then try the following:

● **Hot onion packs.** Hot onion packs are an old-fashioned remedy that really works. Wrap hot sautéed onions in a flannel cloth and apply directly to both ears (one at a time, if desired). Reheat the onions as needed. Leave the hot onion pack on for 30 to 45 minutes, longer if possible.

● **Hot salt packs.** If the onion pack doesn't work, heat some salt in a cast-iron skillet; when the salt is too hot to touch, pour it onto a dishcloth or cotton cloth. Fold it carefully, being sure not to burn yourself. Using other towels to protect against the heat, place it against the ear for at least 30 minutes. Treat both ears.

treating swimmer's ear

Swimmer's ear is an ear infection caused by water in the eardrum. It doesn't respond well to oil applications. Instead, combine several drops of tea tree or lavender essential oil with ¼ cup of rubbing alcohol. Shake well. Using a dropper, apply several drops in each ear. Massage the outer ear. Repeat several times daily, until symptoms subside. Hot salt packs can also be helpful.

● **Echinacea.** Take ½ to 1 teaspoon of echinacea tincture several times a day to activate the immune system.

For information on treating earaches in children, see page 182.

GARLIC–MULLEIN FLOWER OIL

This is a wonderful remedy for ear infections; it relieves the pain and helps eliminate the infection. The flowers of mullein are often difficult to purchase, so gather some in the summer and fall. You can also buy this oil ready-made in most natural foods stores.

> 2 to 3 tablespoons chopped garlic
> 2 to 3 tablespoons mullein flowers
> Extra virgin olive oil

1. Place the garlic and mullein flowers in a double boiler or small saucepan. Add just enough olive oil to cover the herbs. Warm for 20 to 30 minutes over very low heat.

2. Strain well; I generally strain through a fine wire mesh strainer lined with cheesecloth. Store in a tightly covered glass jar in the refrigerator.

3. To use, warm the oil in a teaspoon held over a candle or a stovetop burner. Warm only to body temperature (about room temperature).

4. Suction oil into a dropper and instill 3 or 4 drops into the ear. Massage the outer ear and around the base of the ear after applying the oil.

5. Administer the warm herbal oil every 30 minutes or as often as needed. Any excess oil will drain out on its own within a few minutes.

fevers

Any temperature over 98.6°F, the perfect human body temperature, is considered a fever. Fever is the immune system's natural defense for stopping infection and disease. However, high fevers can be dangerous and should be addressed by your health care practitioner. Low-grade fevers can be treated at home.

Warmth

Make a big pot of herbal tea with ginger and lemon or with a combination of peppermint, elder, and yarrow; drink several hot, steaming cups. Wrap up in blankets, cover yourself with quilts, and sweat out the infection.

Fluids

Drink lots of fluids during a fever, and avoid foods and drinks that are dehydrating, such as coffee, black tea, and soda.

Echinacea

Take ½ to 1 teaspoon of echinacea tincture several times daily to boost the immune system.

WHEN TO CALL THE DOCTOR

Consult with your medical practitioner if, in adults, a fever rises above 104°F or, in children, a fever persists for several days or rises above 101°F.

Catnip Enemas

Catnip enemas are one of the very best techniques for lowering a fever and hydrating the system, especially in children. You will need an appropriate-sized enema bag with a pressure regulator on the tubing. Be sure to use an infant or child's-size enema bag for the little ones. Consult your health care provider before administering enemas, and use them only in extreme cases when liquids are not tolerated. See page 184 for instructions.

Cold Cloths

Wrap the forehead and feet with washcloths dipped in cold water with a few drops of lavender essential oil added to it.

Cold Wraps

Cold sheet wraps are one of the best techniques for treating a fever; they hydrate the system and improve circulation.

Cold wraps are administered in a bed, which will need to be protected with plastic sheeting. Soak a bedsheet in a large pan of cold or tepid

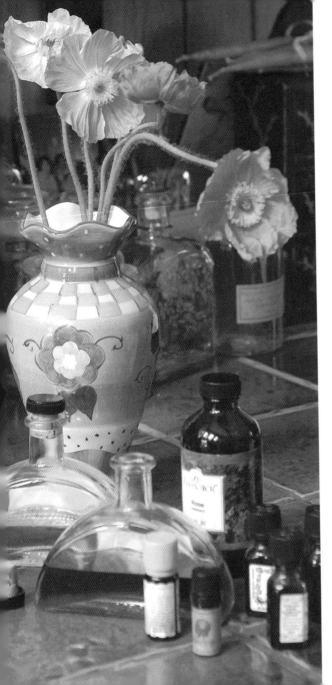

water. Add to the water or sprinkle on the bed-sheet essential oils such as lavender, eucalyptus, tea tree, cajeput, pine, or cedar to enhance the therapeutic value of the wrap. Wring out the sheet completely, then place it on the plastic sheeting. Instruct the person to lie down in the middle of the sheet and wrap it snugly around him or her, from toes to neck — leave only the head protruding. Place a tepid damp cloth on the forehead.

This treatment should be administered for 15 to 20 minutes only. Do not let the person become chilled; be sure the room is warm. After the wrap, serve the patient a large cup of warm ginger tea and put him or her directly into a warm, comfy bed.

headaches

Headaches are thought to be the most common affliction of humankind. In the United States alone, more than half a billion dollars is spent yearly on headache medication. Headaches are the result of a number of problems, including low blood sugar, constipation, toxicity of the blood, allergies, lack of sleep, eye stress, mental stress, and emotional tension. In rare cases, headaches can signal deeper problems, such as brain tumors, but most often they are the body's complaint against the overtaxed mind. Though there are hundreds of drugs promising instant

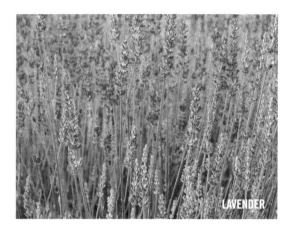

LAVENDER

and Asian grocery stores), brine-cured olives, a cup of miso soup, or a strong alkalizing tea blend. Vascular headaches respond to proper treatment within 15 to 60 minutes.

ALKALIZING HERB BLEND FOR VASCULAR HEADACHES

> 3 parts dandelion root
> 2 parts burdock root
> 1 part yellow dock root
> Skullcap or valerian tincture

headache cures, the cause of the headache has to be corrected before the problem can be solved.

Headaches fall into three categories: vascular headaches, which are caused by dilation of the blood vessels in the head; tension headaches, which are caused by constriction or tension of the muscles in the scalp, neck, and head; and mixed-type headaches, which are combination vascular/tension headaches.

Combine all the herbs. Prepare as a decoction, following the instructions on page 381. Drink ¼ cup of tea with ¼ teaspoon of skullcap or valerian tincture added every 30 minutes until symptoms subside.

Tension Headaches

Tension headaches are usually the result of stress, tension, heat, lack of fluids or food, low blood sugar, salty foods, or excess mental concentration. The next time you get a headache, try to identify the last time you ate, the foods you ate, or the activity you engaged in prior to the onset of symptoms. This will help you determine the best treatment.

Tension headaches may take longer than vascular headaches to respond to treatment, sometimes up to 24 hours. Remedies consist of balancing the contractive condition of the body

Vascular Headaches

Vascular headaches are generally the result of too much cold food in the diet and an overly acidic condition of the body. Foods such as ice cream, cold liquids, alcohol, and sweets can agitate the vascular type of headache.

To get rid of a vascular headache, quickly alkalize the diet with salty, contractive foods such as umeboshi plums (available in natural foods with cooling liquids and cooling, sweet, or sour foods. These include apple juice with lemon, unsweetened cranberry juice, applesauce with lemon juice, and room-temperature herbal teas such as chamomile and lemon balm served with lemon.

Changing your activity is one of the most effective home treatments for tension headaches. If the headache comes on during sedentary activity, such as driving for several hours, working at your computer, or sitting in a meeting, take breaks to do something more active. Take a brisk walk, jog, or find some other form of vigorous physical activity.

General Headache Remedies

Most headaches, whether vascular or tension, respond well to simple care. Try any or all of the following treatments.

Lavender Oil Bath

Baths are soothing, and adding lavender essential oil to the tub water enhances the calming effect. If a full bath is not possible, use lavender essential oil in a hot herbal footbath, or use the recipe on page 58. If you can persuade someone to rub your shoulders while you're soaking your feet, you'll soon kiss that headache goodbye. You can also wrap your head in a cool cloth sprinkled with lavender essential oil and drink a warm nervine tea, such as a blend made with skullcap, feverfew, and chamomile.

Valerian Tincture

Used for stress-related headaches, valerian tincture is extremely effective. Take ¼ teaspoon of the tincture every 30 minutes until symptoms subside. If you prefer tinctures in diluted form, mix the valerian dosage with warm chamomile tea or water.

recurring headaches are a warning

Recurring headaches indicate deeper health issues that need to be addressed. Look first at lifestyle. Allergies can also be a reason for recurring headaches. Are you eating foods that trigger a chemical reaction in your system? Do you have allergies to pollen, mold, grass, or other natural substances? Poor digestion or intestinal infection can cause headaches in susceptible individuals. Is your diet healthful? Do you have regular bowel movements? Is your digestive system functioning properly? If a headache persists or if you have recurring headaches, consult your health care practitioner.

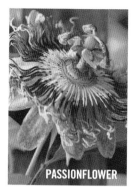

PASSIONFLOWER

Niacinamide

This B vitamin has been very effective for many people suffering from headaches. Take 100 mg three times daily.

Herbal Teas

By drinking an herbal headache tea, not only do you receive the healing benefits of the herbs, but you also help hydrate your system — and dehydration is one of the leading causes of headaches.

HEADACHE TEA

This is one of my favorite tea blends for headaches; it also makes a great tincture. It is even more effective if used in conjunction with a hot lavender oil bath.

> 2 parts lemon balm
> 1 part feverfew
> 1 part lavender

Combine the herbs and prepare as an infusion, following the instructions on page 380. Drink ¼ cup every 30 minutes until the headache is gone.

To make a tincture, combine the herbs and follow the instructions on page 384. Take ¼ teaspoon of the tincture three times daily.

NERVE FORMULA FOR HEADACHES

The mere act of drinking a warm cup of tea often eases a headache. Drink this tea and you'll be even better off. Chamomile and lemon balm soothe the nervous system, while skullcap relaxes the over-anxious mind and passionflower calms the spirit.

> 3 parts chamomile
> 3 parts lemon balm
> 1 part passionflower
> 1 part skullcap

Combine the herbs and prepare as an infusion, following the instructions on page 380. Drink ½ cup every hour until symptoms subside.

SKULLCAP HEADACHE BLEND

Skullcap is a wonderful herb for treating headaches and nervous stress.

> 2 parts lemon balm
> 2 parts skullcap
> 1 part chamomile
> 1 part feverfew

Combine the herbs and prepare as an infusion, following the instructions on page 380. Drink at least ¼ cup every 30 minutes until the headache symptoms are gone.

JETHRO KLOSS'S FAMOUS ANTISPASMODIC TINCTURE

This headache formula was a favorite remedy of Jethro Kloss, a famous herbal doctor of the early 1900s.

> 1 part black cohosh root
> 1 lobelia (seed or leaf)
> 1 part myrrh resin
> 1 part skullcap leaf
> 1 part skunk cabbage leaf
> 1 part valerian root
> ¼ part cayenne
> Brandy or vodka (80 proof)

1. Combine the herbs. Place the mixture in a widemouthed quart jar. Add brandy or vodka until the herbs are covered by an inch or two of the alcohol. Put a tight-fitting lid on the jar and place it in a warm, shaded area for 4 to 6 weeks. Shake the jar occasionally to prevent the herbs from settling on the bottom.

2. Strain and rebottle the liquid. To use, take ¼ teaspoon of the tincture diluted in warm water or tea every 30 minutes or more often until symptoms subside.

Migraine Headaches

Migraines are similar to tension headaches in that they are contractive in nature and are caused by similar imbalances, but they are far more severe and are often recurring. Consequently, they are more difficult to correct. Migraines are a signal from the body to the brain that it has reached its limit; they are often experienced by people who expect much of themselves.

Migraines have been linked to genetic components but more often are the result of allergies, tension, immune suppression, or a combination of all these factors. In the case of allergies, the offending foods may not be linked to the migraine, because symptoms generally do not arise for several hours. Nutrition, or lack of it, also plays a major role in both the occurrence and the treatment of migraines. Follow the dietary suggestions listed for tension headaches.

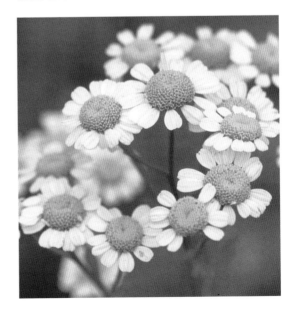

feverfew for migraines

Feverfew is the herbal medicine with the greatest success rate for migraine sufferers. It is not a "quick fix"; it is more effective as a preventive than as a curative for the active stages of the migraine. If you grow feverfew, eat a leaf or two daily. You can also use it ain dried form in tea; drink a cup or two daily. I recommend tincturing this herb with lavender; take 1 teaspoon daily as a preventive.

To be effective, feverfew must be used over a period of at least 3 months, and the quality of the herb must be good. Use organically cultivated feverfew if possible.

Feverfew does not normally have side effects, but pregnant women should not use it. Women who experience cramps or excessive bleeding during menstruation while using feverfew should discontinue its use.

Though there are several classifications of migraines, their symptoms and causes are similar and their treatment is much the same. Many of the commercial drugs available for migraines can have harmful side effects, and though they offer temporary relief, none will cure the condition. Migraines are generally corrected only after a long and serious commitment to alter the lifestyle patterns that contribute to the problem. Incorporating many of the suggestions just given for relieving tension headaches will be helpful. In addition, build into your treatment program the following vitamin protocol: At the first signs of a migraine, begin taking niacinamide, 300 mg daily; vitamin B_6, 200 mg daily; and rutin, 200 mg daily. Divide the doses and take two or three times during the day.

Alacer's Emergen-C (found in most natural foods stores) is also very effective in helping prevent migraines when taken at the onset of the symptoms. Take two packages (2,000 mg) of Emergen-C twice a day.

Some types of migraines respond remarkably well to a potent dose of caffeine. In tension headaches, the veins contract and pressure builds in the head; caffeine quickly dilates the capillaries, initiating a sudden burst of blood through the veins. I have seen this very powerful remedy work several times. When you feel a migraine coming on, mix ½ teaspoon of guarana, a caffeine-rich herb, with two packages of Alacer's Emergen-C. Repeat if necessary. If guarana is not available, take a large dose of coffee. It may keep you up, but often it averts the headache.

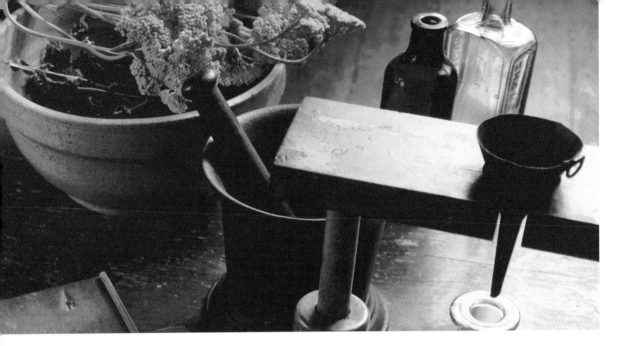

heartburn

This unpleasant burning sensation behind the breastbone — sometimes accompanied by a sulfurlike flavor in the mouth — is caused by spasms and irritation in the esophagus or upper stomach. Heartburn is a sure sign that you are offending your stomach in some manner. Stress, too much food, and a rich diet are common causes of heartburn.

The best herbs to use for treating heartburn are those that calm the nervous system and are good digestive nervines, such as chamomile, hops, and lemon balm. Mucilaginous herbs, such as marsh mallow, licorice, and slippery elm, will soothe the irritated stomach lining.

To prevent heartburn, try the following:

- Drink an infusion of 1 part licorice, 1 part chamomile, and 2 parts lemon balm 30 minutes before and after meals to prevent heartburn.

- Use a digestive bitter such as Swedish Bitters (available in herb and natural foods stores) and/or hops tincture with every meal.

- Drink peppermint tea before and after meals. Try adding a drop or two of peppermint essential oil to water and drinking small sips during the meal.

- Relax during and after meals. Try deep breathing, offering prayer before your meal, and chewing slowly, counting your chews. Don't eat when you're upset; take a walk instead.

herpes

A painful viral infection that can reside dormant on the nerve endings for many years, herpes has recently increased in such epidemic proportions that it has become the second most common venereal disease in the United States. Few people have not experienced it in some form or another, whether as cold sores, shingles, or herpes simplex I or II. I've seen terrible cases covering the bottoms of little children and a painful outbreak hiding the entire face of a beautiful woman.

Herpes simplex II, genital herpes, and herpes simplex I, a less painful though even more common type of herpes that appears as cold sores and fever blisters, are agitated by stress, tension, a compromised immune system, and a sugar-rich diet. Holistic treatment of the nervous system has successfully eliminated many cases and offers not only temporary relief from the virus but lasting results.

The following suggestions for preventing and treating outbreaks are also useful in treating shingles, or herpes zoster, a very painful type of herpes that most often afflicts the elderly.

Heading Off an Outbreak

If you learn to pay attention to your body and the unique signals "your" herpes sends out, you can often prevent an outbreak from happening. It is highly unusual for there not to be a series of "smoke alarms" that the body sends out loud and clear, if we're willing to pay attention.

To prevent a herpes outbreak, follow these guidelines:

- Follow the suggestions given in chapter 3 for supporting the nervous system.

- Drink several cups a day of bitter teas that are cooling to the liver, such as Oregon grape root, dandelion root, and yellow dock root. They will help fight off the infection and alkalize the system.

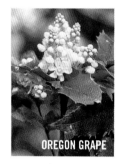

OREGON GRAPE

- Incorporate reishi, maitake, and shiitake mushrooms into your diet. These mushrooms are all indicated for viral infections and help support the function of the immune system. Shiitake, a delicious and tender morsel, should be incorporated into your meals on a weekly basis. Reishi and maitake are most often taken as tinctures (available at most natural foods stores), though they can be cooked in soup and served several times during the week.

- Take echinacea tincture (¼ teaspoon two or three times a day, 5 days a week) for 3 months to build and strengthen immune health. For a tonic immune-system enhancer, blend the echinacea with astragalus tincture.

- Supplement your diet with 500 mg of lysine daily for 3 months. Lysine is an amino acid that aids in the production of antibodies and enzymes and in the healing of damaged tissue.

Treating an Outbreak

Immediately upon the first signs of a herpes out-break, follow these guidelines.

Watch Your Diet

Avoid all sugars and sweet foods, especially chocolate. Herpes thrives on a sugar-rich, acidic system. Also avoid foods high in arginine, an amino acid that is found in excessive amounts in people who have herpes. Foods high in arginine include peanuts, peanut butter, and chocolate. Include foods in the diet that are rich in calcium and B vitamins.

the best herpes remedy: licorice root

Licorice root extract or tincture has been my most successful remedy for clearing up herpes simplex I and II. Licorice inhibits both the growth and the cell-damaging effects of herpes. Amanda McQuade Crawford, an incredible herbalist and a good friend, shared this remedy with me several years ago, and I have recommended it to others many times since. It's best applied several times a day with a cotton ball or swab immediately upon the first signs of the outbreak. I've used it myself on fever blisters, which disappear completely within two days.

Add to your diet lysine-rich foods such as nutritional yeast, eggs, milk, and beans. Many people feel it beneficial to take lysine supplements: three 500-milligram tablets three times a day during the outbreak. However, you should not continue on this high-dose lysine program for longer than a few days.

Support Your Immune System

Begin taking ¼ teaspoon of echinacea tincture every hour throughout the day.

Support Your Nervous System

Drink nervine herbs throughout the herpes outbreak: passionflower, skullcap, chamomile, lemon balm, and lavender. Be kind to yourself. Usually a herpes outbreak is a signal that you're "stressing," so lighten your load, don't add to it.

Treat the Affected Area

There are several simple remedies that soothe the lesions and support quick healing. They include:

- **Ice.** Apply an ice pack directly to the lesion. Repeat several times during the day until all symptoms subside.
- **Aloe.** Aloe vera gel brings a cooling relief and helps gently dry up the herpes blisters. Apply several times daily.
- **Antiviral herbs.** Apply tincture of licorice root — a superb antiviral herb — to the area. Other herbs with a good reputation as antiviral

medications for herpes are lemon balm (especially the essential oil), tea tree essential oil, bergamot (which can cause photosensitivity, so be careful), and St.-John's-wort (helpful for reducing the pain of herpes). A good remedy combines the tinctures of St.-John's-wort, licorice, and calendula. Mix in equal amounts and apply frequently throughout the day, gently dabbing onto the affected area with a cotton ball or swab. This tincture combination should simultaneously be used internally; take ½ to 1 teaspoon three times a day.

- **Kloss's Liniment.** Apply Kloss's goldenseal liniment (see the recipe on page 80) to the affected area. You might wish to add essential oil of lemon balm and extract of licorice root to the liniment for added antiviral effect.

- **Acidophilus.** Apply a mixture of yogurt and acidophilus to genital blisters. This will help heal them, though it may sting a bit at first.

indigestion and poor digestion

The inability to digest foods creates sluggish elimination, gas, and poor assimilation of nutrients. Though they can be caused by lack of digestive enzymes or intestinal flora, poor digestion and pain and gas in the abdomen are usually a result of poor eating habits, poor-quality food, and stress. Therefore, indigestion responds well to lifestyle changes.

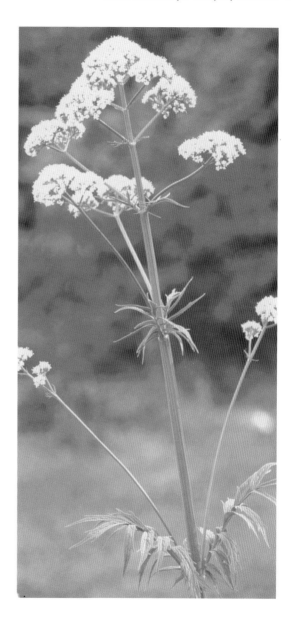

Lifestyle Changes

Before taking supplements and herbs in an effort to curb indigestion, first try these simple suggestions:

• Say a prayer before your meal; honor the food that you're about to eat. Consider carefully the work that has gone into producing your meal, and give thanks for it.

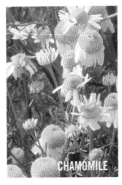
CHAMOMILE

• Chew slowly and thoughtfully. If you are engaging in conversation, keep your voice quiet and the conversation peaceful.

• Don't rush through your meal. Savor its taste, aroma, and presentation. Imagine this as your last meal, and enjoy every bite of it.

• Don't drink cold fluids with your meal. In fact, it's best not to drink immediately before or after a meal.

• Start paying attention to which foods you combine at meals, and the effects that particular combinations have on your digestion. Combining carbohydrates and protein, as American meal plans often do, ensures gas and putrefaction in the system. Ask your health care provider or a nutritional consultant about using food combinations to enhance, rather than obstruct, digestion. There are several good books on the technique of food combining; check them out at your local library or bookstore.

Simple Home Remedies

In addition to changing your habits:

• Drink a cup of peppermint or chamomile tea 30 minutes before and after meals.

• Buy a ready-made digestive bitter such as Swedish Bitters (available at health food stores) or make up a batch of Digestive Bitter Tincture.

• Add ginger and cayenne to your food or make a warm tea with them. Use fresh grated ginger and only a few grains of cayenne.

• Take papaya enzymes (available at most health food stores) with meals to aid digestion.

• Take a daily supplement of acidophilus. This product restores weak intestinal flora and is readily available at every natural foods store.

• Make a mix of carminative seeds, such as anise, cardamom, cumin, dill, and fennel, and chew them at and between meals. These are all very helpful for reducing gas and bloating.

DIGESTIVE BITTER TINCTURE

2 parts fennel

1 part artichoke leaf

1 part dandelion root

1 part organically cultivated gentian

½ part ginger

Combine the herbs and make a tincture, following the directions on page 384. Take ½ to 1 teaspoon before and after meals.

laryngitis and sore throat

Though sore throats and laryngitis are not technically the same ailment, they respond to the same treatments. Laryngitis is inflammation of the throat, resulting in hoarseness and often, though not always, a sore throat. It is generally the result of an infection or stressed vocal cords. Sore throats are always the result of infection and don't necessarily result in laryngitis.

The best thing to do for laryngitis is to rest the voice. Garden sage is often recommended; use it as both a tea and a gargle. In addition, try using an herbal throat spray. Several herbal companies make excellent throat sprays that incorporate echinacea, licorice, slippery elm, and other herbs specific to irritated vocal cords. You can also make your own.

TRIPLE-STRENGTH THROAT SPRAY

1 teaspoon echinacea
1 teaspoon licorice
1 teaspoon sage
1 cup water
A few drops of tea tree or eucalyptus
    essential oil

Make an infusion of the herbs and the water, following the directions on page 380. Add the essential oil to the tea. Put the mix in a mister or spray bottle and squirt into the back of the throat as needed.

THROAT-COAT BALLS

This tasty herbal candy is excellent for sore or strep throat. If organically grown goldenseal is unavailable, substitute Oregon grape root.

1 part licorice root powder
1 part slippery elm or marsh mallow powder
½ part echinacea powder
¼ part organically grown goldenseal powder
A few drops of peppermint essential oil
Carob powder

Make a batch of herbal candy as instructed on page 383. Use enough carob to thicken, and adjust the flavors to suit you. Take 1 marble-sized ball three or four times daily.

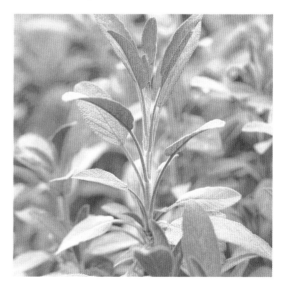

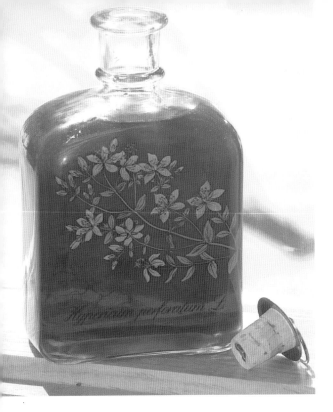

SORE THROAT GARGLE

This is my favorite gargle for sore throats and laryngitis; however, I'm the first to admit that it's not my tastiest recipe.

> 1 cup apple cider vinegar
> 1 cup strong (triple strength) sage tea
> 2 to 3 teaspoons salt
> Pinch of cayenne

Combine all ingredients. Gargle with this mixture frequently throughout the day.

COUGH-BE-GONE & SORE THROAT SYRUP

This syrup for sore and inflamed throats is a much tastier recipe than my Sore Throat Gargle.

> 4 parts fennel seed
> 2 parts licorice root
> 2 parts slippery elm bark
> 2 parts valerian
> 2 parts wild cherry bark
> 1 part cinnamon bark
> ½ part ginger root
> ⅛ part orange peel

Make a syrup as instructed on page 382. Take 1 to 2 teaspoons every hour or two throughout the day, or use whenever a bout of coughing starts up.

THROAT SOOTHER TEA

This tea strengthens the voice and soothes throat irritation.

> 2 parts licorice root
> 1 part cinnamon
> 1 part echinacea
> 1 part marsh mallow root
> ⅛ part ginger

Decoct the herbs as instructed on page 381. Drink several cups of tea a day.

neuralgia/pain

Pain is the result, not the cause, of illness. It is the sensation or feeling that the body sends to the brain to signal that something is awry. Though the underlying problem ultimately needs to be corrected, the very nature of pain calls for immediate attention.

Allopathic medicine certainly offers a wide selection of effective medications that provide quick pain relief. When instant pain relief is needed, these medications are superior to herbal remedies. They work by tampering with the signals of the nervous system. Sometimes they are necessary for relief of severe pain. However, pain is often manageable, and, in fact, it can be a valuable part of the healing process.

At times it may be necessary to utilize the quick-acting pain-relieving drugs, but they are overused and often abused in our society. The following suggestions offer reliable alternatives. Although these herbs are most often used for mild to moderate pain, they can be effective for severe pain when the dosage and frequency of use are increased.

St.-John's-Wort
St.-John's-wort infused oil (see the recipe on the following page; the oil is also available at most natural foods stores) and St.-John's-wort tincture work effectively for relieving pain. Use the oil externally and the tincture internally, several times daily or as often as needed.

harvesting st.-john's-wort

Collect St.-John's-wort blossoms just as they are opening. Pinch a bud and a squirt of bloodlike oil will burst out. If ready, the buds will stain your fingers bright red. Traditionally, people collected the herb on June 24th, the anniversary of the day St. John the Baptist was beheaded.

Although the flowers are preferred, some leaves are useful; I generally suggest roughly 70 percent flowers to 30 percent leaves. The ripening of the buds depends on weather conditions and location. Allow the buds to air-dry in a warm, shaded area for a few hours. Though this isn't always necessary, it allows some of the moisture to evaporate and, most importantly, it's a polite way to give whatever tiny creatures have made their home in the flowers an opportunity to escape.

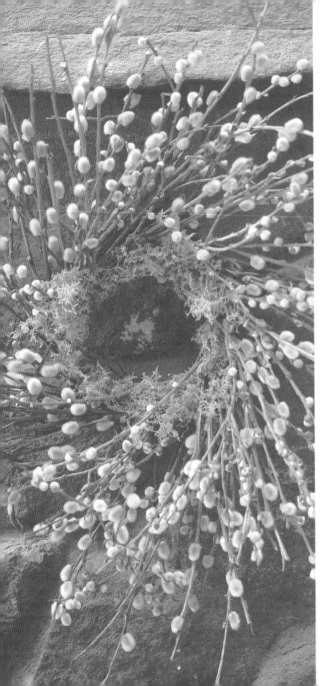

ST.-JOHN'S-WORT OIL

This oil is generally used topically for nerve damage, pain, swellings, bruises, and other types of trauma to the skin. But I like to use St.-John's-wort internally as well. I add it to salad dressings and mix it with stir-fries. I even mix it with my animals' food when they are particularly stressed or anxious.

St.-John's-wort flowers and leaves
Virgin olive oil

1. Place the St.-John's-wort in a widemouthed jar. Pour in enough olive oil so that it rises 2 to 3 inches over the herb. Cover tightly and place the jar in a warm, sunny location for 4 to 6 weeks.
2. Strain the oil through a fine-meshed strainer and rebottle. The oil should be a deep blood red; the redder, the better. Apply topically to sprains, bruises, wounds, swellings, and other areas of tissue trauma.

Valerian

Valerian tincture is an effective pain reliever and has special benefits for pain of the muscles and skeletal structure. Take the tincture frequently until the pain subsides. I have given large doses of the tincture successfully for severe pain caused by second-degree burns. Within 15 minutes, the pain was bearable — though it might have helped that the valerian was in a base of high-quality brandy!

Salicylic-Rich Herbs

Herbs high in salicylic acid, such as willow bark, wintergreen, and meadowsweet (*Spiraea* spp.), have been used for centuries to relieve the pain of inflammation and fevers. These herbs were the original active ingredients in aspirin. They can be powdered and encapsulated or made up as teas or tinctures. I like to combine them with other pain-relieving herbs, such as valerian and wild lettuce.

Herbal Sedatives

Herbal sedatives (see page 48) are effective for relief of pain and should be given in small, frequent doses. For instance, when administering a tincture, give ¼ teaspoon every 15 to 30 minutes until the pain subsides.

Poppy

California poppy, though nowhere near as strong as its exotic Oriental cousin, the opium poppy, nonetheless has effective pain-relieving properties. It is effective for inducing sleep and reducing pain.

poison oak and poison ivy

Contact with these beautiful woodland vines causes a hot, itchy rash; poison oak is the culprit on the West Coast, and poison ivy on the East. This contact dermatitis can be quite severe for some people. There are several simple and effective home remedies for this painful itch.

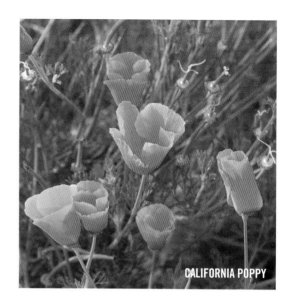

CALIFORNIA POPPY

how to resist the itch

For the irritation, which at times can be unbearable, take large doses of kava-kava and/or valerian tincture. As a distraction, read a good novel or watch some spellbinding videos. If you tend to unconsciously scratch the rash at night, which is common, do what parents do to infants: Cover your hands with socks before you go to bed. When worse comes to worst, remember, this, too, shall pass. The affliction always runs its course.

Itch-Relief Remedy

My favorite remedy for poison oak/ivy was a French-made toothpaste containing green clay, salt, water, and peppermint oil. The company has gone out of business, but the remedy is easy to make.

ROSEMARY'S ITCH-RELIEF REMEDY

Store this wonderful healing cream in a glass container with a tight-fitting lid. If it dries out, reconstitute by adding water.

> 1 cup green volcanic clay
> Water or witch hazel extract
> 2 tablespoons salt
> Peppermint essential oil

1. Mix the clay with enough water or witch hazel extract to make a creamy paste. Add salt and several drops of peppermint essential oil; the paste should smell strong and feel cooling to the skin.
2. Spread the paste directly on the affected area and leave on until it is completely dry. To rinse off, soak a washcloth in witch hazel extract or water and rub gently. Be careful not to scrub the skin, or you'll aggravate the itching.

Cooling Herbs

Since the rash produces a "hot" condition in the body, it is important to use cooling herbs to help with the symptoms. Cleavers, chickweed, burdock, and dandelion are recommended. Make a tea with a combination of these herbs; drink several cups a day. Along similar lines, avoid spicy foods, as they'll agitate the heat condition and make the itch worse.

Kloss's Liniment

I've found, through personal experience, that Kloss's Liniment (see the recipe on page 80) is excellent for stopping the itch and spread of poison oak and poison ivy. Dilute it with water or witch hazel extract so it stings but doesn't burn.

Echinacea

Assist the body in healing by taking echinacea tincture — 1 teaspoon every 2 hours — throughout the day.

Yogurt

In sensitive areas where it's not possible to use Kloss's liniment or a drying clay (such as on the genitals or in the eye area), use unsweetened yogurt instead. This was my grandmother's favorite remedy when I had poison oak as a child — not an uncommon occurrence. She would cover me with her tart Armenian yogurt and leave me to dry. It was a bit uncomfortable, but it worked.

Cool Water

Though it's tempting to take a hot bath or shower, which will temporarily make the rash feel better, hot water will always agitate the condition

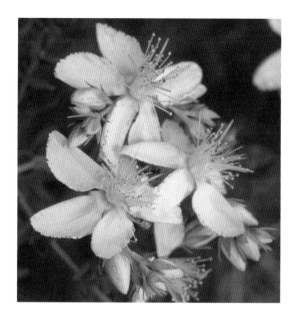

in the long run. Avoid hot baths, showers, saunas, and sweat lodges. Bathe only in tepid water. A drop or two of peppermint essential oil (no more or you'll be flying out of that tub before you get in it!) added to the bathwater will help cool the rash and give temporary relief from the itching and burning.

Saltwater

Ocean water is one of the most healing treatments for these rashes. It both soothes the irritation and encourages healing of the rash. If you don't live near the sea and are unable to bathe in it daily, simulate the ocean waters in your tub: add kelp, baking soda, and sea salt to a tub full of cool water.

toothache

A toothache can be caused by stress or anxiety, but it is generally caused by bacteria infecting the tissue at the base of the tooth. The pain is the irritated nerve sending a signal that something is awry.

When a tooth begins to ache, immediately make an appointment to see a good dentist. In the meantime, you can alleviate and often cure a toothache by applying a poultice of herbs (see the recipe below) directly to the site of infection. Clove essential oil applied topically is an effective analgesic. High dosages of valerian (½ teaspoon of the tincture every 30 minutes) will also ease the pain. In addition, tea tree essential oil can be applied directly to the infection.

TOOTHACHE POULTICE

Substitute chaparral for goldenseal in this formula if organically grown goldenseal is not available.

> 1 part powdered organically grown goldenseal
> 1 part powdered myrrh
> 1 part powdered spilanthes (if available)
> 1 part powdered turmeric
> 1 drop clove essential oil

Combine the herbs with the clove oil and enough water to make a thick paste. Make a small cylinder-shaped poultice and apply directly to the tooth.

HEALING MOUTHWASH

This mouthwash has helped lessen my trips to the dentist.

> ¾ cup water
>
> ¼ cup vodka
>
> 2 dropperfuls calendula tincture
>
> 2 dropperfuls organically grown goldenseal or chaparral tincture
>
> 1 dropperful myrrh tincture
>
> 1 or 2 drops peppermint essential oil

Combine the water and the vodka. Add the tinctures and the essential oil and shake well. Dilute several tablespoons of the mixture in ½ ounce water, and use as a mouthwash.

urinary tract infections and cystitis

Cystitis is an infection of the bladder and urinary system. Symptoms include difficult and burning urination, feeling as though you have to urinate but being unable to, low energy, and sometimes fever. This type of infection can be dangerous, so be mindful and treat it right away.

Cystitis is generally easy to treat with home remedies. Begin treatment at the first signs of infection: a slight burning sensation when urinating or incomplete emptying of the bladder. If you follow even just some of these suggestions, the cystitis should be cleared up in a day or two. If the condition persists for longer than a week, consult a holistic health care practitioner.

Rest

Bed rest is always recommended. Your body is trying to fight off an infection, so slow down.

Cranberry Juice

Cranberry juice prevents bacteria from adhering to the kidneys and urethra and is one of the best preventives and remedies for urinary tract infections. Drink several cups a day. Though unsweetened cranberry juice is best (it is very tart, so you may wish to dilute it with tea or apple juice), cranberry cocktail does work.

Herbs for the Urinary System

Take herbs used specifically for cystitis, such as uva-ursi, pipsissewa, buchu, cleavers, chickweed, nettle, and dandelion leaf. Combine two or more of these to make a tea; drink several cups a day. Take several teaspoons of echinacea tincture daily to boost your resistance.

PRACTICE CAUTION

Do not make love when you have a urinary infection. It is not contagious, but lovemaking can irritate the condition.

CYSTITIS REMEDY

This is an excellent infection-fighting formula.

> **2 parts cleavers**
> **2 parts fresh or dried cranberries**
> **2 parts uva-ursi**
> **1 part chickweed**
> **1 part marsh mallow root**

Combine the herbs and prepare as an infusion, following the instructions on page 380. Drink 4 cups daily, ¼ cup at a time.

Water

Drink adequate amounts of water when you're suffering from cystitis. Fill a quart bottle with water and add the juice of one or two lemons and a squirt of uva-ursi tincture.

Warmth

Keep the kidney area warm. Don't expose it to cold water or cold air. Place a hot-water bottle over the kidneys at night and whenever you're sitting. If you must go to work, take your hot-water bottle with you. Wear long sweaters that cover the kidney area.

Diet

Eat lots of yogurt and miso or chicken soup. Avoid alcohol and sugary foods, which will agitate cystitis.

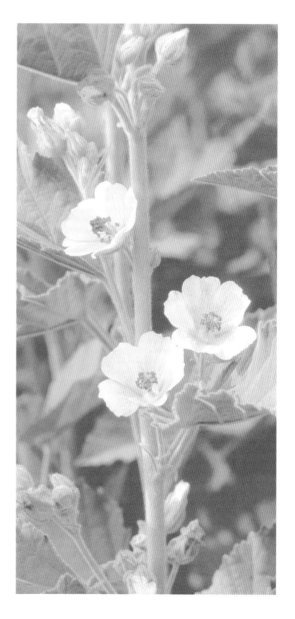

warts

Warts are viral infections that appear as hard, knotty little protrusions on the skin. Although they are unsightly and annoying, they rarely cause serious problems.

Warts are among the most mysterious of all ailments to treat. They can respond to a plethora of approaches — from throwing a beefsteak over your left shoulder to burning them off with chemicals. Sometimes they respond to nothing at all. Over the years, I've heard of a variety of effective treatments. Here's a list of what I've found to be the best:

- **Banana peel.** The inside of a ripe banana peel applied topically is the recommended remedy of Cascade Anderson Geller and David Winston, both renowned herbalists. Tape the peel over the wart; change it several times daily. It may take 2 to 3 weeks, but they swear it works.
- **Celandine juice.** Fresh celandine juice is excellent for getting rid of warts. Crush the fresh plant and apply as a poultice; change the poultice several times daily.

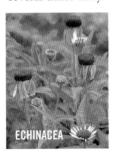
ECHINACEA

- **Anti-wart tincture.** A tincture made with equal parts black walnut, echinacea, and pau-d'arco is effective if warts are of the spreading type; take ½ teaspoon three times a day, and apply topically, as well.

- **Essential oils.** Antiviral essential oils such as tea tree, cajeput, and thuja have been applied topically for several weeks with some success.
- **Kloss's Liniment.** Kloss's Liniment (see recipe on page 80) and cayenne packs applied directly to warts have been successful for me.

Of course, you can also try my self-proved cure for warts. When I was 13, I was awkward, thin, with long dark hair. You can imagine my chagrin when a wart appeared on my chin. I looked at it every day in the mirror, stared it down, and told it to go away. In seven days, it was gone.

first aid at your fingertips

To treat ailments of an everyday nature, we need to be aware of the healing herbs that are a part of our everyday life. In and outside the home, we are surrounded by nature's cures. The food we eat, the spices we season our food with, the plants of the meadows, forests, and swamps just outside our door — all are provided to us in nature's master plan. Consider the case of poison ivy. Touch it and you'll get an awful, itchy rash. The cure? Jewelweed, which, it just so happens, grows most often in and around patches of poison ivy.

Of course, you can best take advantage of nature's gracious gifts by stocking them in your medicine cabinet. But if you find yourself in a situation where you are injured, ill, or just plain uncomfortable and you don't have a ready-made remedy to ease your woes, take a good look around you. Most likely, you'll find the healing power you need right at your fingertips.

The Weedy Wonders

Everywhere, under every footstep, along the road-sides, in empty city lots, in country fields, and thriving beneath the great arching bridges of superhighways, you can find valuable medicinal herbs. These plants thrive in abundance in most regions of North America. These weedy wonders are both versatile and effective medicinal herbs. Make friends with them!

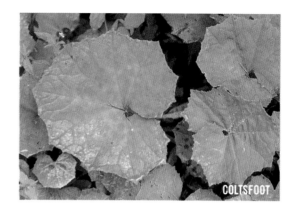

COLTSFOOT

- **Burdock.** Rich in vitamins and minerals, burdock is excellent for the skin and is a superior blood purifier.

- **Chickweed.** Chickweed is rich in calcium, potassium, and iron. With its emollient and demulcent actions, it is an exceptional poultice herb and is excellent for skin irritations and eye inflammation. Chickweed is also a mild and safe diuretic.

- **Cleavers.** Another mild, safe diuretic, cleavers is used to tone and soothe irritations of the kidneys and urinary tract. It is also an excellent lymphatic cleanser.

- **Coltsfoot.** An antiasthmatic and expectorant, coltsfoot is excellent for coughs, colds, and bronchial congestion, helping dilate the bronchioles and expel mucus.

- **Dandelion.** This common weed is an excellent tonic herb, a prized digestive bitter, one of the safest and most effective diuretics, and an excellent source of vitamins and minerals, including calcium, magnesium, iron, and vitamins A and C.

- **Mullein.** Mullein is useful for respiratory infections, bronchial infections, and asthma. The leaves are superb for treating glandular imbalances; the flowers, made into an oil, are excellent for treating ear infections.

- **Nettle.** A superior tonic herb, nettle is rich in iron, calcium, potassium, silicon, magnesium, manganese, zinc, and chromium, as well as a host of other vitamins and minerals. It is a great hair and scalp tonic, an excellent reproductive tonic for both men and women, and a superb herb for the genitourinary system. Nettle is also extremely helpful for treating liver problems and allergies and hay fever.

- **Plantain.** In addition to being a highly nutritional food, plantain is one of the best poultice herbs. It is among my favorite herbs for treating blood poisoning, used externally on the infected area and internally as a tea. The seeds are rich in mucilage and are often used in laxative blends for their soothing bulk action; they are also very effective for treating liver sluggishness and inflammation of the digestive tract.

- **Red clover.** Red clover is one of the best detoxification herbs and respiratory tonics. It is useful for children who have chronic chest complaints such as coughs, colds, and bronchitis. It is also rich in minerals, most notably calcium, nitrogen, and iron.

- **St.-John's-wort.** Well known for lifting the spirits, St.-John's-wort is also valued as an herbal remedy for damage to the nerve endings, such as in burns, neuralgia, and wounds. It is highly effective for relieving stress, anxiety, depression, seasonal affective disorder, and chronic fatigue.

- **Wild raspberry.** Raspberry is a highly nourishing reproductive tonic, providing nutrients that tone and strengthen the genitourinary system. It is incredibly rich in iron and is also a good source of niacin and manganese, a trace mineral used by the body to produce healthy connective tissue such as bone matrix and cartilage.

- **Yarrow.** An excellent diaphoretic, yarrow is often used in teas to promote sweating, thereby helping reduce fevers. It can be used both internally and externally to stop bleeding and is effective for relieving menstrual and stomach cramps. It is often recommended for its beneficial effects on the heart and lungs.

- **Yellow dock.** Yellow dock is one of the best herbs for the digestive system, including the liver. It contains biochelated iron and is useful for treating anemia and fatigue. It is especially helpful for women with PMS and men and women with hormonal imbalances.

Kitchen Aids

Many of my favorite medicinal plants have sneaked into the household via the kitchen door, ushered in by the Mistress of Spices, their healing spirits camouflaged in culinary garb. Most of your favorite kitchen herbs are renowned healers, respected throughout the ages by various cultures. Many are still found in very effective remedies and even pharmaceutical preparations.

Basil

Basil is a favorite tonic for melancholy and low spirits, and it has potent antispasmodic properties,

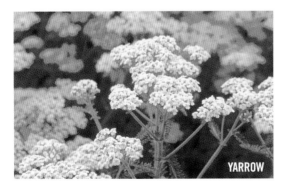

YARROW

making it useful for relieving headaches. It is commonly used to treat stress-induced insomnia and tension as well as nervous indigestion, and it is a well-known aphrodisiac.

Black Pepper

Considered one of the great tonics in traditional Chinese medicine, black pepper is warming, energizing, and stimulating. It is indicated for "cold type" problems such as flus, coughs, colds, slow circulation, and poor digestion.

Cardamom

A divinely sensuous flavor, cardamom belongs to the same family as ginger. It stimulates the mind and arouses the senses. It has long been considered an aphrodisiac, in part because of its irresistible flavor. In Ayurvedic medicine, cardamom is considered one of the best digestive aids. It is often combined as an anticatarrhal in formulas for the lungs.

Cayenne

This herb is as esteemed for its medicinal value as for its culinary fire. It is a supreme heart tonic and has long been used for poor circulation and for irregular or weak heartbeat. It is specifically indicated for colds and flus, used to increase circulation to the extremities, and to improve digestion and sluggish bowels. It is also used internally and externally to halt bleeding.

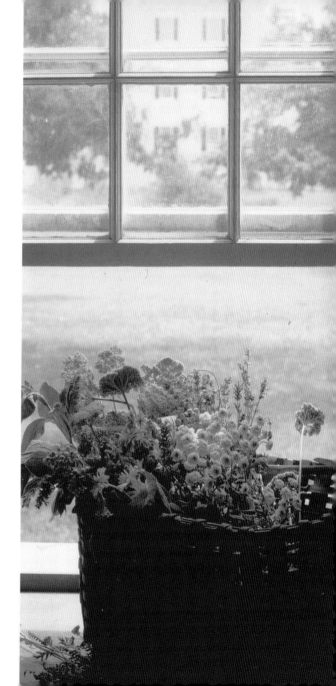

Chives

Similar to garlic, though not as potent, chives have the same antiseptic properties as garlic. They help in the digestion of rich foods and protect the respiratory system. People sensitive to garlic can often enjoy the medicinal and culinary benefits of chives.

Cinnamon

Highly valued in traditional Chinese medicine as a warming herb, cinnamon is used to build vitality, stimulate circulation, and clear congestion. It is a well-respected digestive aid and has powerful antiseptic actions as well. Indicated for poor digestion, colds, and the flu, cinnamon is often used in medicinal formulas to flavor the less tasty herbs.

Cloves

Clove oil is most famous as an analgesic herb for toothaches, but the entire clove bud, powdered and applied directly to the gum, is as effective. Aside from its analgesic properties, clove is stimulating, warming, and uplifting. It is used for sluggish digestion and nausea.

Dill

Dill is one of the most famous of old English remedies for infant colic. Nursery songs were made up about it and sung to the children. Dill's warming and comforting qualities are indicated for gas and colicky digestion.

Garlic

Were I forced to have only one herb in my kitchen, garlic would be it. There's nothing that enhances the flavor of foods or improves health more than garlic. It is the herb of choice for colds, the flu, sore throats, and poor digestion. It stimulates immune activity, improves circulation, and lowers cholesterol. It has a long reputation as a culinary herb and an even longer reputation as a medicinal plant. Garlic, the infamous "stinking rose," may be nothing less than one of the world's greatest medicines.

Ginger

Ginger runs a close second to garlic in my estimation. It is one of the finest herbs for nausea, morning sickness, and motion sickness. Ginger is a warming, decongesting herb used for cold-type imbalances such as poor circulation, sore throats, colds, the flu, and congestion. It is a wonderful herb for the reproductive systems of both men and women and is often used in formulas for cramps and PMS. As if that weren't enough, ginger is quite delicious.

Horseradish

What better remedy is there for sinus congestion and head colds? This is my number one favorite. The root is rich in minerals, including silica, and in vitamins, including vitamin C. Its warming antiseptic properties make it the herb of choice for asthma, catarrh, and lung infections. Horseradish is also prized as a digestive aid and is especially useful when eating heavy, meaty meals.

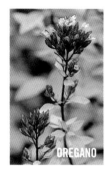

Marjoram and Oregano

Calming and soothing herbs, both marjoram and oregano are used for nervousness, irritability, and insomnia due to tension and anxiety. They are excellent in tea, either in combination or singly, to soothe the nerves or to calm butterflies in the stomach. These delicious herbs also have antispasmodic properties that can be used advantageously for digestive and muscular spasms.

Mint (Peppermint, Spearmint, and Lemon Balm)

Rich in vitamin C, beta-carotene, and chlorophyll, mint is stimulating to the mind and creates "wakefulness." Whiffs of the essential oil, and sometimes even the tea, will improve alertness and awareness, so it's useful when driving, when studying, and during times of stress. It is an excellent antispasmodic and is indicated for cramps and spasms. A terrific remedy for nausea, mint is recommended for travel sickness and some cases of morning sickness. It's also great for tummy aches in children and adults. The flavor of mint cleanses the palate and can be used to rinse the mouth after a bout of vomiting.

Parsley

This superb garnish should never be left slighted on the side of your dinner plate. It may be, in fact, the most nourishing item on the plate. High in iron, beta-carotene, and chlorophyll, parsley is used for iron-poor blood, anemia, and fatigue. It enhances immunity and is indicated for those prone to infections. A primary herb for bladder and kidney problems, it is a safe, effective diuretic. Parsley is used to help dry up a mother's milk during the weaning process and is effective as a poultice for mastitis or swollen, enlarged breasts. Because of this, you should not use parsley in any quantities when nursing, as it may slow the flow of milk.

Rocket (Arugula)

Imagine my delight when I discovered that arugula, my favorite salad green, was a famous sexual stimulant and tonic. I'm not sure whether to indulge more or to be more temperate in my servings.

Rosemary

As rosemary is my namesake, I must admit that I have some preference for this herb. It is legendary as a cerebral tonic and stimulant to the brain. Powerful for those states of debility that are accompanied by loss of memory, loss of smell, poor vision, strain, and nervous tension, rosemary also enhances the cellular uptake of oxygen. It is useful for relieving respiratory congestion and for maintaining liver function and digestion.

Sage

Sage is another remarkable culinary remedy. It aids in the digestion of fatty meats, lowers cholesterol levels, and is a tonic for the liver. It has antiseptic properties and helps with colds, sore throats, and ear infections. It is one of the best remedies for laryngitis and sore throats, often used as a spray or a gargle.

Thyme

This is the best herb we have for stimulating the thymus, a major gland of the immune system. Thyme is a great pick-me-up for low energy. Its antispasmodic properties are useful for lung problems and for convulsive coughs such as whooping cough. It's an excellent remedy for sore  throats (combined with sage), head colds (combined with horseradish), and stiffness related to chills. Thyme also helps stimulate the body's natural defense and, combined with echinacea, boosts the immune system.

Turmeric

This is one of the best herbs for immune health and is often overlooked because of the huge popularity of echinacea. But it has upheld its reputation for its immune-enhancing properties for centuries and is highly regarded for its antitumor and antibiotic activities. In East Indian medicine, it is valued as a blood purifier and metabolic tonic. It is used to regulate the menstrual cycle and relieve cramps, reduce fevers, improve poor circulation, and relieve skin disorders. It is highly valued as a first-aid item for boils, burns, sprains, swelling, and bruises.

Making a First-Aid Kit

You may find, as many others have, that herbs become a passion. Slowly but surely, they take over the entire house: First it's only a small space in the bathroom closet, then a cupboard in the kitchen is cleared, next the entire basement is given over to your herbal wares, and the cars are parked in the driveway because the garage is filled with bottles of odd-looking preparations. About this time, your family may be saying, "No more." But let's assume you're a long way from there and you just want to organize a small kit of useful herbal remedies.

First assess the needs of yourself and your family, and the situations that may arise requiring first aid. Do you have young children? What maladies is your family prone to? A good kit consists of items that can be used for a variety of purposes.

Keep your herbal first-aid kit in one place so it is readily available to you and your family. Baskets, sewing boxes, small suitcases, travel pouches, cosmetic bags, and fishing tackle boxes make great containers for first-aid kits. Be sure everything is clearly labeled so that others can use it.

A NATURAL FIRST-AID KIT

Plenty of herbs work well for minor emergencies. Some of the most versatile herbs and preparations are listed below. In addition to these and your favorite medicinal teas, stock an assortment of powdered herbs; they are easy to mix for poultices and to encapsulate as needed.

Item	Form	Use for
All-purpose/ burn salve	Salve	Cuts, wounds, burns, sunburns
Aloe vera	Gel	Cuts, wounds, burns
Antifungal salve	Salve	Cuts, wounds, burns, sunburns
Cold-care capsules	Capsules	Colds, sluggish digestion, infections
Echinacea	Tincture	Colds, flus, infections, weak immune system
Eucalyptus	Essential oil	Congestion (added to steams), achy muscles, insect repellent, cuts and abrasions, warts, cold sores
Garlic	Oil	Ear infections, parasites, colds
Green clay	Powder	Splinters, wound disinfectant, poultices for poison oak/ivy, skin infections
Kloss's Liniment	Tincture/liniment	Splinters and slivers, poison oak/ivy. For external use only. See recipe on page 80.
Lavender	Essential oil	Headaches, minor burns and sunburn, insect bites, congestion
Licorice root	Tincture	Sore throats, bronchial inflammation, herpes simplex I and II
Mullein flower	Oil	Ear infections, pain
Peppermint	Essential oil	Digestive problems, burns, mouthwash, stimulant
Rescue Remedy	Flower essence	Trauma, both emotional and physical; can be used externally and internally for adults, children, and pets
St.-John's-wort	Oil	Burns, swellings, pain, bruises, sunburn, achy muscles
St.-John's-wort	Tincture	Burns, pain, nerve damage, depression, anxiety
Tea tree	Essential oil	Congestion (added to steams), achy muscles, insect repellent, cuts and abrasions, warts, cold sores, toothaches
Valerian	Tincture	Pain, insomnia, stress and nervous tension, achy muscles

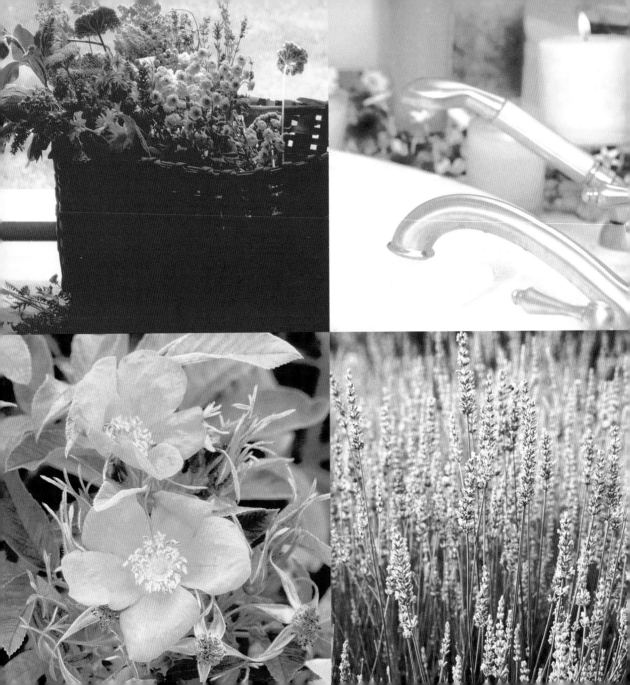

5

Recipes for Radiant Beauty

A mythical Greek goddess whose name meant harmony and balance, Cosmeos gave to mortals the gifts of0 herbs, flowers, and other simple pleasures to nourish the body and the soul. She personified radiant health that flowed from a core of harmony and balance. Cosmeos never sought to mask what she was or how she looked; rather, she fed her inner fire with the eternal gifts of the earth. Her beauty was as abundant as the flowers growing wild on the hillside and as powerful as the granite bones of the mountain.

The modern word *cosmetic* stems from the Greek word *kosmeticos,* meaning "skilled in adornment." This is precisely what Cosmeos was all about; it was never her intent to cover up; she used her creations to revel in who she was. She is one of my favorite goddesses. I envision her as a wild woodland creature running freely through the forests with her sister herbalist Artemis, whose name also has been immortalized in the name of a plant.

Cosmeos, though much misunderstood in the modern-day world of beauty, still yearns to flower in each of us. Her life force is in the rare and unique beauty that resides in the heart, that inner sparkle of the eyes and the radiant glow of the skin. Her teachings are not about what makeup to paint your face with or how to arch the curve of the eyebrow but are, instead, lessons rich with the lore of plants, of health, and of playfulness.

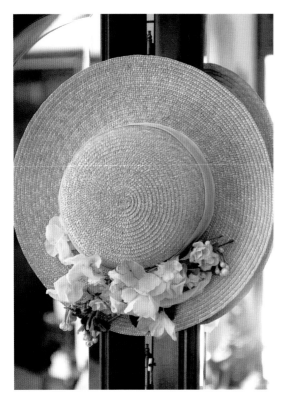

learning the lessons of the goddess

Cosmeos has been a special teacher to me all these years. She has taught me to "take time to smell the flowers" and, furthermore, to rub the juice of those flowers all over me! From her I've learned not to take my herbal work too seriously, and that medicine is found in many expressions. The gentlest cup of tea can often be a potent remedy for the toughest medical cases. She has shown me that nourishing ourselves with lovely herb baths and medicinal oils is often just as healing as the swallowing of tinctures and pills. And, most of all, she has taught me that beauty is as personalized as the profusion of flowers found growing wild on the hillside.

Nowhere in the garden or in the wild do you find an ugly flower. There are odd ones, unusual ones, crazy and outrageous ones, bright ones, dull ones, loud ones, and shy ones. But never have I seen a collection of flowers and proclaimed a single flower in it less than beautiful. Each is unique and so perfectly divine that it has its own beauty. Why can't we see this same unique beauty in one another?

Beauty at Any Cost?

The ethereal concept of beauty and cosmetics has created a rather bizarre fashion industry, one in which beauty means self-manipulation, starving oneself in the name of fashion, and actual surgical restructuring of the body to please somebody else's sense of style. There is little contentment in the profound sense of beauty anymore; rather, it has become a restlessness to achieve something unattainable.

We've replaced simple, old-fashioned truths such as "beauty is in the eye of the beholder" with the new adage "beauty at any cost." Whether that cost is the depletion or destruction of rare and precious resources or the inhumane use of animals to test cosmetics hasn't seemed to matter. But beauty cannot exist long alone. It needs balance and harmony, Cosmeos's gifts, to truly emerge and endure.

The Healing Power of Beauty

When I was a young child growing up on my parents' farm in California, I would often walk into the fields and lie in the tall grasses. I would take off my clothes and lay my body right on top of the bare ground, feeling the earth beneath me. It nourished me and filled me with a deep sense of beauty. I would look up at the blue sky and ask that I be a reflection of all that I saw in nature, so that when people looked at me, they would see the fields and the wildflowers and the depth of the sky in my eyes. It is this early sense of beauty that has permeated and inspired me all these years.

Though much of my work as a community herbalist has been concentrated on creating medicinal formulas and helping people with their illnesses, I always find a way to weave "the beauty way" into my healing work. I want Cosmeos's hand in the pot!

When I mixed and blended my early medicinal tea blends, they always contained a few herbs "just for beauty." My tinctures and elixirs, likewise, had a sweeter taste, a touch of the beauty way complementing the healing powers. All of the medicinal formulas I produce for Frontier, a large herbal cooperative, are infused with a sense of aesthetic. I'm a firm believer that beauty aids in healing and, in fact, that it is one of the greatest healers. It seduces and induces people back to wellness, back to that place of balance and harmony that is the soul of life. Without beauty, why would you want to get well? The flowers, the fresh air, the running waters, and the loving

a wish for wellness and beauty

As you experiment and play with the recipes in this chapter, perhaps inviting friends and family to join you, may you also experience the fullness of life that comes from sharing Cosmeos's gifts. We're often told that the way to the heart is through the stomach, but I think that the heart is most truly reached through the art of touch. Use these earth-inspired recipes, all gifts from nature to the human race, to gently touch the hearts of those you love. It's a wonderful way to practice the art of healing, and your children, partner, and other loved ones will love you the more for it.

hearts of those who care for us — this is the beauty of life, and this is what nourishes the soul and invites it back to wholeness.

Over the years, I delighted in making wonderful "all natural" cosmetics and skin-care products. It was a fun respite from making medicinals for an ever-growing clientele of family and friends who were discovering the healing power of plants. I'd spend my evenings playing with and perfecting recipes for herbal masks, baths, shampoos, and creams, then share these recipes with others. We'd stage "facial parties," gathering friends together to treat one another to herbal hand baths and footbaths, facial steams, and masks. After the "works," we'd finish with a gentle massage using my very favorite facial cream. Pure heaven!

I'd often take the show on the road, packing up baskets of materials to take to workshops. I'd treat everyone there — and you can bet those classes were well attended. When I first moved to New England and was invited by Rick Scalzo to speak at the annual Gaia Herbal Symposium, I offered to do a cosmetic workshop. Rick was very hesitant; he wasn't sure anyone would be interested in cosmetics at a conference that featured herbal medicines. But I felt that even if a few people showed up, it would be worth it. So the cosmetic workshop was included on the schedule, and Rick, still thinking it would be of limited interest, assigned me a small room in which to give my presentation. When it came time for the workshop, it was apparent that we would have to do some quick maneuvering; there were more than 150 people in attendance.

I've often thought that if I had not been so busy with my other herbal work, I would have opened a natural beauty spa dedicated to health and healing. I would open my doors to all those who were sick and full of pain. I'd treat them with salt scrubs, soak them in aromatic herbal baths, and wrap them in sheets scented with delicate essential oils. I would serve them delicious garden teas and wholesome foods. I would even henna their hair, because a correctly applied henna brings transformation even to the most sickly. I'd name this little shop after my first herb shop, Rosemary's Garden of Earthly Delights, which is still thriving 25 years later in northern California.

> **"Here in the body** are the sacred rivers; here are the sun and moon, as well as the pilgrimage places. I have not encountered another temple as blissful as my own body."
>
> **— Sahara**

making your own beauty potions

The recipes that follow are among my favorites. Most are my personal creations; a few have been enhanced by the creative suggestions of others. Many of these recipes came to me in those moments of inspiration when I was out among the flowers. Others I've labored long over to get the exact proportions and effects. And some of them were garnered from students, who often took a simple suggestion I made and added the oh-so-perfect ingredient to create a product of excellence.

Many of my recipes have become quite well known. I see them mentioned in other books and find them for sale at craft fairs and herb shows throughout the country. It gives me a tremendously satisfying feeling!

Gathering the Ingredients

It is wise to assemble ahead of time all the ingredients and utensils you need. There have been times when I haven't followed this little bit of advice and in the middle of a project found I was out of a necessary ingredient. This can be either a big or a little inconvenience, but it's always annoying.

As with any recipe, you can substitute ingredients and experiment with the formulas to create a more personalized product, but be sure you understand what the particular ingredient in the formula is "doing," so that you can substitute for

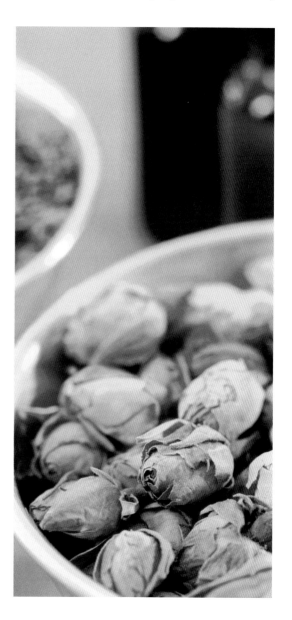

All of these skin-care programs and recipes are offered in the high spirit of Cosmeos. May they serve to enhance your sense of inner harmony and may you become enchanted with your own unique, radiant beauty.

one product another that has similar properties; otherwise, the product may not turn out as hoped for. Ask yourself the basic questions. Is this ingredient an emulsifier? Does it help thicken the product? Does it add moisture? For instance, if you substitute liquid oil for a solid oil in the cream formula on page 132, the cream may turn out runnier than you'd like.

In these recipes, there is always lots of room for creativity. I am one of those people who get frustrated with exact proportions. Coffee mugs are my most usual measuring cups, and spoons from my silverware drawer serve as measuring spoons. When adding essential oils, I lose count somewhere after the fourth or fifth drop and proceed forward by scent and common sense alone. Nothing is exact in my world, and, needless to say, things don't always turn out exactly the same. But I've learned to follow my intuition, and generally

it leads me in its own creative process. Using my common sense rather than exact measurements has often produced exquisite results.

Not to worry, however, if you prefer to follow exact directions! I have carefully formulated each of these recipes so that you can follow them step-by-step with assurance. I strongly suggest that you make the recipes as directed the first couple of times so you get a feel for how they develop. Later, you can try adding your own scent, substituting one type of vegetable oil for another, or using different herbs in the formula. Be sure to write down each of the ingredients and the proportions, so that you can re-create the formula at another time. Don't make the common mistake of thinking that you'll remember. I still lament the many times I've made a perfect product but couldn't recall the scents I'd added or the proportions of oil to water.

Helpful Kitchen Tools

No special tools are needed for creating any of the wonderful cosmetics mentioned in this book. A kitchen with all its normal gadgets will supply you with most of what you need, and the ingredients called for are mostly found in supermarkets or natural foods stores. If not available in your local grocery store, these items are easily acquired from mail-order sources (see Resources). Although you don't need many specific items in order to create your natural beauty products, these everyday tools are helpful to use during recipe making:

- Blender — indispensable in making body lotions and creams
- Fine-mesh strainers
- Hand grater reserved for grating beeswax (beeswax is edible, but it is almost impossible to remove the wax)
- An assortment of glass bottles and jars
- Stainless-steel or glass mixing bowls
- Measuring cups

Selecting Ingredients

Following is a list of some of the more popular cosmetic ingredients and what they are used for. Not only is this practical knowledge, but it gives you greater ability to formulate your own recipes.

If you are familiar with the result each ingredient produces in a formula, you will be able to substitute one item for another. This knowledge comes in handy when you either run out of or don't care for a particular ingredient.

Almond Oil

What it is: Made from the kernels of almonds, this sweet oil is one of the most versatile oils for skin-care products.

What it does: A liquid oil, almond oil is light and works well for most skin types. It smells delicious, too.

Availability: You can find almond oil in natural foods stores.

Aloe Vera

What it is: Native to Africa but common around the world, aloe vera is an excellent plant to keep around the house.

What it does: The gel from the large, succulent leaves of aloe vera is used to treat and soothe burns, rough or irritated skin, and wounds. Aloe is a wonderful moisturizer that also firms and tones the skin. It is a common ingredient in many natural cosmetic products.

Availability: Aloe gel and juice are readily available in natural foods stores and some pharmacies. I keep aloe as a potted plant in my home; when I need fresh gel, it's right there. Though fresh aloe gel is wonderful for use in products that you'll be using up in a few days, for those

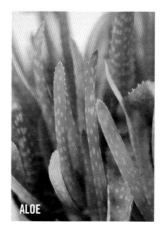

ALOE

that need a longer shelf life, use aloe gel that has at least 1 percent citric acid added as a natural preservative.

Caution: Aloe vera gel should never be used on staph infections. It can lock in the infection and make it worse.

Apricot Kernel Oil

What it is: Derived from the cold-pressed apricot pit, apricot kernel oil is a versatile moisturizer.

What it does: This is another of those perfect, odorless liquid oils that are excellent for skin-care products. It is a light emollient and is suitable for most skin types.

Availability: You can find apricot kernel oil in natural foods stores.

Borax

What it is: Imagine the surprise when women discover that those lovely bath salts they love contain the same ingredient as that popular laundry soap 20 Mule Team Borax. Borax, more commonly called sodium borate by the cosmetic agencies, is a natural mineral mined from only a few places in the world.

What it does: This mineral softens the water, is a cleansing agent, and has the unique ability to suspend soap particles in water so they don't adhere to the skin or clog the pores. The skin is left cleaner and softer because of it.

Availability: Borax is found in almost every grocery store across the country. If not stocked at your local stores, ask them to order it for you.

Castor Oil

What it is: Castor oil is thick, viscous oil extracted from the toxic beans of the castor plant. This oil is not used in cooking but does have a great reputation as a medicinal oil. It's well known for its purging properties and its ability to dissolve cysts and tumors.

What it does: This oil can be used in cosmetic preparations for deep emollient properties. Castor oil is perfect for dry and mature skin.

Availability: Castor oil is widely available in pharmacies and grocery stores.

Clay

What it is: Clay is another wonderful substance mined from the earth. It is the essence of mountains ground down through the ages into a smooth powder. It has been blessed by thousands of sunrises, sunsets, windstorms, and rainstorms. When we use clay in our cosmetics, we are mixing the energy of thousands of years and using it as a beauty aid.

Europeans have used clay for thousands of years both as a medicine and as a cosmetic. Clay baths, facials, and body-care products are popular throughout Europe and are only just catching on in America, where fancy spas now offer a variety of clay-based treatments.

What it does: There are many types of clay, each used for a different purpose. The concentrations of minerals are what determine the color and effect of the clay.

Availability: All the different kinds of clay can usually be found at natural foods stores and spa shops. Look for the following popular varieties:

• *Bentonite.* This softer, more mucilaginous clay has mild properties good for most skin problems. Bentonite can also be taken internally to help supply minerals to people lacking them. It aids in binding toxic minerals, making them insoluble, so they can be more easily eliminated.

• *Green Clay.* High concentrations of plant material and volcanic matter give this clay its

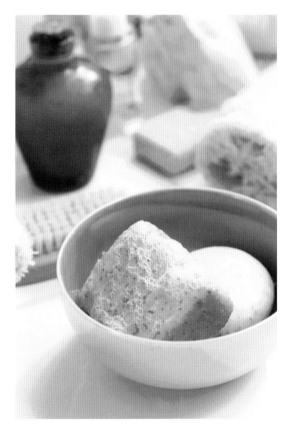

rich mineral content and green coloring. It is my favorite clay for medicinal purposes, but I also find it excellent for most cosmetic purposes. It is fairly mild and can be used successfully for most skin types. However, its green color isn't appropriate for some body powders.

• *Red Clay.* Rich in iron, red clay sports a rusty ✓ color. It is very drying and drawing and is primarily used in medicinal preparations for poison oak/ivy, rashes, and wounds. Red clay is also useful in skin preparations for oily skin, acne, or other problem skin. BOILS ?

• *White Clay.* This is the most versatile of all clays and the one used most often in cosmetics. Because it's milder and less drying than other clays, white clay is used in skin masks, body packs, powders, and bath salts. The white clay generally used in cosmetics is called kaolin. It is available in natural foods stores but can also be purchased at a much lower price in ceramic supply stores.

Cocoa Butter

What it is: Cocoa butter is the fat surrounding the cacao bean. No wonder it smells heavenly; in fact, everything that's made from it has the possibility of smelling like chocolate milk if you are not careful in the formulation.

What it does: A thick, solid oil, cocoa butter is one of the richest oils available. Use sparingly in formulas intended for oily skin! On the other hand, cocoa butter is excellent for dry, mature skin.

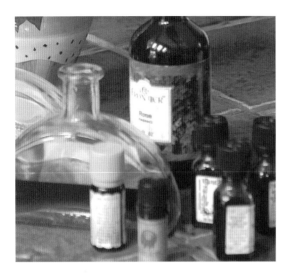

Along with its emollient properties, it will help thicken body-care products. If you get small tapioca-like kernels in your cream, this is an indication that you've added too much cocoa butter to your base.

Availability: Cocoa butter is found in most natural foods stores, some pharmacies, and mail-order catalogs.

Coconut Oil

What it is: This is probably the most-used oil for cosmetic purposes. Long treasured for its protective emollient properties, coconut oil was prized by tropical island dwellers as a cosmetic aid. It was liberally smeared on the body to protect against dryness and combed into the hair to ensure healthy, shiny locks.

What it does: Coconut oil is a rich emollient. Not as thick or fatty as cocoa butter, this oil is more suitable for most skin types. It is commonly used as a moisturizer for skin and hair.

Availability: Found in most natural foods stores, herb stores, and some pharmacies, coconut oil is also available through mail-order catalogs. The best source, though, is the local people who make it and sell it on the beaches of tropical islands.

Grapeseed Oil

What it is: This fixed or liquid oil is one of the lightest and best oils available.

What it does: Considered a "non-oily" oil, grapeseed oil is quickly absorbed by the skin and leaves no oil residue. It's perfect for oily or blemished skin, and especially for teenage skin. It's also odorless.

Availability: Grapeseed oil is readily available in natural foods stores and some grocery stores.

Lanolin

What it is: Lanolin is the protective oil found on the wool of sheep. It helps keep the sheep warm and makes their coats somewhat weather-resistant.

What it does: This thick, viscous substance is the oil most like our own skin oil, making it one of the best moisturizers for humans.

Availability: Hydrolyzed lanolin, which is odorless but heavily processed and often laden with synthetic chemicals, is readily available in pharmacies.

Though it is a bit more challenging to use, I always recommend pure or anhydrous lanolin. Use only small amounts or the sheeplike odor will permeate everything you make. Anhydrous lanolin is available in some pharmacies, as well as in most natural foods stores.

Rose Water

What it is: You must be careful when purchasing rose water to buy only the 100 percent pure form. Often what is available in pharmacies and even some natural foods stores is synthetic rose oil and water with preservatives added. Pure rose water is the distilled water of roses. It is usually made by steam distillation, and it smells heavenly and tastes delicious.

What it does: Rose water is used in cosmetics mainly for its lovely scent, but also because it has light astringent properties. It is often used as toner for fair and dry skin.

Availability: Rose water is available in most health food stores and herb shops. You also can often find rose water in delicatessens; it is used as a flavoring in Greek pastries, puddings, and cakes. Try

RUGOSA ROSE

ordering this ingredient from some of the companies listed in Resources, or make your own (see the recipes that follow).

ROSE WATER, METHOD #1

Though distilling fresh rose petals generally produces rose water, the following method is simple and effective, and it ensures a perfect rose water every time. Be sure you use fresh roses that have just begun to open; they are at their prime and will yield the strongest water. The more fragrant the roses, the stronger the scent of the rose water. Using roses that have been sprayed with insecticides will result in the toxins' being extracted into the water.

> **3 parts witch hazel extract, vodka, or gin**
> **1 part distilled water**
> **Fresh, organically grown roses or rose petals**

1. Mix the witch hazel extract (or vodka or gin) with the distilled water. Place the fresh roses in a quart jar. Completely cover the roses with the alcohol mixture, adding enough extra that the alcohol mixture rises 2 to 3 inches above the flowers. Cover tightly and place in a warm shaded area. Let the mixture sit for 2 to 3 weeks.

2. Strain out the roses and rebottle the water for use. Rose water does not need refrigeration, though storing it in a cool place will prolong its shelf life.

ROSE WATER, METHOD #2

This recipe is the more traditional way to prepare rose water. Though it's a little more involved, it's fun to do and the results are outstanding. You can make a quart of excellent-quality rose water in about 40 minutes. However, if you simmer the water too long, you will continue to produce distilled water, but the rose essence will become diluted. Your rose water will smell more like plain distilled water than like heavenly roses.

Be sure you have a brick and a heat-safe stainless-steel or glass quart bowl ready before you begin.

2 to 3 quarts fresh rose petals
Water
Ice cubes or crushed ice

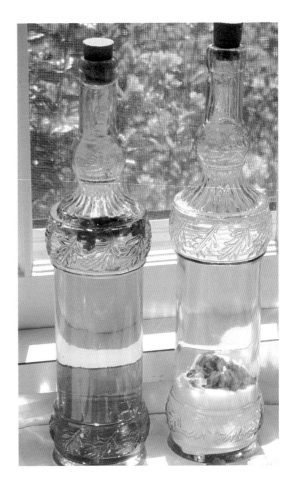

1. Place a brick in the center of a large pot with a rounded lid (the speckled blue canning pots are ideal). Place the bowl on top of the brick. Put the roses in the pot; add enough flowers to reach the top of the brick. Pour in just enough water to cover the roses; it should rise to just above the top of the brick.

2. Place the lid upside down on the pot. Turn on the heat and bring the water to a rolling boil. Then lower the heat to a slow, steady simmer and toss two or three trays of ice cubes (or a bag of ice) on top of the lid. You've now created a home still! As the water boils, the steam rises, hits the top of the cold lid, and condenses. As it condenses, it flows to the center of the lid and drops into the bowl.

3. Every 20 minutes, quickly lift the lid and take out a tablespoon or two of the rose water. It's time to stop when you have between a pint and a quart of water that smells and tastes strongly like roses.

Witch Hazel Extract

What it is: This is an old-fashioned herbal product made from the bark of the witch hazel plant, a small, shrublike tree native to North America. It is produced by steam distillation.

What it does: Witch hazel extract is used in many cosmetic products for its light astringent and firming properties. Witch hazel also has mild antibacterial properties, making it an excellent treatment for acne and skin problems.

Availability: The extract can be found in most pharmacies and natural foods stores. You can make your own witch hazel extract by purchasing witch hazel bark from an herb company and soaking it in alcohol (use rubbing alcohol for extract to be used externally and brandy or vodka for extract to be used internally). However, the commercially available extracts are of good quality, so I usually find it simplest to buy witch hazel extract.

it's not just a girl thing

Don't hesitate to undertake a beauty session with your male friends. They'll resist it at first, but once you get going, they'll love it. If you have your eye on a particular guy, or if you'd like to spice things up with your husband, invite him into your herbal beauty parlor. Turn on the red light, bring out all the silky, smooth, aromatic potions you've been making, and treat him to a special man's night out.

When I began dating my boyfriend, Robert, I was quite impressed with him. Aside from being a skilled carpenter and owning his own construction company, he was charming, kind, handy, and handsome to boot. On his birthday, I decided to give him the special treatment and invited him to my house for the afternoon. He came — a little suspiciously, I might add.

I seated him in the biggest, most comfortable armchair I own and proceeded to untie his shoes. I placed each foot and each big carpenter hand into a pot of steaming water filled with aromatic herbs. I gently covered his face with a moisturizing clay mask, and, while he sat there, hands and feet in steaming water, face covered, eyes closed, I began slowly to massage his feet, his shoulders, and, finally, his head. Well, quite frankly, that man was in heaven — and has been there ever since. Though he did command me, "Don't you dare tell my friends!" And, of course, I never did. . . .

my favorite
skin-care recipes

These are my all-time favorite cosmetics recipes. They're simple to make, fun, and inexpensive. Best of all, they work wonders. All of the following recipes are made with the finest of natural ingredients; each of the ingredients contributes to the integrity of the final product. One of the wonders of making your own skin-care products is that you can have the finest quality for the least amount of money. You also have control of what goes into the product and onto your face.

Do not be fooled by the many "natural" ingredients used in commercial skin-care products. Many of these ingredients are added only so that the consumer is impressed. (*Consumer* is the somewhat derogatory title bestowed on us by the manufacturers of products. I'm starting a small rebellion and asking that we be called the conscious public.) Notice how far down the list of ingredients the natural ones are. The farther down the list, the smaller the amount the ingredient is in the total product. Also, note how many ingredients listed are preservatives, coloring agents, synthetic scents, and chemicals.

It is true that not all chemicals and ingredients with "synthetic" names are harmful. But most ingredients in their totally natural state are called by names we recognize. If a natural ingredient has received a manufactured-sounding name, it is often because it's been manipulated to be something less than natural. My best advice is if you don't know what something is or what it does, don't smear it on your face.

Important Advice

Before you get started on these recipes, remember to have fun, enjoy the process, and be creative! These recipes are meant to be played and tampered with. Add the extra pinch of herb, a new exotic scent, a touch of this or that. Just as a good cook follows an exact recipe only once, then adds her own spark of inspiration, so these formulas are best awakened with your own dreams.

A few words of advice about experimenting with these beauty-care recipes:

- Always experiment in small batches, so that you won't waste a lot of precious ingredients.
- Know what each ingredient does in the formula, so that you can substitute something that works similarly.
- Keep a collection of your favorite recipes. These may be passed down to your grandchildren or be the base of your own book someday.
- All herbs used in these recipes are dried, unless otherwise specified.

Cleansing Grains

A perfect soap replacement, cleansing grains are mild, nourishing, suitable for all skin types, and can be used daily. I've tried most cleansing grains on the market. Some are quite nice, but my own simple recipe remains my favorite. I can mix and blend it to suit myself. It's inexpensive enough that I can use it as a total body scrub. And it's completely biodegradable and even quite tasty — I could eat it in a pinch!

Many commercial cleansing grains are far too harsh; they feel like sandpaper on the skin. Teenagers with acne often use these rough cleansers, thinking that somehow they can scrub that acne away. Not so! Most types of skin, and especially blemished skin, must be treated gently. Harsh cleansers will only further irritate the

already inflamed condition. By contrast, these light grains are perfect for blemished skin. They gently cleanse, distribute excess oil, remove dead cells, and improve circulation.

MIRACLE GRAINS

There are many items you can add to this basic formula, such as seaweed, vitamins A and E, and other combinations of herbs. Be creative! You may design a truly unique and wonderful formula personalized for your skin type.

You may wish to add a few drops of essential oils such as lavender, rose, or lemon balm to enhance the scent and the effect of the grains. The oils must be pure, not synthetic; synthetic oils can burn or irritate the skin.

quick grains tip

You will want to grind the ingredients for Miracle Grains very finely, but remember to leave just a touch of "grit" in them. This is what serves as the cleansing "grains." You won't have any trouble achieving this with the lavender and roses, because they always retain a somewhat coarse feeling.

I have found that electric coffee grinders work best for grinding small amounts of herbs, flowers, and spices. However, do not use the grinder you use for coffee; your herbs will smell like coffee beans, and your coffee will forever smell and taste like roses and lavender.

> 2 cups white clay
> 1 cup finely ground oats
> ¼ cup finely ground almonds
> ⅛ cup finely ground lavender
> ⅛ cup poppy seeds or finely ground blue corn (optional)
> ⅛ cup finely ground roses

1. Combine all the ingredients. Store the grains next to the sink in a glass container or in spice jars with shaker tops.
2. To use, mix 1 to 2 teaspoons of the cleansing grains with water. Stir into a paste and gently massage on the face. Rinse off with warm water.

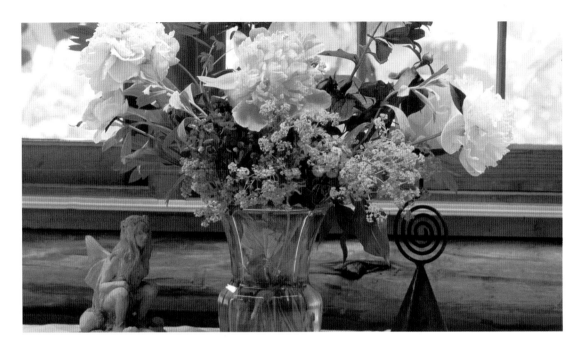

MOIST MIRACLE GRAINS

I prefer the dry cleansing grains for storage purposes and usually package them that way for gifts; but for my personal use, I always make them moist. They're so much easier to use when made up already, and they have the addition of a couple more yummy ingredients.

Honey serves as a natural preservative for the grains, as well as adding its wonderful moisturizing quality. Though it may seem as though the honey would make the grains very sticky, it doesn't.

I usually mix only enough moist grains for a week or two to prevent spoilage. If the grains do spoil, it's because the ratio of honey to distilled water was off. The distilled water is added to give a smoother consistency. Don't use much.

Miracle Grains (see recipe on page 127)
Honey
Pure distilled rose water (or plain
    distilled water)

1. Combine the dry Miracle Grains with enough honey and rose water to form a paste.
2. Gently massage onto the face. Rinse off with warm water.

Herbal Facial Steams

Following are two of my favorite recipes for facial steams. Everybody who makes these steams has his or her favorite recipe that is, I suspect, often based on whatever herbs may be on hand. When blending your own formulas, use herbs that have been traditionally used for the care of the skin. Know also whether the herb is slightly drying (astringent) or moisturizing (mucilaginous). Add flowers for color and texture; it is lovely to be steaming your skin over a big pot of simmering roses, marigolds, chamomile and lavender blossoms.

To perform a facial steam, bring 2 to 3 quarts of water to a boil in a large pot. Toss in a healthy handful of herbs, cover, and let simmer for just a couple of minutes. Then remove the pot from the heat source and place it on a heatproof surface at a level that will enable you to comfortably sit and place your face over the pot. Leaning over the

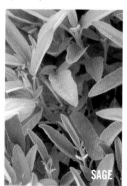

pot, drape a large, thick towel over both your head and the pot, capturing the steaming herb water. It will get very hot under the towel. To regulate the heat, raise or lower your head or lift a corner of the towel to let in a little cool air. You can come out occasionally to catch a breath of cool air, if necessary. Steam for 5 to 8 minutes.

STEAM FOR DRY TO NORMAL SKIN

3 parts comfrey leaf
2 parts calendula
2 parts chamomile
2 parts roses
1 part lavender

Combine the herbs, adjusting the amounts to suit your skin type. Store in an airtight glass bottle. Use as instructed at left for a facial steam.

STEAM FOR NORMAL TO OILY SKIN

3 parts comfrey leaf
2 parts calendula
1 part raspberry leaf
1 part sage
¼ part rosemary

Combine the herbs, adjusting the amounts to suit your skin type. Store in an airtight glass bottle. Use as instructed at left for a facial steam.

Astringents

Astringents, also known as toners, are used to remove excess oil from the skin. They are usually applied after cleansing; they remove any residual cleanser and tone the skin, helping prepare it for moisturizing. While astringents are especially appropriate for oily skin, all types of skin can benefit from their pore-tightening effects.

THE QUEEN OF HUNGARY'S WATER

This wonderful astringent lotion has been hailed as the first herbal product ever produced and marketed. Legend has it that the early Gypsies formulated it and claimed it to be a cure-all. Whether or not it is I hardly know, but I do know that it is an excellent astringent for the face and a great rinse for dark hair.

This is one of the world's finest cosmetic formulas. It combines gentle common herbs in a masterful way, it's easy to make, and it's a versatile formula that serves many purposes. The Gypsies used it as a hair rinse, mouthwash, headache remedy, aftershave, footbath, and who knows what else! I have seen this formula sold in department stores in exotic little bottles for a fancy price. You can make it for the cost of a few herbs and a bottle of vinegar.

> 6 parts lemon balm
> 4 parts chamomile
> 4 parts roses
> 3 parts calendula
> 3 parts comfrey leaf
> 1 part lemon peel
> 1 part rosemary
> 1 part sage
> **Vinegar to cover (apple cider or wine vinegar)**
> **Rose water or witch hazel extract**
> **Essential oil of lavender or rose (optional)**

1. Place the herbs in a widemouthed jar. Fill the jar with enough vinegar that it rises an inch or two above the herb mixture. Cover tightly and let it sit in a warm spot for 2 to 3 weeks.

2. Strain out the herbs. To each cup of herbal vinegar, add ⅔ to 1 cup of rose water or witch hazel. Add a drop or two of essential oil, if desired. Rebottle. This product does not need to be refrigerated and will keep indefinitely.

BAY RUM AFTERSHAVE AND ASTRINGENT

This recipe is inspired by the gorgeous aromatic bay tree, which grows in abundance around my home in the California coastal range. This wonderful all-natural tonic is a bracing astringent or perfect aftershave to tighten and firm pores. It also makes a great gift.

Fresh bay leaves are really the best to use; the dried leaves maintain little of the pungent intensity.

> **Bay leaves (fresh, if possible)**
> **Allspice, ground or grated**
> **Whole cloves**
> **Ginger, grated or ground (grated is preferable)**
> **Rum**

1. Pack a widemouthed jar with bay leaves, leaving some room at the top. Add the desired amount of allspice, cloves, and ginger to give the product a bit

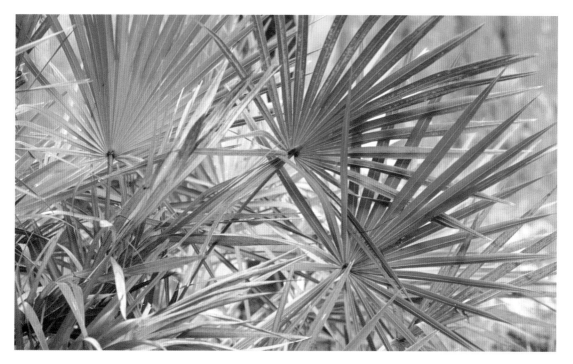

of a spicy aroma. Fill the jar with enough rum that it rises about an inch or two above the herbs. Cover tightly and let sit for 3 to 4 weeks in a warm place.
2. Strain out the herbs and rebottle the herbal liquid. You may wish to add a drop or two of essential oil of bay to strengthen the scent, especially if you have used dried bay leaves to make the astringent.

Facial Cream

The following recipe makes the most wonderful facial cream I have ever experienced. I have used it in its many variations for many years, smoothing it over every inch of my body, and my skin — now heading into its sixth decade — is still soft and supple as a child's. (Well, this may be stretching the truth a bit, but it still feels wonderful to me!)

The cream is rich with natural ingredients. Deeply moisturizing, it provides nourishment and moisture for the skin. And for the final stroke, it is relatively inexpensive to make. This basic formula, though excellent as is, can be further embellished with your own creative spirit. There is plenty of room for creative input. Feel free.

ROSEMARY'S PERFECT CREAM

Though this recipe appears easy, it is also a bit challenging. You are attempting to combine water and oil; they don't normally mix. Follow the recipe closely. If it doesn't turn out right the first time, don't be discouraged. Try again; the luscious cream is well worth your time and effort.

Package your cream in glass jars. It doesn't need to be stored in the refrigerator.

WATERS

⅔ cup distilled water (or rose water)

⅓ cup aloe vera gel

1 or 2 drops essential oil of choice

Vitamins A and E as desired

OILS

¾ cup apricot, almond, or grapeseed oil

⅓ cup coconut oil or cocoa butter

¼ teaspoon lanolin

½ to 1 ounce grated beeswax

1. Combine the waters in a glass measuring cup. (Tap water can be used instead of distilled water, but it will sometimes introduce bacteria and encourage the growth of mold.) Set aside.

2. In a double boiler over low heat, combine the oils. Heat them just enough to melt.

3. Pour the oils into a blender and let them cool to room temperature. The mixture should become thick, creamy, semisolid, and cream colored. This cooling process can be hastened in the refrigerator, but keep an eye on it so it doesn't become too hard.

4. When the mixture has cooled, turn on the blender at its highest speed. In a slow, thin drizzle, pour the water mixture into the center vortex of the whirling oil mixture.

5. When most of the water mixture has been added to the oils, listen to the blender and watch the cream. When the blender coughs and chokes and the cream looks thick and white, like buttercream frosting, turn off the blender. You can slowly add more water, beating it in by hand with a spoon, but don't overbeat! The cream will thicken as it sets.

6. Pour into cream or lotion jars. Store in a cool location.

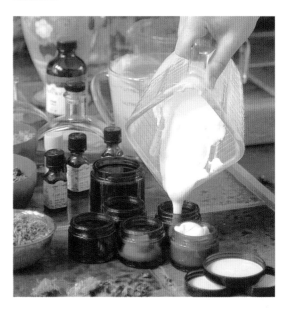

Tips for Making and Using Perfect Cream

For many years, I'd first put the waters into the blender and then add the oils, until one of my students told me she had reversed the process and never had any more problems with separation. It is wonderfully simple suggestions like this that have made this cream so successful. So keep playing with the recipe, and keep me informed of your findings.

Unlike many commercial creams that only coat the surface of the skin, this cream penetrates the epidermal layer and moisturizes the dermal layer of the skin. Because it is extremely concentrated, a little goes a long way. Take a tiny drop on the end of your finger and gently massage it into your face. There will be a temporary feeling of oiliness, but it will disappear within a few minutes as the cream is quickly absorbed. Though I recommend just a small amount on your face, you can be generous on the rest of your body.

The only real "rule" about this cream is that it never can be used with any negative thoughts about the body it's being used on. When smoothing it over the creases and maps of the skin, do so with love. Do it as if you're anointing yourself with precious balm. You are! This is part of the cream's magic.

Followed exactly, the cream recipe should work for you. If the waters and oils separate, it is most likely because they weren't at the correct temperature; the waters must be at room temperature and the oils must be completely cooled. If the waters and oils separate, you can separate them entirely and begin the process again. Or just put a little note on your package that says SHAKE BEFORE USING.

Rosemary's Perfect Cream should never become moldy or go bad. If it does, you'll find it's generally because of one or more of the following:

Recycled lids. If you reuse a container, be sure the inner cardboard ring in the lid has been removed. It's a perfect host for bacteria.

Food ingredients. Many foods support bacterial growth. For instance, if you decided you wanted a strawberry-scented moisturizer and blended fresh strawberries in your cream base, you'd develop mold on your "Strawberry Delight" within days.

Improper storage. Don't store the cream in a warm location. It's best to store any extra in the refrigerator or a cool pantry.

what makes it "perfect"?

What makes our skin dry out is lack of water, so a good moisturizing cream contains a large percentage of water. The oil you put in the formula coats, soothes, protects, and, most important, holds in the water. A perfect cream is an approximately equal balance of water and oil. But because water and oil don't mix well, getting them to cohabitate in a cream can be a wee bit challenging.

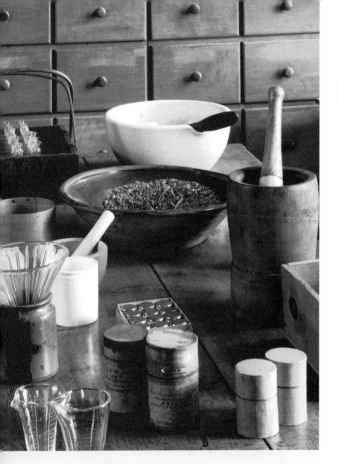

getting the right proportions

Proper proportions are essential to the success of Rosemary's Perfect Cream. The proportions should be roughly 1 part waters to 1 part oils. The oils should be approximately ½ cup liquid oil (such as almond and apricot) to ⅓ cup solid oil (such as cocoa butter, coconut oil, beeswax, and lanolin).

regular skin-care routine

Follow this regular skin-care routine for beautiful skin.

Daily
- Cleanse with cleansing grains.
- Close pores with an astringent.
- Massage in a light cream.
- Finish with a light mist of rose water or an astringent.

Weekly
- Use a honey or clay mask suitable for your skin type.

Monthly
- Treat yourself and a friend! Follow the entire five-step program that follows for radiant skin!

a five-step skin-care program for perfect skin

This treatment takes about 45 marvelous minutes and, for best results, should be done at least once or twice a month. By following this simple, inexpensive treatment, you can be assured of healthier, glowing skin within 2 to 3 months. But you can also be assured of being everyone's favorite "party girl." Invite friends over for a facial party. Take your "facial kit" with you to parties and family gatherings. You'll always be invited back.

My tea parties are highly popular. I invite friends over for tea in the gardens and when the moment is just right, after tea and light laughter, I bring out the cosmetics. Before long, everyone is involved in the giving and receiving of facials. This is healing work. It makes people happy, lets them have fun and enjoy life's sweet blessings. And it makes them feel better.

Step One: Miracle Grains

Lightly cleanse your face and neck with Miracle Grains (see the recipe on page 127). Use the grains to gently massage and stimulate the skin. The grains will massage off dry, dead skin, increase circulation to the facial surface, and provide a nourishing "meal" for your face. Rinse off the grains with warm water.

Step Two: Herbal Facial Steam

Select an herbal facial steam that's best for your skin type (see the recipes on page 129). Bring the herbs to a boil in a large pot of water. Remove from heat source; steam for 5 to 8 minutes.

A facial steam is the best possible way for deep pore cleansing, and each of the herbs used is rich in nutrients that nourish and tone the skin. The aromatic oils of the plants are released by the heat and are absorbed by the skin. And best of all, it feels so good!

Immediately after you complete your facial steam, rinse your face with cold water and gently

> "**Anyone** who keeps the ability to see beauty never grows old."
>
> — **Franz Kafka**

pat with The Queen of Hungary's Water (page 130) or rose water (pages 123 and 124). Gently pat dry. Your face will feel smooth and will glow with radiance.

Step Three: Facial

Facials are excellent for stimulating circulation to the skin by drawing fresh blood to the surface. They promote deep pore cleansing and help heal blemishes and acne. Facials also help tone and firm the skin.

There are several kinds of facials available. My favorites are made with a base of cosmetic clay, which is particularly suitable when you want a drawing, firming type of facial. Clay is very high in minerals and nourishes the skin. More important, the mineral deposits are thousands of years old. These unique deposits of earth have seen a million sunrises and moonsets; they've been washed by powerful rainstorms and impregnated by lightning and thunder. We mix that clay with a little water and put it on our faces in the name of Cosmeos. Now that is pretty powerful medicine!

Honey, too, has its magic and is another of my favorite facials. It is a marvelous cosmetic aid for the skin. A natural humectant, honey both moisturizes and cleanses the skin. Furthermore, bacteria cannot live in honey. Applying a honey pack to your face is a bit messy, but the results are well worth the trouble.

If choosing a clay facial, mix it with just enough water to make a nice paste. The thicker the clay/water mix, the more drying the facial. Apply, and leave on until completely dry. It is

personalized clay facials

For a more individualized clay facial, you can add many other therapeutic ingredients to the mask. Mashed ripe avocado, yogurt, banana, a small amount of almond or grapeseed oil are but a few suggestions. Each will add its own special healing touch. When I first started to do facials, one could find me towel-turbaned in the kitchen, wearing on my face whatever was going into the dinner pot. It created lots of funny reactions, but I learned quite quickly with this hands-on approach what was perfectly divine for my skin type.

tempting to want to rinse it off beforehand, especially as it starts to tighten, but you will not receive the full benefits from a clay facial if you rinse it off before it is completely dry.

For dry skin, choose a white cosmetic-grade clay. White clay, though lightly drawing, is very gentle to the skin. For a more nourishing facial, mix with yogurt or avocado, or both.

For oily skin, choose green, red, or yellow clay. These clays are much more drying than the white variety. They also are very high in minerals and are excellent for problematic, blemish-prone skin. In natural therapeutics, these clays are often used for soothing poison oak and poison ivy, bee stings, and insect bites.

For all skin types, honey makes an excellent facial pack. It draws fresh blood to the surface of the skin, removes impurities, and smooths and softens.

If you choose to use the honey pack, apply a fingerful of honey to skin that is completely dry. It won't work well if the skin is wet or damp. Be sure all your hair is out of reach; it gets very sticky when full of honey! Gently massage, pat, and rub honey into the skin. Let your senses tell you what strokes to use. I usually enjoy a rather vigorous rubbing and patting motion, but others prefer a gentle stretching and light patting. Either way, your skin will be so invigorated and stimulated it fairly glows. Rinse the honey off with warm water. It comes off very easily, but be sure to rinse off completely or you will feel sticky for the rest of the day. The fresh flow of blood brought to the surface of the skin by the honey facial will create a deep, warm, lasting glow.

Step Four: Tonic Astringents

When the facial is completely dry, rinse off with warm water. Be gentle to your skin while rinsing off the facial material. Honey will rinse off easily and quickly, but clay may take a bit more effort. Use soft, circular motions. Massage your skin; do not scrub it. Immediately after rinsing the facial, apply an astringent preparation to tone and close the pores. Use a cotton pad for application, or mist the skin with a spritzer bottle. Choose from the following treatments:

- For dry skin, use rose water, a very light, gentle astringent.
- For normal to oily skin, use The Queen of Hungary's Water or Bay Rum Aftershave and Astringent (see the recipes on page 130).

Step Five: Massage and Cream

The finishing touch is a light, delicate facial massage using your specially formulated Perfect Cream (see the recipe on page 132). This is usually everyone's favorite part, especially when someone else does it for you and you can just sit back and enjoy.

Spread a small amount of cream on your palms and gently circle the outer edges of the face, always stroking upward and outward. Follow the contours of the face, using your fingers to trace the structure. You can use gentle motions, circular motions, and sweeping motions up and away from the face.

May your body be **blessed**.

May you realize that your body is a **faithful** and **beautiful friend** of your soul.

May you recognize that your senses are **sacred thresholds**.

May you realize that holiness is mindful gazing, **mindful feeling**, mindful listening, and mindful touching.

May your senses always enable you to **celebrate the universe** and the mystery and possibilities in your presence here.

May Eros bless you.

May your **senses gather you** and bring you home.

— **Celtic blessing**

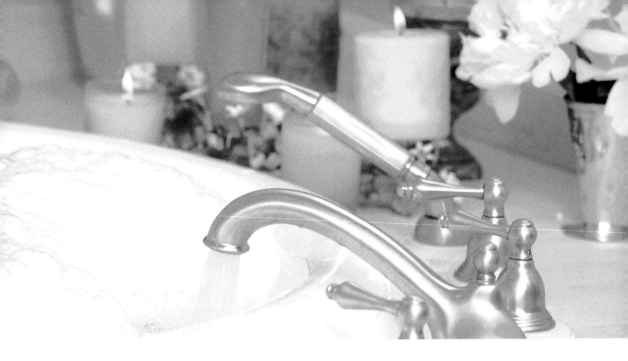

beauty and the bath

Beauty begins in the bath. A centuries-old ritual, herbal bathing not only is a soothing cosmetic affair but also has important therapeutic applications. I've used herbal baths with great success for people suffering from terrible headaches, stress, and skin problems. The worse case of shingles I've ever seen responded well to herbal baths prepared with oats, sea salt, and essential oil of lavender.

It's unfortunate that the bath has been replaced with the shower, another of those quick conveniences of modern times. Though certainly a quick way to freshen the body, showers are no replacement for a long, luxurious soak. I've heard people reflect that they don't like the idea of soaking in their dirty bathwater. Heavens, rinse off first if you're so dirty! But don't forgo the pleasures of a bath.

Making a Special Bathing Place

Aside from lack of time, I think a major reason people don't allow themselves the therapeutic benefits of bathing is the bathtub itself. Tubs have grown smaller and smaller over the years, while the human body keeps growing larger. There's nothing quite as comfortable as an old-fashioned claw foot tub. You can find them, a bit beat up but still serviceable, at many barn sales; with a fresh application of ceramic, they're as good as new. Those old claw foots — or anything else as deep and long — make herbal bathing a divine pleasure.

If you have a country place or even a garden in town that's well protected, you can create an outdoor bathing pavilion that's fit for the queen or king in you. Place a claw foot tub in a private location in the yard. Plant all manner of flowering vines around it, supporting them with an arbor or trellis. If you prefer to gaze at the stars while bathing, leave the space above the tub open. On warm evenings, enjoy cool baths surrounded by your aromatic jungle of plants. On cooler evenings, fill the tub with great pots of hot water and sink into the delicious warmth as your lungs savor the crisp air. Don't tell too many people that the tub is there, or you'll never get the chance to soak in it yourself.

Years ago, when I lived in the beautiful Carmel Valley off the Pacific Coast Highway, I met a delightful older woman. I happened to be hitchhiking back "home" (to my camp on the banks of the Carmel Valley River), when she picked me up in her large, late-model car. She told me about the days when she was a young woman living in Carmel. There was an old farmer down the coast who had hot springs on his land. He had moved several old claw foot tubs onto the cliffs above the sea and ran the natural hot mineral water into them. He rented those tubs out by the hour, and she and her friends would go there on dates, making out madly in the hot tubs while watching the sun go down. Those were the early days of Esalen, now a famous hot springs resort in Big Sur.

Therapy in a Tub

Herbal baths can be extremely therapeutic. When you are immersed in water, the pores of the skin are open and receptive to the healing properties of the herbs; it's a highly effective method of treatment. In fact, there have been several well-known herbalists whose preferred method of treatment was via the bath.

On the following pages, you'll find some of my all-time favorite recipes for the herbal bathing ritual. Use them, make them your own, and enjoy!

"**When I wash my face** in the sink, splash water from a fountain, take a bath, I am always reminded of the stream or river or ocean that these drops of water flow from."

— **Svevo Brooks**

RELAXING BATH BLEND

The ingredients in this bath blend encourage a peaceful state of mind. Use the blend whenever you need to relax.

2 parts chamomile

2 parts lavender

2 parts roses

1 part comfrey leaf

1. Mix the herbs. Place a large handful or two of the herbal mixture in a muslin bag or handkerchief and tie the container onto the nozzle of the tub.
2. Turn the tap on hot and let it pour through the herbal bath bag, turning the tub water into a strong herbal infusion.
3. Run enough cold water into the tub to bring the water to the desired temperature.

Note: For a shower, tie the herbal container onto the showerhead. When it is soaked through, untie it and use it as your washcloth. It's not quite as effective as an herbal bath, but it will do in a pinch.

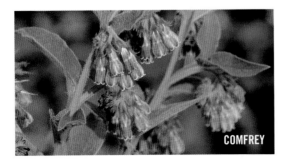

COMFREY

STIMULATING BATH BLEND

Bathing in herbs is like immersing one's body in a giant cup of tea. All the pores are open and the skin, our largest organ of absorption and elimination, absorbs the healing essences of the herbs. You emerge renewed, refreshed.

I prefer using cloth bags for the herbs so I can use the herbal bag as a washcloth while bathing.

3 parts peppermint

2 parts calendula

1 part bay leaf or eucalyptus

1 part rosemary

1 part sage

1. Mix the herbs. Place a large handful or two of the herbal mixture in a muslin bag or handkerchief and tie the container onto the nozzle of the tub.
2. Turn the tap on hot and let it pour through the herbal bath bag, turning the tub water into a strong herbal infusion.
3. Run enough cold water into the tub to bring the water to the desired temperature.

Note: For a shower, tie the herbal container onto the showerhead. When it is soaked through, untie it and use it as your washcloth. It's not quite as effective as an herbal bath, but it will do in a pinch.

BODY POWDER

This is the nicest powder recipe I know of. Smooth and silky, it serves as a natural deodorizer because of its absorbent properties. It can be given any scent or combination of scents. And best of all, it's simple and inexpensive to make.

This recipe is a favorite one for young children to make. They can make a nice mess, end up with a great product, and have lots of fun doing it. (Sounds just like me when I'm playing with herbs!)

Package the powder in traditional shaker powder containers, spice jars with shaker tops, or fancy tins. You can make beautiful feather dusters by collecting small feathers and gluing them together, then tying ribbon around the base. If feathers are difficult to find, visit a fly and tackle shop. They always have an exotic collection.

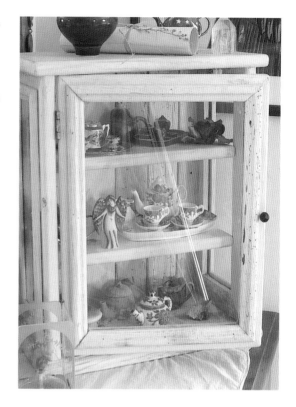

> 1 cup white cosmetic-grade clay (kaolin clay)
> 2 cups arrowroot powder or cornstarch (or a
>   combination of both)
> Essential oil of choice (optional)
> Lavender and rose flowers (optional)

1. In a large bowl, using a wire whisk, mix the clay and arrowroot or cornstarch. Add essential oil. (Because of its absorbent properties, the powder will absorb far more than you imagine. Buy your essential oil in 1- to 4-ounce bottles. Though the initial expenditure may seem high, your savings will be significant.)

2. If you wish to use lavender and roses in the powder, grind them (or other herbs of your choice) to a fine powder using a coffee mill or seed and nut grinder. Sift, then grind again. The herbs must be as finely powdered as possible or they will make the powder feel gritty. Add the herbs to powder and mix well.

3. Cover the body powder with a porous cloth and let it sit for several hours to dry. Package it in small containers.

BATH SALTS

A simple, delightful recipe, bath salts add valuable trace minerals to the bathwater, soften the water, and gently cleanse the skin. Bath salts are made from a combination of mineral salts. Most people are surprised, and some mildly offended, to learn that the major ingredient in most bath salts is borax. But borax is quite a wonderful substance. A natural mineral salt found only in a few places in the world, borax is incredibly versatile: Packaged in a large box with a picture of a mule team on the front, it is used for laundry; placed in a small, fancy jar, it's used as a cosmetic.

Presented in glass bottles or fancy tins with a rounded seashell as a scoop, these homemade bath salts make wonderful gifts. The original inspiration for this recipe came from a dear old friend, Warren Raysor, affectionately known as "Dr. Astrology." Warren is the founder of Abracadabra, a wonderful all-natural cosmetics company.

> **2 cups borax**
> **⅛ cup sea salt**
> **⅛ cup white clay**
> **Essential oil of choice**

1. Combine the borax, salt, and clay. Use a wire whisk to mix the ingredients evenly. Scent with essential oil. (The mix will absorb a lot of oil.) Ideally, your bath salts should smell about twice as strong as you'd like your bath to smell. If you put your nose down to the container and inhale and think, "Oh, this is nice," then it's not really strong enough. You should be thinking, "Ooff, this is strong," because the salts are going to be really diluted when you mix them in the bathwater.

2. Cover the mix with a porous cloth and let sit several hours to dry. Again, blend well with the wire whisk. Add 4 to 6 tablespoons of the salts to bathwater, allowing the salts to dissolve in the water before bathing.

Note: Using salts in the bath is a very good old-fashioned remedy for aching muscles, flu, congestion, and sinus pressure. In these cases, use essential oils that have a deep, pungent odor, such as eucalyptus, thyme, and pine.

"I began to reflect on Nature's eagerness to **sow life** into everywhere. Into every empty corner, into all forgotten things and nooks, Nature struggles to **pour life,** pouring life into the dead, life into life itself. That immense, overwhelming, relentless, **burning** ardency of Nature for the stir of life."

— **Henry Beston**

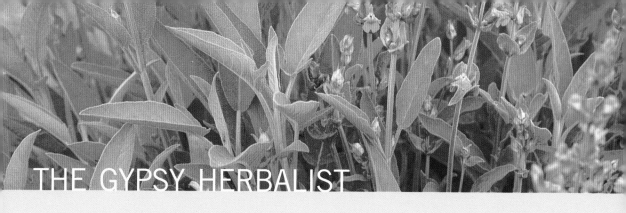

THE GYPSY HERBALIST

Though she has spent her life as a nomad, living among the Gypsies and peasants of the world, Juliette de Bairacli Levy has, I believe, had a larger influence on American herbalism than any other individual of the past several decades. She is a prolific writer, a pioneer of holistic veterinary medicine, and a lifelong scholar, and her teachings permeate the field of herbalism.

I "met" Juliette in the Sonoma County library, where I stumbled across her book *Traveler's Joy.* I was immediately taken with it, and her. Who was this Gypsy scholar who wandered the world with her hounds, her bags of herbs, and small children by her side? So I decided to write to her.

I was just 22 when I sent that passionate letter. I don't remember what I wrote, but I'm sure I bared my heart, sharing with Juliette my love of the green world. Several months later, much to my surprise, I received a lovely reply. And thus

began a correspondence that continues to this day, and a friendship that has changed my life.

After corresponding with Juliette for several years and reading as many of her books as I could find, I decided it was time for a visit. My dear friend Svevo Brooks and I organized an herbal tour of Greece, with a stop on Kythera, Juliette's island home. But by a few weeks before our departure date, I hadn't heard from her regarding our visit. I was getting nervous. The trip included many points of interest, but for me and many others, the highlight was meeting Juliette. Finally, just two days before we planned to leave, I received an airmail envelope with that familiar scratchy handwriting. Of course we could come see her, she said.

Over time I learned that this is the way things are with Juliette; nothing is ever certain, and everything is an adventure. A couple of years later, I invited her to be the featured speaker at a large herb conference, and she accepted. But as the days passed, Juliette had not made arrangements for her airline ticket. We were paying for it, but she had insisted that she get it herself so she could decide which days to leave and return. I began to worry. Finally, with less than two weeks remaining and no confirmation of a ticket, I decided to call her.

Now, calling Juliette is never an easy affair. She prefers to live in remote areas, as far from signs of civilization as she can muster. And she does not have a phone. She was still on Kythera at this time, so I called the local taxi driver, Tarzan (his real name), whom I knew from previous visits, and begged him to find her and bring her to the nearest village's pay phone, which I'd call in a couple of hours. Bless his heart, he did. So there was Juliette on the phone, explaining to me in her kind, cockney English accent, "Rosemary, I've decided not to come, but instead I am sending you some tapes to play to the audience. They are very good, my favorite stories." I tried to imagine telling 600 conference attendees who were thrilled to finally meet Juliette that she had decided to send tapes instead. So I said to her, "Juliette, pack your bags, because I'm coming to get you." Then I flew over there and brought her back with me.

Bringing Juliette to North America and the people who adored her may be the best thing I ever did. For the first time she had the opportunity to experience the effect her work had had on people and how much they appreciated it; the gratitude they showered on her was amazing. At that conference and at subsequent gatherings, people lined up, sometimes several generations of one family, to meet her, holding in their hands dog-eared copies of books that Juliette had authored. I heard over and over again how her sage advice had saved their pets, their farm animals, their children, or themselves.

Renowned around the world, friend to kings, queens, peasants, and Gypsies alike, Juliette truly is one of the great herbalists of our time. Now in her late 80s and living in the Azores, she still travels the world, teaching about animal rights and herbs and advocating for a simpler and saner way of life. She has been a teacher to me not only through her words, which often ring like poetry, but also, and perhaps more so, through her life. She is a wonderful, beautiful, eccentric woman and one of my greatest mentors.

SALT GLOW

This recipe is far too easy for the remarkable benefits it gives. Again, it is the simple gifts of life that are often the best. A salt glow is one of my favorite exfoliating treatments. It leaves the skin feeling silky soft and renewed, relaxed but refreshed.

I first had the opportunity to experience this wonderful body therapy while camping in southeastern Ohio. Two women friends were insistent on treating me, and being the glutton I am for goodness, I acquiesced. As they rubbed salt and oils over my body, massaging and gently scrubbing it in, then rinsing it off with warm water, I knew I had reached heaven. If you think I'm exaggerating, just try it!

Similar recipes are a favorite treatment at many famous and expensive spas. But it's so wonderfully simple, inexpensive, and easy to do that you should try it at home. Invite a friend over for a "salt glow exchange." It's nicest to do it outside, where you can rinse off the salt and not worry about getting it everywhere.

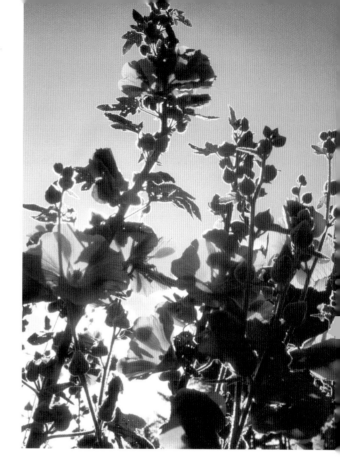

        2 cups fine sea salt
        4 cups grapeseed, apricot, or almond oil
        25 drops essential oil of choice

1. Place the salt in a widemouthed jar and cover with grapeseed, apricot, or almond oil. Scent with essential oil. For best storage, place it in a cool area.

2. To use, dampen your entire body. Using either your hands or a loofah mitt, vigorously but gently massage the salt-and-oil mixture into your skin. Begin at your feet and work upward in a circular motion. Be careful to avoid any scratched or wounded areas. When you have massaged your entire body, rinse with warm water. Finish with a dry-towel rub.

the cleaner, the better?

When I was in my early 20s, I spent a summer backpacking in the Olympic National Forest in the Pacific Northwest. I was young and wild, carefree, with only a pack on my back for my belongings. The rivers ran straight from the snow-covered Olympic peaks and were mighty cold. Though I swam often, the thought of washing my hair in glacier water was another matter. Besides, I didn't want to degrade that crystal-clear water with soap.

So I ended up not washing my hair for several months, or at least very infrequently. I noticed a peculiar sequence. About a week after washing, my hair would begin to feel oily and dirty, always a signal in the past that it was time to wash again. But I waited, and I noticed that my hair would reabsorb its own oils. Instead of getting dirtier and greasier, it would "self-clean." The less I washed it, the less dirty and oily it became.

Though I've never again spent a summer not washing my hair, I certainly learned from that experience. I wash my hair, which is thick, dark, and glossy, much less frequently than most people, and it seems to get dirty less often than the hair of people who wash all the time.

glorious hair

No matter if your hair is long or short, light or dark, coarse or thin, it is a garden alive. Hair grows in response to nutrients and the energetics of the world around it. It is an "antenna," a connection to the energy forces of the world.

Animals express themselves, in part, through their hair. Have you ever seen an angry or frightened cat, its hair literally standing on end, a clear statement to all who come near? In comics and children's stories, people are often depicted expressing themselves through or how they wear their hair: flat against their face, standing on end, swirling around them electrified with energy. Even our great stories tell the power of hair: Samson, for example, knew where his strength lay. Unfortunately, so did Delilah!

Caring for Your Hair — Naturally

Since I was a child, my hair, too, has been my garden. I tend to wear it long and often loose, so that it flows down past my shoulders. The times I've cut it short and styled it in a half-honest attempt to look modern or younger, I've felt a bit lost. Even though I enjoyed the bobbed hair and soft curls, I bided time until it grew again, determinedly and unstoppably, like a weed, down my back. Caring for this mass of hair has taught me a great deal about natural hair treatments, and I'm delighted to have the opportunity to pass my recipes on.

The biggest mistake that people make with their locks is overwashing them. There are plenty of good hair-care products available these days. But even the best shampoo, if used too often, will tend to dry your hair and wash away important natural oils, no matter how much conditioner you apply afterward.

Have you ever noticed how few people over 50 have shiny, healthy hair — hair you'd die for? There aren't very many of them. Though it may be part of the natural aging process to lose some of your crowning glory, it's not a natural process for it to lose its gleam and glow. What we often see is hair that hasn't weathered well. This lack of life is almost always due not to aging but to the unhealthy practices of overwashing, blow-drying, and using chemical products such as sprays, perms, and gels.

ESSENTIAL OILS FOR HAIR CARE

Essential Oil	Hair Type	Effect or Treatment
Basil	Oily	Promotes growth
Chamomile	Fine to normal	Gives golden highlights
Clary sage	All types	Dandruff treatment
Lavender	Normal	Scalp treatment for itchiness, dandruff, and even lice!
Lemon	Oily	Gives golden highlights; treatment for dry scalp, dandruff, lice, and underactive sebaceous glands
Myrrh	Dry	Treatment for dry scalp, dandruff, lice, and underactive sebaceous glands
Patchouli	Oily	Dandruff treatment
Peppermint	Dry	Promotes hair growth
Rose	Fine	Soothes scalp
Rosemary	Oily	Dandruff treatment; promotes hair growth
Tea tree	Oily	Treatment for dry scalp, dandruff, lice, and underactive sebaceous glands
Ylang-ylang	Oily	Dandruff treatment

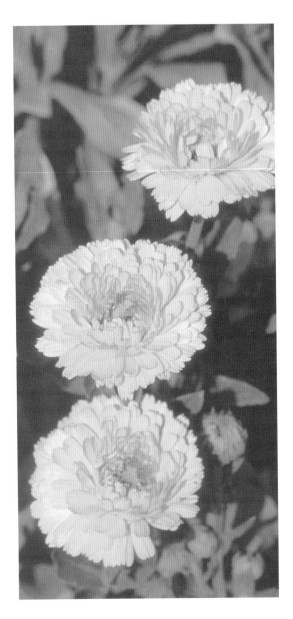

Healthy, natural hair care is basically a very simple undertaking. Here are some tips for your daily routine:

- Eat a healthy, balanced diet. The same good diet you eat for glowing skin will feed the garden of your hair.

- Use only gentle, non-detergent-based shampoos. The herbal shampoo recipe on the facing page is an excellent gentle cleanser.

- Rotate between two or three favorite shampoos. Even the best shampoo will tend to create imbalance if used continuously.

- Wash your hair infrequently, only once or twice per week. At first this will feel uncomfortable. But the "squeaky clean" feeling we have been taught to achieve is, in essence, hair that has been stripped of its natural protective oils.

- Condition your hair monthly with a natural herbal rinse (see the recipes that follow).

- Massage your scalp thoroughly every few days, or at least once weekly. A good scalp/hair massage can be almost as sensuous as a full-body massage, and it's also a good bonding ritual for parents to use with their children.

- Brush your hair as often and for as long as you can each day. Be sure that your hairbrush is kept clean; a good rule to follow is to wash your brush each time you wash your hair. As with scalp massage, hair brushing is tremendously enjoyable when shared with children or a partner.

Herbal Shampoo

Herbal shampoo is incredibly easy to make, and you can tailor the ingredients to meet your needs. There's a wide variety of essential oils to choose from, depending on whether you want to give your tresses a delicate aroma, treat dry scalp, or promote hair growth.

MAKE-IT-YOURSELF HERBAL SHAMPOO

All of the ingredients can be found in natural foods stores. If your hair is exceptionally oily, you may find it better to replace the jojoba oil (a wonderful nongreasy nutrient) with rosemary essential oil.

> 8 ounces distilled water
> 1 ounce herbs (choose from the combinations given at right)
> 3 ounces liquid castile soap
> ¼ teaspoon jojoba oil
> 25 drops of pure essential oil (see the chart on page 147)

1. Bring the water to a boil. Add the herbs, cover, and let simmer over low heat for 15 to 20 minutes. Strain and cool.
2. Slowly add the castile soap to the tea, then mix in the jojoba oil and essential oil. Store in a plastic container with a flip-top lid in the shower or bath. Shake before using.

GOLDIE LOCKS INFUSION

Use this formula for golden highlights.

> 2 parts calendula flower
> 1 part chamomile flower
> 1 part comfrey leaf

DARK OF THE NIGHT INFUSION

To effect dark highlights, try this formula.

> 2 parts garden sage leaf
> 1 part black walnut hull, chopped
> 1 part comfrey leaf

DESERT BLOOM INFUSION

Desert Bloom is an excellent formula for dry hair.

> 1 part calendula flower
> 1 part marsh mallow root
> 1 part nettle leaf

RAPUNZEL'S LOCKS INFUSION

Bothered by oily hair? Use this astringent recipe.

> 1 part rosemary leaf
> 1 part witch hazel bark (not extract)
> 1 part yarrow leaf and flower

Hair Rinses and Conditioners

Most hair conditioners available on the market are used as detanglers and help "tame" our wild locks. Unfortunately, most conditioners, including those found in health food stores, contain glycerin. Though a wonderful natural substance, glycerin coats the hair shaft and, while making it feel smooth and shiny, draws dust and dirt from the air onto the hair. I prefer to use herbal hair rinses or herbal vinegar rinses.

My mother, named after the exotic night-blooming jasmine and now in her late 70s, embraces the beauty of Cosmeos. Her hair, though streaked with bits of silver, is still blue-black. Her secret? Those fabulous Armenian genes — and her famous vinegar rinse.

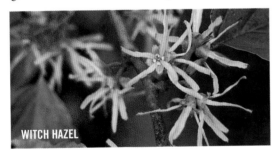

WITCH HAZEL

VINEGAR HAIR RINSE

This rinse will keep indefinitely, so I make it by the gallon. Vinegar is especially suited for oily hair, though it can be used effectively for dry hair as well. Apple cider vinegar is usually the best vinegar for the hair, but wine vinegar is milder and more appropriate for dry hair. Vinegar rinses are also good for itchy scalp, dandruff, and dull hair, and they help restore the natural acid of the scalp. You can use any of the herbal formulas and essential oils listed in the shampoo section, or formulate your own favorite blends. If the smell of vinegar is not appealing to you, don't fret; the essential oils help lessen the strong odor, and the scent won't linger.

Herbal blend of choice (see page 149)
Apple cider or wine vinegar
A few drops of essential oils of choice
Distilled water

1. Fill a quart jar halfway with your herbal blend. Completely cover the herbs with the vinegar and cap tightly. Place the jar in a warm spot for 3 to 4 weeks. Shake it daily to keep the mixture agitated.
2. Strain the vinegar through double cheesecloth or a fine-mesh strainer. Add the essential oils, rebottle in a plastic bottle, and store in the bathtub or shower.
3. Before you bathe, dilute the rinse with distilled water. Generally, for oily hair, dilute 1 part rinse with 4 parts water; for dry hair, dilute 1 part rinse with 6 parts water. After shampooing and rinsing, pour the vinegar rinse slowly through the hair, massaging it into the scalp. Rinse with warm water and then, if you can stand it, cold water. (Rinsing with warm and then cold water stimulates the scalp and leaves your hair with an even glossier sheen.)

HERBAL HAIR RINSE

The oldest hair rinses were made from fresh botanicals and pure water. It's curious to me how many people still prefer these simple and effective rinses, in spite of all the fancy new products that are forever coming out in the marketplace.

> **1 to 2 ounces herb blend of choice (choose
> from blends in the shampoo section
> or formulate your own)**
> **1 quart water**
> **A few drops of essential oil of choice**

1. Simmer the herbal mixture in the water for 15 to 20 minutes. Strain well. Add a drop or two of essential oil to cooled tea.

2. After shampooing and rinsing, slowly pour the cooled mixture through the hair and massage into the scalp. Do not rinse.

"Flowers do not spread their fragrance; it is an **effortless** happening. When the heart opens, **love awakens** and spreads like the fragrance of a blooming flower."

— **Amrit Desai**

HAIR CONDITIONING TREATMENT

Though I enjoy nutrient food packs such as the Herbal Hair Rinse, my favorite conditioner is a hot oil treatment. These are best for dry hair, though they can be adapted for oily hair as well. Your hair may feel a bit more oily than usual at first, but your smiling hair will quickly absorb any extra oil. This is a wonderful treatment to do before going into a sauna or steam room.

> **A small amount jojoba, olive, or coconut oil**
> **Herb mixture of choice (optional)**
> **Essential oils of choice (optional)**

1. Warm the oil to 100 to 105°F in a double boiler. If using, add herbs and essential oils.

2. I usually dampen my hair before the treatment, though most people don't. Long or thick hair will require 1 to 2 teaspoons of the oil mixture. Short or fine hair will require less than ½ teaspoon of the mixture. Begin by massaging the oil into the scalp, and then work down through the strands of hair, covering all of the hair completely. Put a shower cap or plastic bag over the hair, then cover with either a towel or a wool cap. If possible, sit in the sunshine or by a woodstove or fireplace; heat facilitates the conditioning process. Leave it on for an hour or two, then shampoo and rinse.

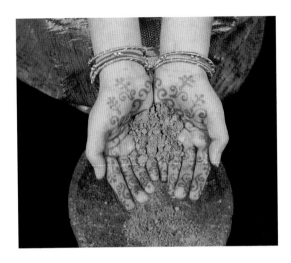

coloring your life with henna

No book on cosmetics and skin care would be complete without mentioning henna, one of the most marvelous and magical of skin- and hair-care herbs. When I was in high school, I began a love affair with henna that has endured for several decades, and so I have more than a little to share on the subject.

Henna, or Egyptian privet *(Lawsonia inermis)*, is a plant with a rich and varied history. Its use dates back to time immemorial: No one knows for sure where or when it was first used. However, records dating back more than 5,000 years specify its use as a medicine, talisman, ceremonial substance, and cosmetic used to color hair and paint the body. Originally found in North Africa, Australia, and Asia, henna has spread and naturalized in many areas of the world, including the subtropical regions of the United States.

Though we generally tend to think of it as a colorant, henna has a long list of medicinal properties and is still used in many parts of the world as an astringent for headaches, as a gargle for sore throats, and to treat stomach upset and pain. Though I've used henna primarily as an external coloring agent for hair, I've long suspected its powerful medicinal properties.

I noticed early on that whenever I used henna on people, their energy changed, brightened, they seemed refreshed and renewed. It was different from going to the beauty salon and having their hair colored. People seemed to feel better. It definitely relieved head tension and seemed to help people relax (except, perhaps, for their temporary anxiety waiting to see how bright their hair would turn once the henna was washed out).

Choosing the Right Henna

It is essential to get henna from a good source. Poor-quality henna will not yield the dramatic lights that a good-quality product will. Undoubtedly, there are several good hennas that I don't know about, but I have found that Rainbow henna and Persian henna are consistently good. (These can be purchased through Frontier Herbs, Wild Weeds, and Mountain Rose Herbs; see Resources.)

The basic shade of henna is red, and all henna has a whisper of red in it. But by carefully blending different parts of the plant that are harvested at different times, a whole range of colors is created. Colors range from neutral to blond to the reddest of reds to black. I further like to blend these shades to get more specific colors. It does take a little knowledge, but I will share with you what I have discovered.

I have found that people are a little wary of choosing a bright shade the first time they try henna, but they often later wish that they had. Trust your intuition — and your hairdresser — and be brave!

Blond Hair

I don't recommend using henna on blond hair unless you want to go red. Even then, I would exercise caution. Since all henna — even the neutral and blond shades — has an undertone of red, blond hair and other light shades will pick up this red shade. And so-called blond henna doesn't

a "magical" herb

A wise old man told me that henna aligned with the polarities of the earth and attracted *lay lines,* powerful magnetic forces of the earth. I mentioned this in class to a group of people I had just anointed with their first henna. One of the participants went to her psychic healing class shortly after we had done the henna. The instructor approached her, saying, "All the energy lines in this room are running around you, in fact, right through your hair." She laughed and said she was a believer after that.

I use henna as a transformational tool, not to cover natural hair color but to enhance it; to change not the way you look but the way you feel about yourself. I often take pounds of various shades of henna with me when I travel.

You never know when transformation and magic may want to happen.

I've taken henna with me to the Swiss Alps and to South and Central America. I'll never forget sitting around the campfire with the famous enthnobotanist and healer Dr. Rosita Arvigo, at her home at Ix Chel, Belize. We had been traveling for several days through the jungles and were looking for a bit of comfort. Soon we had the campfire going, with good food cooking, and out came the henna. By evening's end, Rosita's dark brown locks had been transformed to shades of burgundy and red. The henna got everybody going, so that soon the entire camp was covered with green goop, red hair, and laughter.

necessarily make blond hair blonder. It often makes the hair redder or darker. So if your hair is a light shade of blond, do not expect henna to lighten your hair — even if the package says blond henna.

Neutral henna or blond henna can be used to condition blond hair, but it will often darken it a bit. And strawberry henna adds wonderful shades of gold, burnt red, and copper to blond hair. Again, henna will not make the hair lighter or "blonder"; it does not contain bleaches of any sort, and therefore will not strip the hair of its natural color.

Dark Blond to Light Brown Hair

You must be careful when selecting henna for light shades of hair, because the hair picks up the henna tones readily. If you want to just highlight your natural color, choose a shade that best describes your hair. For example, if you have dark blond hair, use blond henna. If your hair is light brown, use light brown henna. A color selection that seems to be everyone's favorite, and the one I certainly like the best, is a mixture of shades that creates a warm, coppery glow. I mix the following shades, but remember to adjust for your own natural coloring:

- 1 part neutral henna
- 1 part light brown henna
- 2 parts copper henna (use less copper to tame down the color)

Medium Brown to Dark Brown Hair

These shades are fun because you can be more daring and do so much more than you can with the more tentative, lighter shades of color. Look at the hair to determine the natural highlights, and select a shade of henna that accentuates the natural color. I find shades of red mixed with different tones of brown are beautiful. If the hair color has a lot of gold and copper tones, use copper henna. Here are some suggested formulas:

For reddish tones:
- 1 part medium brown
- 1 part red
- 1 part copper

For copper tones:
- 2 parts copper
- 1 part medium brown
- 1 part neutral to be conservative or 2 parts red to be wild!

Dark Brown to Black Hair

Black hair is similar to blond hair from a henna point of view. It generally has so much of its own light that henna adds little coloring, but it does condition and adds body. However, for a person with dark brown hair, adding shades of bright red henna can be just stunning.

People always react with "I don't want my hair to be orange!" I can certainly appreciate that sentiment. Shades of dark brown hair will never turn orange but will blend with the red henna to create rich auburns, fiery copper tones, and many other stunning colors. There are several shades of red henna available, such as burgundy and wine. They all have red as a primary color but shimmer with different highlights. Play and have fun with the shades. Experiment to find which color or combination of colors most suits you.

You might wish to begin by using only one color, then try combining shades. Leave the henna on for 2 full hours if you have dark brown hair. You need not worry about its being too bright. It won't be. Henna was made for dark brown hair. It colors it gorgeously. If anything, upon washing it out, you'll wish it were brighter!

Gray Hair

Most books and "experts" warn against using henna on gray or graying hair. It can, if done incorrectly, turn the hair shockingly orange. But applied correctly, henna can transform even the dullest silver hair into soft tones of gold and light strawberry red. The trick is to mix the right colors and to leave the henna pack on for only about 30 to 45 minutes. If your hair is predominantly gray, use only subtle shades of henna, such as neutral mixed with a little light brown and a dash of copper. Leave it on for about 30 minutes at first. The next time you do it, you can fine-tune the shades and decide if you wish to leave the pack on a bit longer. For gray hair that has not turned completely white but still has some of its original color, mix together:

- 2 parts neutral
- 2 parts light brown
- ⅛ part copper or blond

Note: Use less copper if you have more gray hair or prefer less coppery red tones.

Applying Henna to the Hair

Not an instant dye nor a neat and easy process, henna requires time and patience. It also makes a bit of a mess. Whenever possible, I host henna parties outdoors with a hose hooked to the

how much and how often?

It is much better to mix too much henna than to run short. So mix a little extra — you can use it on your dog's tail or your husband's beard. Short hair requires 2 to 3 ounces of henna; long hair (falling below the shoulders) requires 4 to 6 ounces.

My recommendation is not to henna your hair more than once every 10 to 12 weeks. In Indian and Arab tradition, henna is used far more often; however, that history does not also include frequent shampooing, permanents, and blow-drying. If henna is used too often by those who employ these Western "traditions," it does tend to dry the hair.

hot-water faucet for rinsing. An all-natural substance, henna is good for the garden, but in quantity it is not so good for the bathroom drain!

I've found the following to be the simplest and least messy steps, and they yield fantastic results.

Step 1: Prepare the Henna Paste

With a wood or plastic spoon, mix the henna with very hot water in a glass, ceramic, or plastic bowl to make a thickish paste. A perfect henna paste is neither too dry nor too wet. If it's too dry, it will be difficult to apply and will flake. It will also tend to dry the hair out. If it's too wet, it will be running down your face and generally making a mess. So aim for the perfect mix, somewhat like a bowl of cooked oatmeal — easy enough to put on but not so loose that it will run down your face. Getting the right consistency is tricky at first. Keep mixing it with water until it's smooth and creamy. It takes far more water than you'd imagine.

Step 2: Prepare the Hair

There's no need to shampoo hair before a henna treatment unless the hair is dirty. In fact, I discourage it; too much washing is one of the major causes of dry, unmanageable hair. Try applying henna just before you're ready to wash your hair. The natural oils in your hair and scalp will help moisturize your hair and prevent dry, flyaway hair.

Dampen the hair thoroughly and towel dry. Massage a small amount of olive or jojoba oil into the hair, especially the ends.

admiring your henna lights

The term for describing henna-treated hair is "henna lights." It truly does light up the hair in sunlight. (You can see it in the photo at right; Juliette and I just had our hair hennaed.) But hair must be completely dry to fully reflect henna's beauty. So don't be disappointed when you first wash out the henna and run to the mirror to look at your hair. It will probably just look wet! You must wait patiently (or impatiently) until it is dry. Now look!

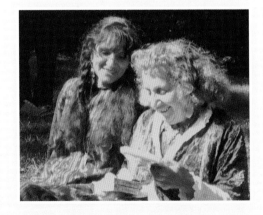

Step 3: Apply the Henna

Put on plastic gloves, or you'll have bright orange hands for about 2 weeks. Section hair and cover each section completely with henna paste. If you don't get all the hair evenly covered, blond and gray shades will end up with a streaked appearance. Short hair is easy; long hair takes time. It goes faster if two people are working on it at the same time.

When all the hair has been completely covered, take more henna and "grease" it thickly over the hair. Pat it on thickly! You'll look like a greaser and feel as though you have a thick skull.

Step 4: Cover Your Hair

If you have long hair, pin it up in a bun. Cover with a shower cap, plastic wrap, or a plastic bag. Then wrap with an old towel to hold it all in place.

Step 5: Check the Time

The longer the henna pack is left on, the richer and darker the color will be and the longer the color will last. The times given here are just suggested as guidelines. Everybody's hair is different and will take the color differently.

Dark shades (medium brown, dark brown, black) should leave the henna paste on for 2 hours.

Light shades (light brown, slightly or predominantly gray) should leave the paste on for 30 to 60 minutes. The longer it's left on, the stronger the color will be (not always a desirable effect!).

Predominantly gray hair (more than ¾ of the natural hair color) should be allowed to dye for approximately 30 minutes the first time. Gray hair can be successfully hennaed, but careful color selection and timing are essential.

Step 6: Wash Out the Henna

When rinsing out the henna, you may feel as though you're washing out 15 pounds of mud and that it is never all going to come out. In the meantime, all that shampoo is undoing the fine conditioning you have just given your hair.

I have found that the very best way to get the henna out is to wash once just as you regularly do. If you normally follow with a detangling rinse, do so. Then, even though you can still feel henna in your hair, let your hair dry naturally. Any henna left in the hair will brush out as soon as your hair is dry. It is so much easier and better for your hair. (I hate to admit that it took me years to figure out this little trick!)

Remember, for the full effect, let your hair dry completely before racing to the mirror. Of course, you'll do it anyway, but at least you'll be warned. You generally don't see much until after the hair dries. And then — watch out — you may be hooked! It will be beautiful, you'll feel divine, and you'll be another henna "junkie"!

Henna will fade dramatically after one or two washings, and then it pretty much "fixes" itself and will fade gradually after 2 or 3 months.

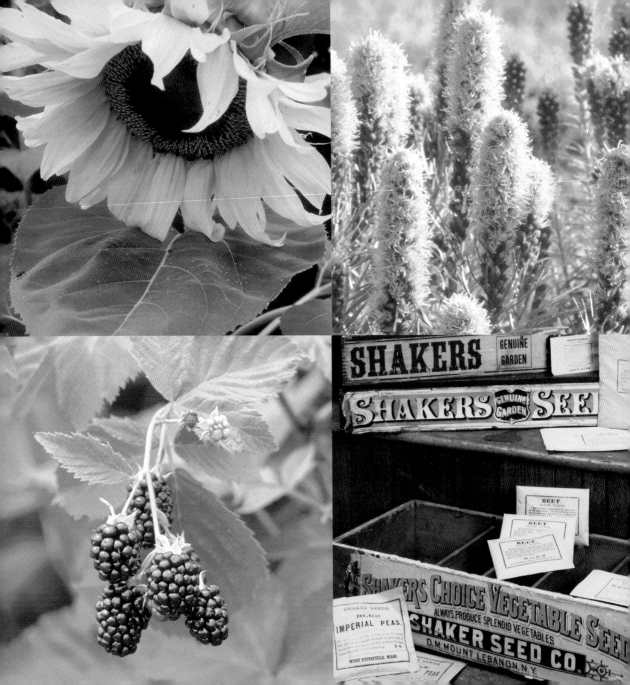

6

For Children

As I sit here writing, I am looking forward to my sister-in-law and her two beautiful daughters, Samantha, 10, and Lindsey, 6, coming for an overnight visit. They are bringing along their friend Marissa, who is 11 and already filled with the love of plants. For the girls, this will be a special "herb visit" with "Aunt Rosie." I have been planning for the past few days the things I wish to do with them. It's hard to choose — there's so much that's green and beautiful. We'll make my famous herbal face cream, and maybe we'll do herbal steams and give each other facials. I've collected some great little blue glass containers for handmade lip balms that we'll color red with the root of alkanet, a flower I grow in my garden.

It's autumn, and the golden leaves of New England have woven a rich tapestry upon the forest floor. Though it's raining outside, we'll undoubtedly take a long walk through the forest, drinking in the colors once again before the long winter sets in, seeing if there's still a plant here and there to identify and harvest. I'm thinking, too, of stories that will be fun to tell by the campfire tonight. We're going to camp out in the yurt, a round tent with a woodstove that will keep us warm and snug, for the weather is already beginning to turn cold in these Vermont mountains.

It is at times like these that I am most reminded of my own childhood and my early encounters with plants. I am forever thankful for the lessons my grandmother taught me as a child in her gardens. No matter how little — or how much — you think you know about the plants, that knowledge is a gift to pass on. What we learn to love as children, we will love and respect as adults.

plants and children

A long time ago, when I was just a child, my grandmother took me into her gardens and introduced me to her weeds. When we walked in the scented oak forest, she would rub my skin with fresh bay leaves, assuring me it would prevent poison oak and would keep the insects from swarming over us. When I fell in the nettle patches, she soothed the painful welts with the fresh juice of that plant.

She showed me how to knit with chicken feathers and taught me special games to play with the shiny, smooth bones she kept on the mantel. Her teachings were without fuss. Strong and powerful, like her, her words sank deep and took root in this young child's heart. That magic my grandmother taught me in the garden of my childhood stayed with me throughout my life, and I have continued the journey into the green.

I've studied the healing power of herbs with many gifted teachers, traveled to many botanically rich areas, come to know a great many plants, spent many years gaining experience as a community herbalist, and studied the science as well as the art of herbal healing. Still, the things I learned as a child with my grandmother have remained some of the most powerful teachings of my life. It is her simple, strong wisdom that I seek to pass on to you and your children.

Herbalism instills in a person a deep appreciation for Mother Earth and knowledge of natural healing and well-being. Teach children early this love of the earth, the respect for plants and nature. All children benefit from a close association with nature and from the use of herbs and the ancient tradition of herbalism. What one learns to know and love as a child is often what is treasured most as an adult.

Herbs offer tremendous benefits for children's health. Most of the simple woes of childhood respond quickly to herbal therapies. Cuts, scrapes, burns, bee stings, colds, and runny noses become opportunities for you and your children to see how effectively herbal remedies work. Even the more tenacious childhood illnesses, such as chicken pox and measles, the flu, fevers, and allergies, respond to the healing power of herbs. When it's necessary to resort to allopathic medication, herbs provide a wonderful complement, helping support the child's system while the medication does its work. A simple knowledge of herbs and a well-stocked herbal pantry can considerably lessen the trials of childhood illnesses.

using herbs wisely

Children's bodies are sensitive and respond naturally and quickly to the gentle, effective, healing energy of herbs. I believe this is because there is an inborn wisdom that is still strongly connected; the "umbilical cord" is still deeply entwined with the body of Mother Earth and the many gifts that flow like a life-giving stream from her core. Administered wisely, herbs do not upset the delicate ecological balance of children's small bodies as does much of modern medicine but, rather, work in harmony with the young child's system.

When to Use Herbs

Herbs can be used with confidence for simple ailments such as colds, colic, and teething, as well as the many common childhood illnesses that children often contract. Herbs can also be used as

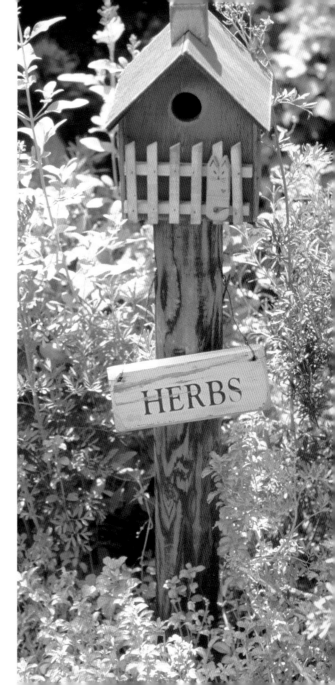

supplements to our modern system of allopathic medicine when dealing with more complicated health problems. Contrary to popular opinion, herbs and orthodox medicine are not at odds, but are two systems of healing that can complement each other. Consult your physician or holistic health care provider for guidelines on using allopathic drugs and herbal remedies in combination.

When to Seek Medical Help

Allopathic medicine is an excellent crisis-oriented system, and it is important to know when your child's injury or illness warrants immediate emergency intervention. While your child is well, establish a good relationship with a pediatrician, preferably one who is holistically minded. Then, should your child have a serious injury or an acute illness, you will feel comfortable bringing

children's connections with the plant spirits

Mary, a practicing herbalist who lives in Tahoe, California, had a beautiful herb garden. Her youngest daughter, Amber, loved being in the garden. When Amber was three years old, she became enthralled by the fairies and flower spirits that lived in the garden. She persuaded her mom to make miniature garden settings for the fairies, to set up tea parties with tiny greeting cards and little flower-covered archways.

Mary delighted in this summer pastime and her daughter's sense of enchantment. But then, suddenly, Amber started having trouble sleeping at night. Around midnight, she would go to her parents' doorway and ask to sleep with them. "The fairies won't leave me alone," she'd tell them. "They are stringing lights all over my room and waking me

with their singing." And father and mother, half asleep, would let their little daughter crawl under the covers with them.

One night, they decided enough was enough and Amber must go back to her own room to sleep. But when they got to the door, Mary tells me in a voice still hushed after these many years, they heard ringing and singing. And when they opened the door, there were miniature lights dancing about the room.

I love this story, because there are still many children who hear the songs of the plants. They talk to the plants and the plants "talk" back. They seem to know what to pick to put on their "owies." And they'd much rather be out in the garden than sitting mindlessly in front of the TV.

your child to him or her and accepting his or her recommendations. Seek medical help if the child:

- Is not responding to the herbal treatments you are using.
- Shows signs of serious illness, such as fever greater than 101°F, low-grade persistent fever, hemorrhaging, delirium, unconsciousness, and severe abdominal pain.
- Is lethargic and weak, unresponsive, or difficult to awaken.
- Complains of stiff neck and headache and is unable to touch his or her chin to the chest. In babies, the fontanel (soft spot on top of the head) may bulge. These are possible early signs of meningitis and require immediate medical assistance.
- Contracts recurring ear infections.
- Shows any signs of choking on a foreign object; these include difficulty breathing, sucking in breath, and turning blue.
- Becomes dehydrated. Warning signs are dry lips, dry mouth, and no urination in 6 hours.
- Has bee stings or insect bites that cause allergic reactions and shock. Extreme anxiety, difficulty breathing, and other unusual responses can be warning signs.
- Has red streaks on the skin emanating from the point of infection; this could indicate blood poisoning.
- Has burns that cover areas on the body twice the size of the child's hand or that are infected. Also look for signs of shock and third-degree burns.

Safety Precautions

Contrary to what you may have heard or read, my experience has been that almost any herb that is safe for an adult is safe for a child as long as the size and weight of the child are accounted for and the dosage is adjusted accordingly. People often express concern about using strong medicinal herbs such as goldenseal, valerian, or St.-John's-wort for children, but I've found them to be extremely useful and effective. However, use them in small amounts for short periods of time only, and use them in conjunction, or formulated with, the milder herbs listed in this book.

Any herb, even the safest and most researched of herbs, can affect different people differently. Much in the same way that some people get horrendous allergic reactions to strawberries, milk, and plant pollen, some people are adversely affected by even the most benevolent of herbs. Though it is a rare and unusual occurrence, whenever such a reaction is reported, it makes national headlines. Were drug reactions reported with the same fervor, we'd all be terrified of aspirin and cough syrup. However rare these reactions to herbs may be, though, it is always wise to be cautious when using an herb for the first time.

Perform small-dose tests. Use the herb in small amounts at first, to see how it works for you and your child. A good safety measure is a patch test. Make an herb tea, then "paint" a small amount onto the skin of the inner arm. Wait 24 hours; if you do notice any adverse reactions — a skin rash, itchy eyes, throat swelling, itchiness — discontinue use immediately. If the child does not experience an adverse reaction, you may administer a very small amount internally. Discontinue immediately if any signs of allergic reaction appear. You may wish to try the herb again, prepared in the same manner and administered in the same amount, after a few days. If the child again experiences discomfort, then I would attribute the effects to the herb or herbal formula and look for another, more compatible herb.

Store preparations in childproof containers. Store medicinal preparations — herbs as well as homeopathic or allopathic medications — out of reach of children. One of the problems with many medicinal preparations, including herbal remedies, is that they are made to taste appealing. Thankfully, most of your herbal remedies won't be harmful if used in larger amounts than intended. Still, keeping preparations out of reach and in well-sealed containers is a good general rule.

herb preparations just for kids

Once in a while, you'll find that unusual child who will eat every herb you give him or her, no matter how bitter or unpleasant tasting. Both my son and my grandson were like that, eager to consume whatever formula they were given.

Andrew, my grandson, seemed to thrive on the flavor of bitter herbs. Whenever he had respiratory problems, we would give him a goldenseal formula, strongly diluted yet still bitterly potent, in a 1-ounce dropper bottle. Andrew would run around with his herbal remedy in hand, drinking it as readily as he would apple juice.

More often, getting herbal preparations into children will be a creative challenge. The flavors of medicinal herbs are unfamiliar and sometimes bitter, pungent, or sour, and children are often unwilling to try them. In fact, when children are ill, they sometimes refuse to eat anything, even their favorite foods. Since consistency, when treating both adults and children, is the key to any herb's effectiveness, it is important to develop preparations and recipes that are pleasant tasting and easy to persuade children to take.

Following are some of my favorite ways to administer herbs to children. These suggestions come from years of observing what children will and will not accept. Each child, of course, is unique; what is acceptable for one may not work for another. Each age group brings with it a different set of challenges. Be innovative and willing to work with the individual nature of each child.

Herb Candy

I make a candy I call "jump for joy" balls. They are one of my favorite ways to administer herbs to children (and adults), because they taste delicious

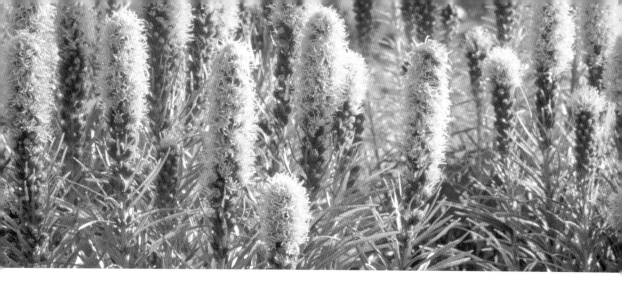

and are very effective. The herbs are powdered, then mixed into a paste made with ground fruits and nuts or nut butters and honey. You can flavor herb candy in so many ways. Be creative and invite your children to help you in the process. They'll love their herbal medicine. Just be sure to keep it out of reach.

Once, and only once, I made the mistake of leaving my Super Zoom Balls, a high-energy herbal formula and not a formula for children, on top of the refrigerator. My ambitious and very mischievous grandson managed to maneuver a chair to the counter, climb to the top of the refrigerator, and promptly consume half of the herbal candy before he was discovered. That night, we were all up far later than we cared to be.

To determine the daily dosage, it is necessary to know how much powdered herb you included in the total recipe and how many herb balls this amount made. Determine the dosage of herb by using charts provided on page 168. Divide the candy into once-daily dosages.

To make herbal candy:

1. Grind raisins, dates, apricots, and walnuts in a food processor or grinder. Alternatively, you can mix nut butter (such as peanut, almond, or cashew) with honey in equal portions, then proceed with the rest of the steps.

Note: If you're concerned about the use of honey in small children (due to reports of botulism poisoning), use maple syrup, rice syrup, or maple cream.

2. Stir in shredded coconut (the unsweetened type) and carob powder.

3. Add the herb powders. Mix well.

4. Roll the mixture into balls. Roll the balls in powdered carob or coconut. Store in the refrigerator.

Herbal Pops

Herbal pops are a fun and easy way to get a child to take his or her prescribed tea formula. They are refreshing in the summertime and provide the wonderful healing properties of the herbs in a delicious and fun form. Because they are so cold, I do not recommend them for cold types of imbalances such as flu, colic, ear infections, or respiratory infections. The cold makes them excellent for teething babies, however.

To make herbal pops:

1. Make a strong tea following the directions on page 380, but triple the amount of herb you would normally use. Strain.

2. Dilute the tea with an equal amount of apple juice or any other favorite juice. Pour into ice-pop trays; freeze.

Glycerin-Based Tinctures

Personally, I feel that glycerites (glycerin-based tinctures) are much better suited for children than alcohol-based tinctures are. When properly made, they're quite strong enough. Because of the sweet nature of glycerin, they taste far better than alcohol tinctures. And they have a long shelf life. See page 384 for instructions on making your own glycerites. My dear friend Sunny Mavor developed an excellent line of herbal tinctures just for children and made them all with a glycerin base. Her product line, Herbs for Kids, can be found in most health food stores.

Syrups for Children

Syrups are delicious, concentrated extracts of the herbs cooked into a sweet medicine including honey and/or fruit juice. Vegetable glycerin may be substituted for honey. It is an excellent medium for the herbs and is very nutritious.

To make syrup:

1. Add 2 ounces of herb mixture to 1 quart of cold water. Over low heat, simmer the liquid down to 1 pint. This will give you a very concentrated, thick tea.

2. Strain the herbs from the liquid. Compost the herbs and pour the liquid back into the pot.

3. To each pint of liquid, add 1 cup of honey (or other sweetener such as maple syrup, vegetable glycerin, or brown sugar). Most recipes call

a spoonful of sweetness

There are many delicious and naturally sweet herbs that can be used to flavor the bitter and less familiar flavors of other herbs. For instance, try adding to formulas herbs like anise seed, Chinese star anise, cinnamon, fennel seed, ginger, hibiscus, licorice root, marsh mallow root, mints, or stevia. Teas can also be sweetened by mixing them with fruit juice. Warm apple juice mixed with most teas is very good, especially if you add a stick of cinnamon.

for 2 cups of sweetener (a 1-to-1 ratio of sweetener to liquid), but I find this far too sweet. In the days when refrigeration wasn't common, the added sugar helped preserve the syrup.

4. Warm the honey and the liquid together just enough to mix well. Most recipes call for cooking the honey and tea together for 20 to 30 minutes more, but this method cooks the living enzymes out of the honey.

5. Remove from the heat and bottle for use. You may wish to add a fruit concentrate or a couple of drops of essential oil such as peppermint or spearmint to flavor, or a small amount of brandy to help preserve the syrup and aid as a relaxant in cough formulas. Syrups will last for several weeks, even months, if refrigerated.

Herbal Baths for Children

Soothing and calming, an herbal bath can work wonders on a child's nervous system (and the parents' as well). The warm water opens the pores of the skin, the largest organ of elimination and assimilation, and the herbal nutrients flow in. It is like immersing your child in a giant cup of tea.

The temperature of the water will affect the healing quality of the bath. Cool to tepid water is excellent when trying to lower a fever. A warm bath relaxes and soothes the child. My favorite herbs for baby's bath are calendula, chamomile, comfrey, lavender, and rose.

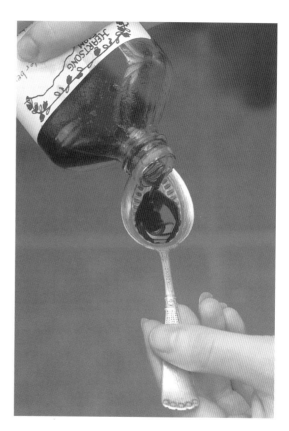

To make an herbal bath:

1. Place a handful of herbs in a cotton bag, nylon sock, or strainer and tie onto the nozzle of the tub. Let the hot water run through it for a few minutes, turning the tub water into a strong herbal infusion.

2. Release the container into the tub. Run enough cold water into the tub to bring the water to the desired temperature.

SUGGESTED DOSAGES FOR CHILDREN

When adult dosage is 1 cup (8 Oz.)

Age	Dosage
Younger than 2 years	½ to 1 teaspoon
2 to 4 years	2 teaspoons
4 to 7 years	1 tablespoon
7 to 11 years	2 tablespoons

When adult dosage is 1 teaspoon, or 60 grains/drops

Age	Dosage
Younger than 3 months	2 grains/drops
3 to 6 months	3 grains/drops
6 to 9 months	4 grains/drops
9 to 12 months	5 grains/drops
12 to 18 months	7 grains/drops
18 to 24 months	8 grains/drops
2 to 3 years	10 grains/drops
3 to 4 years	12 grains/drops
4 to 6 years	15 grains/drops
6 to 9 years	24 grains/drops
9 to 12 years	30 grains/drops

determining dosages for children

There are several different techniques for determining the proper dosage for a child. Like parents who have grown accustomed to the needs and peculiarities of each of their children, most herbalists rely on years of experience and intuition. When I recommend herbs for small children, I base my suggestions on the child's size, his or her general constitution, the nature of the illness, and the herbs I intend to use. Then I pray and let the spirit of the herbs guide me. (My prayer, of course, is balanced with a thorough understanding of the herbs I am using, plus many years of experience using herbs with children.)

If you are just beginning your herbal work or if you are using herbs you are not familiar with, use the charts at left to help you determine dosages. They provide sound guidelines for prescribing the proper amount of herbs for children of all ages.

However, remember that these charts are simply guidelines; it is equally important to consider the weight and overall health of the child. Also consider the nature and strength of the illness and the quality and strength of the herbs being used. These are all-important considerations, especially if you are using stronger herbs in a child's formula.

Administering Herbal Medicine to Infants

Mother's milk is the most effective and the safest way to administer herbs to infants. It is necessary for the mother to drink at least 4 to 6 cups of the tea daily. Not only will the baby have the benefits of the gentle healing herbs, but the mother will as well. If a mother is not nursing, herbal teas and tinctures can be added directly to the young one's bottle.

determining dosages by young's and cowling's rules

These rules for determining dosage rely on mathematical calculations based on the child's age.

Young's Rule: Add 12 to the child's age. Divide the child's age by this total.

For example, the dosage for a four-year-old: $4 \div 16 = .25$, or ¼ of the adult dosage.

Cowling's Rule: Divide the number of the child's next birthday by 24.

For example, the dosage for a child who is three, turning four years old: $4 \div 24 = .16$, or ⅙ of the adult dosage.

herbal remedies for common childhood ailments

By closely observing your child, you can usually detect when he or she is stressed, anxious, or out of balance, and thus more susceptible to illness. Illness rarely just occurs. Usually, it is a result of a stressed immune system, emotional imbalance, lack of sleep, poor hygiene, or poor nutrition.

Sometimes illness occurs because the child is just having too much fun whirling through life. Children live in passion, and the great abundance of energy required to maintain such high levels of activity can leave even the most exuberant of spirits exhausted and depleted.

All children are born with inherent strengths and weaknesses. Watch for these patterns early in life. Pay close attention to the energy levels of your child. Observe him or her through the seasons, noting which season brings with it its own special challenges for your child. Note when and to what he or she is most susceptible. This will help you become more aware of your child's health patterns.

I share this information in the hope that it may assist you in helping your child work his or her way through the common illnesses of childhood. It is not meant to replace the professional advice of a holistic health care provider or a family physician but, rather, to complement such advice.

Teething

Unavoidable, teething affects all children, with varying degrees of discomfort. Though not an illness, it generally is a time of great frustration for both parent and child — for parents because it seems no matter how hard they try, they can't remove the pain, and thus feel helpless; for the child because he or she is experiencing one of the early pains of life, and it hurts!

Often when a child has difficulty teething, various symptoms will arise. Intermittent fever, 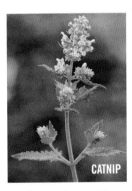 diaper rashes and other skin irritations, extreme crankiness, and diarrhea are not uncommon. Treat each symptom appropriately, following the guidelines suggested in this book, but keep in mind that support is the primary lesson called

CATNIP

for here. The teething process is natural, like many of the other cycles we'll go through in a lifetime. It marks the child's first experience of "biting in," her ability to deal with the stress of life, to call on her own powers as well as the support of family and friends. Rather than isolating or protecting the child, support and reassure her (along with yourself, if needed) that this is a natural process. Thousands of human babies have gone through this before, and yours can, too. The rewards will be a shining set of healthy teeth and the ability to enjoy another of life's great pleasures: the art of good eating.

Catnip Tea

This is an old standby for both child and parent during the teething times. Catnip is soothing to the nervous system and helps relieve acute pain. It is also helpful for teething-related fevers. Administer as tea or tincture in frequent small doses. The tea itself is not tasty, so you may wish to formulate it with other gentle nervines such as chamomile, roses, passionflower, or lemon balm. Dr. Jethro Kloss, a famous herbalist and doctor of the early 1900s, spoke impassionately of catnip: "If every mother would have catnip on her shelf, it would save her many a sleepless night and her child much suffering." It was particularly thoughtful of him to consider the mother and, following his advice, I always suggest catnip and passionflower tea for the parents of teething children.

Calcium-Rich Tea

A calcium-rich tea is very helpful for children throughout the teething period. It is most effective if it is given several weeks or even months before teething begins. It supplies necessary calcium in a form that the body can easily digest and assimilate; use it to supplement a natural diet rich in calcium.

HIGH-CALCIUM CHILDREN'S TEA

An excellent blend of herbs that add high quality, naturally biochelated calcium and other important minerals to the diet, High Calcium Children's Tea is excellent for babies who are teething. It is also beneficial for children who are undergoing growth spurts or who have had a bone or muscle injury.

3 parts rose hips
2 parts lemon balm
2 parts lemongrass
2 parts oats
1 part nettle
1 part raspberry leaf
½ part cinnamon
A pinch of stevia to sweeten (optional)

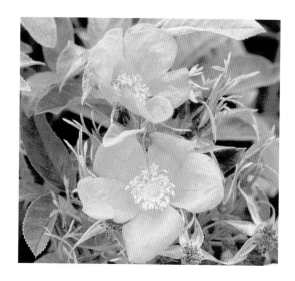

Combine the herbs and store in an airtight container. To make a tea, prepare as an infusion, following the directions on page 380. Use the dosage chart on page 168 to determine the amount to use.

Rose Hip Syrup

Giving frequent doses of a syrup made from rose hips can often relieve teething symptoms. Give 4 to 6 drops of the syrup every hour for infants. For older children, give 100 to 200 mg vitamin C in acerola tablets daily along with frequent teaspoon doses of rose hip syrup. Follow the directions on page 166 for making an herbal syrup.

calcium supplements

Most calcium tablets are difficult to digest and are expensive substances that your body must find a way to eliminate. There are some fine natural calcium supplements on the market. They usually have low dosages of calcium and are made of 100 percent natural food substances such as sesame seeds, dark-green leafy vegetables, sea vegetables, and herbs. Take your reading glasses along with you even to the natural foods store and inspect those labels carefully, especially the small print.

Hyland Teething Tablets

Hyland Homeopathic Pharmacy makes a wonderful herbal teething tablet for children. Interestingly, most parents have reported that although the teething formula Hyland's manufactures works well, the formula for colic is even more effective for teething babies. So I generally recommend Hyland's colic formula for teething difficulties. Try both and let me know which works better for you.

Herbal Pops

Frozen catnip or chamomile pops are excellent for teething children to suck on. The cold helps numb the gums and relieves the pain. Children generally love these pops and they'll suck intently on them until the pain subsides and they're gurgling away happily again.

Clove Oil

Though clove oil is often recommended for sore gums and tooth decay, I generally do not recommend it for teething babies; the oil is far too strong for a child's mouth. If you decide to use it because nothing else is working, dilute it in a vegetable oil base: 1 drop of essential oil of clove to ½ ounce of olive (or any other vegetable) oil. Test it on your own gums. Remember that your gums are much less sensitive than babies' gums. You should barely feel it. Massage gently into the gum

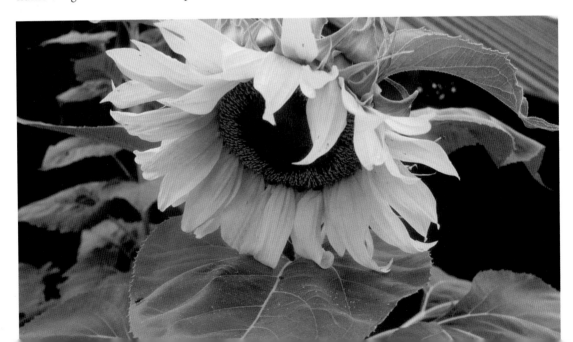

area. It can be comforting to a teething baby; it will numb the area and help relieve any inflammation. Never let children put clove oil on their own gums and always use it highly diluted.

Colic

Colic, a term used to describe an infant's tummy ache, can be a heart-wrenching experience for both the parents and the infant. It is generally caused by painful spasmodic contractions of the infant's immature digestive tract or by air and gas trapped in the intestines. The digestive tract of an infant generally takes about 3 months to mature. This is the time period in which most colic clears up.

Depending on the degree of sensitivity, mealtime can be a painful ordeal. Generally, with a little patience, some simple dietary changes, and the addition of a few gentle, time-tested herbal remedies, even the most persistent colic clears up or is at least lessened.

However, I recently encountered my first colic cure failure! A dear friend and herbal apprentice had just had her first baby. But shortly after birth, Dylan developed one of the worst cases of infant colic I have ever witnessed. His parents tried every remedy and suggestion offered by well-meaning friends, parents, their herbal community, and their fellow churchgoers. Nothing seemed to work. Fortunately, after several months, the colic disappeared as mysteriously as it had come. Dylan is now the epitome of cheerfulness, and his tummy aches are gone. Once again, the lesson here seems to be that support is something we all need every time we go through a life process.

The following suggestions are all gentle and effective and work in harmony with the sensitive nature of the infant.

Create a Relaxed Environment

Often colicky children are extremely sensitive to their environment. Since you, the parent, are a child's primary environment and source of emotional and physical nourishment, your well-being can contribute to the presence or absence of colic. Quiet, peaceful music during mealtimes is often helpful. Mothers should drink warm nervine teas before nursing. Feeding time should, whenever possible, be a time of quiet, restful sharing. Turn off the TV; whatever is being aired is part of the feeding process for your baby. If you are feeling stressed out and tense, the infant will often respond with similar energy. This does not mean that all colicky babies have stressed-out parents, but it is important to note that a peaceful environment is conducive to creating well-being for the child.

Avoid Irritating Foods

Women who are nursing should avoid foods that are irritating to the infant's digestive tract. While every child's system is different, some foods are common digestive-tract irritants. The Brassica family, for example, which includes cabbage, broccoli, cauliflower, kale, and collards, is high in sulfur, which creates gas in the intestines. Avoid hot, spicy foods; an infant's system just isn't ready for them yet. And avoid chocolate, peanuts, peanut butter, and foods high in sugar. Such foods slow down digestive action, cause congestion in the digestive tract, and add to the spasms and contractions of colic. Regularly monitor your child to determine which foods are irritating to him or her.

Avoid Caffeine

Though the amount of caffeine in your daily coffee or tea may not seem to have a big effect on you anymore, it is nonetheless a powerful stimulant. Your child's young system will respond readily to caffeine's stimulating properties, causing him or her to become nervous and highly excitable. Can you imagine anything worse than colic combined with the caffeine jitters? In addition, coffee is very acidic and will adversely affect the immature digestive system of the infant, adding to the difficulties of colic.

old-fashioned colic techniques that still work

In the midst of a colic attack, there are a couple of old-fashioned and effective techniques to try. Place your baby in a warm chamomile or lavender bath. If bottle-fed, the baby can enjoy his feeding from the comfort of this soothing bath. You may relax the child's stomach muscles by placing a towel that was soaked in hot herb tea — such as chamomile or lavender — over the stomach area. Be certain the towel is adequately warm, but not hot. The combination of warm water and herbal essence will often be just what's needed to stop the muscle spasms.

A drop or two of lavender or chamomile essential oil in the bathwater or on the towel will often work wonders.

And there is always the old reliable burping technique. Pad your shoulder and place the child's head against it. Pat his or her back gently. Children seem to become hypnotized into forgetting the problem. What is really happening, of course, along with distracting the child from his grief for a few moments, is that you are helping move the gas deposits along with a steady movement.

Supplement with Acidophilus

Acidophilus and Bacillus Bifidus are highly recommended for infant colic. They are naturally
occurring flora found in the human intestines,
and supplements will help build up healthy intestinal flora and support the growth of digestive
enzymes. There are special preparations of each
of these substances for children, available in most
natural foods stores. Be sure you get an active,
viable form of acidophilus. I generally recommend Natrin, a brand name that seems to be consistently good. To treat colic, double the amount
suggested on the label. A standard dose for colic
would be ¼ teaspoon four or five times daily.

If the child is eating solid foods and is not
lactose-intolerant, include daily servings of
yogurt, kefir, and buttermilk, which contain
acidophilus. If nursing, the mother should eat
several servings a day of these foods.

Use Hyland Colic Tablets

Hyland Pharmacy produces an excellent homeopathic colic tablet. It is available in most natural
foods stores. A safe, all-natural product, this remedy has provided relief for countless colicky babies.
Follow the dosage guidelines on the bottle.

Drink Herbal Teas

The most helpful herbs for treating colic are
anise, catnip, dill, fennel, and slippery elm. Try
these teas to relieve the acute symptoms of colic.

SLIPPERY ELM GRUEL

This gruel (thick tea) is wonderfully soothing and
healing. It is also extremely nourishing. Since the
herbs are powdered, there's no need to strain this
gruel. Slippery elm and marsh mallow root are both
extremely mucilaginous. This makes them very
soothing and healing to the intestinal tract.

1 part marsh mallow root, powdered
1 part slippery elm bark, powdered
⅛ part cinnamon, powdered
⅛ part fennel seed, powdered
Water
Maple syrup

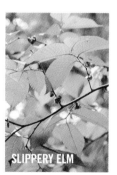

SLIPPERY ELM

1. Combine the herbs. I like
to prepare this herb mix in
large batches and store the
extra in an airtight container
until I'm ready to use it.
2. Use 1 tablespoon of herbs
per cup of water. Bring the
water to a boil. Stir in the
herb mixture, cover, and
simmer over low heat for 10 to 15 minutes.
3. Sweeten with maple syrup to taste. Store the
tea in the refrigerator.
4. To serve, warm the tea and add to juice or
cereal. Infants may drink as much of this tea as
desired. If the infant is still nursing, the mother
should drink 3 to 4 cups daily.

Cradle Cap

Cradle cap is neither a serious nor a contagious problem, and children outgrow it in due time. The sebaceous glands of most infants are not developed and may oversecrete, causing a yellowish, oily crust on the child's scalp. You can remove the "cap" and help regulate the activity of the sebaceous glands by gently massaging a mixture of herbs and olive oil into the scalp two or three times daily. Leave the herb/oil mixture on overnight. The next morning, the crust can be easily removed by gently massaging. Be sure not to pick at the scab or be too rough. Shampoo with a mild baby shampoo only when necessary.

CRADLE CAP TEA

If cradle cap continues to be persistent, give the infant this warm herbal tea.

> 1 part burdock root
> 1 part mullein leaf
> 1 part red clover flower

1. Mix the herbs and store in an airtight container until ready to use.
2. Add 1 cup of boiling water to 1 teaspoon of herb mixture and steep for 30 minutes. Strain.
3. Give the infant 2 teaspoons of the tea three or four times daily for several weeks.

CRADLE CAP OIL

> 1 part chamomile flowers
> 1 part mullein leaf
> 1 part dried nettle leaf
> Olive oil
> Lavender essential oil

1. Combine the herbs in a double boiler. Cover with olive oil. Cook over very low heat for about 1 hour. Strain and bottle.
2. Add 1 drop of lavender essential oil for each ounce of herbal oil. Store in the refrigerator. Warm to room temperature before applying.

Diaper Rash

Most diaper rashes respond readily to natural therapy. Follow the suggestions listed with good faith; all have been used successfully by countless mothers. If the rash is persistent and does not respond to natural therapies, it could be a herpes-related virus or a yeast type of fungus. Consult your health care practitioner or pediatrician in such cases.

One or more of the following are generally the culprit in cases of diaper rash.

• Strong detergents can leave an irritating soap residue on diapers. Simply change soaps. Use mild soaps such as Ivory or a liquid soap such as Heavenly Horsetail or Basic H. Do not use ammonia or bleach. As harmful as bleach is for the environment, it is even worse for your baby.

• Spicy foods, citrus fruits, and other high-acid foods are major irritants for the digestive system of small children, whether they eat them themselves or absorb them through the mother's milk. Digestive problems in turn can lead to diaper rash.

• Teething, fever, and other stress-related incidents cause toxins to be released in the child's system, which can sometimes be manifested as diaper rashes or other skin-related problems.

To get rid of diaper rash, try any of the following suggestions.

Give Acidophilus Preparations

Administer ¼ teaspoon acidophilus culture (available in natural foods stores) three times daily. Use a preparation that's formulated especially for children. You can even try spreading acidophilus diluted in plain unsweetened yogurt directly on the rash.

Take Off Those Diapers!

Leave diapers off as much as possible. The more exposure to air and sunlight the better, though you must be sure to protect your child's delicate skin from sunburn. If the weather is uncooperative or the diaper rash persists, consider using an herbal preparation. Prolonged or recurrent diaper rash should be examined by a pediatrician or holistic practitioner.

covering baby's bottom

Use only 100 percent cotton diapers and change after every bowel movement. Rinse the baby's bottom frequently and dry thoroughly.

If your child is prone to diaper rash, you may choose to do away with plastic pants, a prime contributor to rashes (not to mention landfills). Instead, use a natural wool soaker. These are nonirritating, highly absorbent, and widely available. Denise, my grandson's mother, made all of her own cloth diapers and wool soakers for Andrew. He had the cutest ones on the block. And, again, never a diaper rash in his entire infancy or toddlerhood.

Apply Herbal Powders

Use arrowroot powder or a clay/herb mix for your baby powder and as a remedy for diaper rash. Cornstarch is also very effective but is not recommended for use on yeast-related diaper rashes, as it may encourage the growth of certain bacteria. Commercial baby powder is made with talc, which is a possible carcinogen. It also contains synthetic scents, which can be irritating to an infant's sensitive skin. Make your own baby powder (see page 194) or buy those that are made with natural ingredients.

Apply Herbal Paste

For a more serious rash, mix the clay/herb powder with water or comfrey tea to form a thin paste. Smooth over the rash and leave on for 30 to 45 minutes. To remove, gently rinse with warm water or soak off in a warm tub. Don't attempt to scrape or peel off the paste, as you may further injure the child's irritated skin.

Apply Herbal Salve

The Bottoms-Up Salve (page 195), made with calendula, comfrey leaf and root, and St.-John's-wort, is one of the best remedies I know of for diaper rash. This is a famous old-time formula that I've been making for more than 25 years. It remains one of the best recipes out there and is a superior remedy for diaper rashes. Wash and dry

bare buns

During much of the time that my son was growing up, we lived in the mountains, as close to nature as possible. He seldom wore diapers — or any clothes, for that matter — as there was simply no reason to, and the less I had to wash, the happier I was. Jason never once had a diaper rash. He does, however, have a stigma about nakedness, and I wonder if it isn't a result of his wayward mom's habits.

the baby's bottom after each bowel movement, apply the herbal salve, and follow with a light dusting of clay/herb powder. This salve, used in conjunction with the other suggestions listed, will generally clear up the worst diaper rash, unless herpes or staph is involved.

Diarrhea

There are few children who have not had a bout of diarrhea, or its counterpart, constipation. Diarrhea can be caused by a number of problems, the most common being reactions to or excesses of certain food groups, reactions to bacteria and viruses, teething, fever, emotional upset, or an infection elsewhere in the body.

The primary concern with diarrhea is dehydration, which can occur quickly if fluid intake is not being carefully monitored, and can be fatal if severe. Ensure that the child's fluid intake is adequate. Don't just guess; monitor the amount of liquid the child drinks and give him warm baths. These will help in the absorption of liquid.

Though liquid intake is essential, it is not necessary that the child eat solid food. It is actually best if he or she consumes only warming liquids such as herb teas, vegetable broth, and chicken or miso soup. Eating solid food will make the already stressed digestive system work overtime. It also means more runny diapers, as everything eaten will quickly come out. If the child wishes to eat, allow foods such as yogurt, kefir, buttermilk, cottage cheese, potato soup, mashed potatoes (no gravy or butter), and Slippery Elm Gruel (see the recipe on page 175). These foods are easy to digest and will contribute to healing the irritated digestive system. Though milk products will often exacerbate diarrhea, cultured milk products such as buttermilk and yogurt add beneficial bacteria that aid the system. Also, administer ⅛ teaspoon of acidophilus culture every hour until diarrhea stops. In addition, commercial pediatric electrolyte solutions, such as Pedialyte, are very helpful in preventing dehydration.

BLACKBERRY ROOT TEA

Along with a high fluid intake, herbal baths, and a very simple diet as suggested above, this tea should help remedy diarrhea. Unfortunately, and for reasons I've never fathomed, blackberry root tincture is hard to find. You may have to make your own. It's simple:

> **1 part dry or fresh blackberry root, finely chopped**
> **Alcohol or vegetable glycerin**
> **½ cup warm water**

Follow the directions for making a tincture on page 384. Mix 1 teaspoon of tincture in ½ cup of warm water and administer ¼ teaspoon of this preparation every hour.

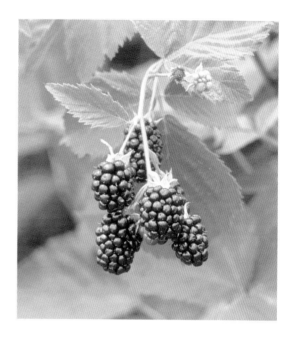

DIARRHEA REMEDY TEA

To make this tea more palatable, you can add a small amount of maple syrup or blackberry juice concentrate (available in natural foods stores) for flavor.

> **3 parts blackberry root**
> **2 parts slippery elm bark**
> **⅛ part cinnamon**

Mix the herbs and store in an airtight container. Simmer 1 teaspoon of the herb mixture in 1 cup of water for 20 minutes. Strain and cool. Administer 2 to 4 tablespoons every hour, or more often as needed.

Constipation

Constipation is one of the most common problems adults suffer. Witness the number of products in any drugstore; we have become a constipated society. Constipation is frequently associated with emotional factors or habits learned at an early age that do not support healthy elimination. Be alert for such behavior when assessing your child's toilet habits. Often, simple habits learned at an early age will eliminate the need for stronger medications later on, and catching the problem in its early stages will eliminate a lifetime of stressful elimination.

Children experience constipation for the same reasons adults do. How many adults do you know who can't go to the bathroom because they don't have the time, are unfamiliar with the bathroom, are uncomfortable with bodily functions, or are stressed out?

If your child develops constipation, the first step is to avoid foods that contribute to the problem. High-fat dairy foods, cheese, wheat, eggs, and refined, processed foods are generally the most common food culprits; watch your child for signs of constipation after consuming these foods. If the child is nursing, the mother should avoid these foods in her diet as well, until the constipation clears up. If the child is bottle-fed on cow's milk, switch to goat's milk or soy milk. Cow's milk can be constipating to some children as well as adults.

Include in the diet those foods that contribute to good elimination: fruits, vegetables, whole grains, water, fruit and vegetable juices, molasses, dried fruit, and foods that supply bulk to the system. There are several herbs that should be included in the diet of a child who is prone to develop constipation: carob powder, slippery elm, flaxseed, psyllium seed, licorice root, and Irish moss. These plants can be powdered in a coffee grinder and added to the child's meals. Use 1 to 4 teaspoons three or four times daily, or as often as needed during bouts of constipation. For children under 10, use the smaller dose. These herbs are not laxatives but provide the bulk necessary in the diet for proper elimination.

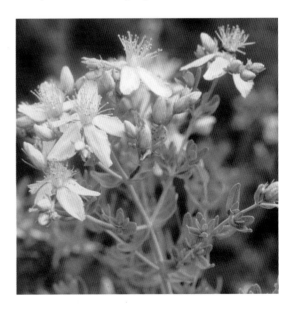

The following suggestions combined with the dietary recommendations should bring relief to the child plagued by constipation:

• Administer ½ teaspoon of acidophilus with meals. Acidophilus adds friendly bacteria to the digestive tract and aids in good digestion.

• Grind equal amounts of slippery elm, flaxseed, and psyllium seed to a fine powder. Mix 1 teaspoon of the mixture with food at each meal.

• Make a special "candy" by grinding together prunes, figs, apricots, and raisins. Mix in powdered psyllium seed, slippery elm, and fennel seed. To flavor and thicken, mix in carob powder, which is made from an herb that's useful for treating constipation. Roll into balls and serve daily as a delicious, nourishing snack.

• Be sure the child drinks plenty of room temperature water. When the child is constipated, upon rising, give him or her a cup of warm psyllium seed water. (To make the water, soak 1 teaspoon of psyllium seed in 1 cup of water overnight. Add lemon juice to taste.)

• Exercise is critical for regular bowel movements. For most children, exercise is not a problem, but you may choose to make a regular time to do some activities together. A nice morning walk is a good way to get the energy moving and is also a nice opportunity to spend time together. The primary goal is to provide some centered, peaceful activity that moves the body while relaxing the mind and the spirit.

TEA FOR CONSTIPATION

4 parts fennel seed

2 parts psyllium seed

2 parts spearmint

1 part licorice root

1 part marsh mallow root

½ part cinnamon

¼ part orange peel

A pinch of stevia

1. Combine all ingredients and store in an airtight container.

2. To make tea, in a saucepan over low heat, simmer 1 teaspoon herb mixture in 1 cup boiling water for 20 minutes. Strain and allow to cool. Administer ⅛ to ½ cup tea with meals or as often as needed.

Note: If constipation persists, add ⅛ part senna pod or leaf to the recipe.

"Every blade of grass has its **Angel** that bends down and **whispers over it,** 'Grow! Grow! Grow!'"

— **The Talmud**

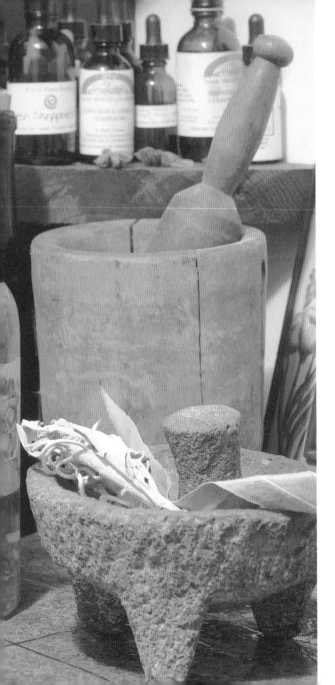

Earaches

Until a child is three or four years old, the ear canals are not fully formed and, consequently, do not drain well. When a child gets congested or has a cold, the ear canals get plugged up with excess mucus, which then cannot drain properly. Bacteria begin to grow in the moisture of the accumulated secretions and infection often occurs.

Ear infections can result from allergies. If your child has recurring ear infections despite your best efforts, consider the possibility of allergies. Wheat, citrus, and dairy products, including milk, cheese, and ice cream, are the most common offenders. If allergies are suspected, don't despair. There are effective natural remedies for them.

Ear infections can be serious. Treated improperly, they can leave a child with impaired hearing or permanently deaf. It is important to treat an ear infection at the first sign of it and to work in conjunction with a holistic health care practitioner and your family pediatrician. Watch for the early signs: congestion, colds, runny nose, fever, excessive rubbing or pulling of the earlobe, combined with irritability and fussiness. If your child wakes up screaming in the night and pulling at her ears, an infection has eked its way into the ear canals and will need to be attended to immediately.

The use of antibiotics, though sometimes effective for acute situations, does not correct the cause of the problem. Because antibiotics (which means "against life") can create such havoc in the young child's system, disrupting the immune cycle and making the child further susceptible to disease, it is important whenever using antibiotics to follow the suggestions outlined in this section.

Avoid Congesting Types of Foods

These include eggs, dairy, wheat, sugar, orange juice, and all refined, processed foods.

Enforce Rest and Recovery

It is imperative that a child with an ear infection gets plenty of rest and does not go out into the cold air prematurely. It is a common mistake to think a child has recovered from an ear infection and send him out to play. So many times have I heard that "Johnny kept me awake crying all night with a bad ear infection. Come morning, he was fine, so I sent him off to school. But, wouldn't you know it, that ear infection was back in full force again in the middle of the night." Ear infections have a way of doing that. Usually, what happens is that the child is just happy to be feeling better and wants to get out and play. Seriously consider keeping the child housebound for at least a few days until recovery is complete.

Give Acidophilus

Acidophilus culture, given in doses of ½ teaspoon several times daily, can be very helpful for ear infections.

Give Warming Tea

A tasty tea of fresh grated ginger, fresh squeezed lemons, and honey or maple syrup is a refreshing decongesting blend.

Support the Kidneys

Be certain the child's kidneys are working well and he is taking in sufficient fluid. Warm packs placed over the lower back (the area of the kidneys) can help relieve ear infections. This technique stems from traditional Chinese medicine, in which the health of the kidneys is directly connected to the health of the ears. Note, however, that this treatment should be combined with other therapies for optimal results. And give the child cranberry juice, which is a strengthening tonic for the kidneys.

Apply Garlic–Mullein Flower Oil

See the recipe on page 82; this oil is also available in most natural foods stores and herb shops. This oil is one of the best herbal remedies for ear infections. It's important to treat both ears; the ear canals are connected and the infection can move from one to the other. The oil not only helps fight the infection but also relieves pain. Be certain the oil is warm, not hot.

Dose with Infection-Fighting Tincture

Doses of Ear Infection Tincture (see the recipe on page 184) help the body fight off the infection.

EAR INFECTION TINCTURE

The herbs in this recipe can also be powdered and capsulated to administer to older children.

> 1 part echinacea root
> 1 part fresh garlic
> 1 part usnea
> ¼ part ginger root
> ¼ part organically grown goldenseal root

Make a tincture following the directions on page 384. Administer ⅛ teaspoon of the tincture diluted in warm water or juice three times daily.

Fevers

A fever is a natural mechanism for fighting infection and is a sign of a healthy immune system. It is only when a fever is too high or lingers too long that it can be dangerous. If your child's fever reaches 101°F or lasts for several days, contact your health care provider or pediatrician immediately.

It is imperative to keep your child's intake of fluid high during bouts of fever. Dehydration, not the actual temperature of a fever, is the greatest danger of childhood fevers.

Use the following techniques to control a fever.

Apple Cider Vinegar Treatments

To lower a fever, bathe the child in a tepid bath with ¼ cup apple cider vinegar added to the bathwater. Be certain there are no drafts in the room.

After the bath, quickly wrap the child in a warm flannel sheet.

Another treatment is to wrap the child's feet in a cool cloth that has been dipped in a mixture of apple cider vinegar and water. Keep the child bundled warmly.

Catnip–Elder Tea

This is a traditional formula for childhood ills that involve fever and stress. Catnip and elder are strong but gentle diaphoretics, and catnip also has nervine pain-relieving properties.

CATNIP–ELDER FEVER-REDUCING TEA

> 2 parts catnip
> 2 parts elder blossoms
> 1 part echinacea root
> 1 part peppermint

1. Mix the herbs and store in an airtight container.
2. To make tea, pour 1 cup of boiling water over 1 teaspoon of the mixture and steep for 1 hour. Strain. Administer every 30 minutes. See the dosage chart on page 168 for guidelines.

Catnip Enemas

A warm catnip enema will bring down a child's fever and provide necessary fluid to the system in extreme cases when the child cannot keep down fluids. It is an excellent way to administer the healing essences of herbs into a sick and feverish body. Though unfamiliar to most people these days, enemas are a time-tested home remedy. They should not be used in children under the age of three unless recommended and supervised by a health care practitioner or pediatrician.

It is absolutely essential that you be properly trained to administer an enema. If you've never given this treatment before, consult your pediatrician or health care provider for instructions. Do not use this treatment unless recommended by your health care professional.

To prepare an herbal enema:

1. Combine 1 pint of water and 3 tablespoons of catnip. Warm over low heat for 15 minutes.

2. Remove from heat and let the liquid cool to an appropriate temperature. Enemas to reduce fevers should be cool but not cold. Strain well and pour less than 1 cup of liquid into an enema bag (one that lets you regulate the flow of liquid).

3. Place the enema bag at shoulder height so that the liquid can flow smoothly. Lubricate the tip with herbal salve or oil and insert into the rectum. Slowly release a gentle flow of liquid. You would be wise to have the child in a tub for this process.

The longer the child holds in the liquid, the more effective the enema is. But even if the child holds it in for just a couple of minutes, the medicine will be effective. It is helpful, after withdrawing the tip, to fold a towel and press it firmly over the anus for a few minutes to aid in retention.

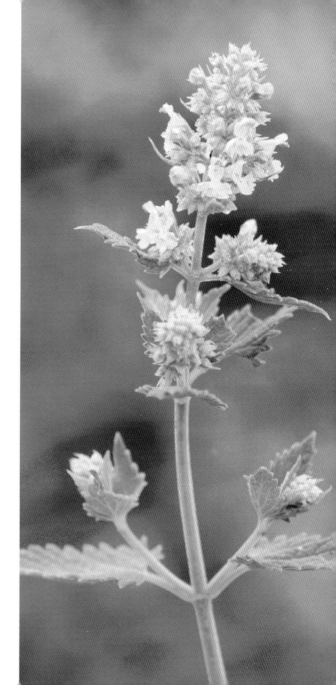

Chicken Pox, Measles, and Other Skin Eruptions

Though chicken pox and measles are distinctly different, treatment is similar. When treating these common disorders of childhood, you want to aid the body's natural defense mechanisms. Though these illnesses are a great discomfort, most children sail right through them. My son, Jason, avoided these "natural" childhood illnesses. I'd dutifully take him around the neighborhood, exposing him whenever possible, knowing that the earlier a child gets these illnesses, the better able he is to cope with them. But his immune system seemed resistant to them, and to my surprise, he never got them.

The following treatments are geared toward helping the body's natural immune system and its inherent ability to respond to these childhood disorders. However, be sure to involve your pediatrician if the child is under two years old, and always treat measles more cautiously.

SUPER IMMUNITY SYRUP

Super Immunity Syrup assists the body in warding off infection and lessens the uncomfortable effects of the rash. It will help your child endure the chicken pox and the measles more comfortably and recover from them more quickly. This formula can also be made into a tea, but you'll need to add some pleasant-tasting herbs such as lemon balm and lemongrass for palatability.

> 2 parts oats (milky green tops)
> 1 part astragalus root
> 1 part burdock root
> 1 part echinacea root and tops

Make an herbal syrup following the instructions on page 166. At the onset of infection, administer 1 teaspoon of the syrup every hour. After the first 24 hours and through the course of the infection, administer four to six times daily, until the symptoms clear.

oatmeal bath

Nothing is as soothing to itchy, irritated skin as a warm oatmeal bath. Prepare a big pot of oatmeal, adding three times as much water as usual. Cook for five minutes. Strain. Add the liquid to the bathwater. For extra comfort, place the strained oatmeal in a cotton bag or sock and add it to the bathwater.

Add to the water a couple of drops of lavender essential oil, which in addition to being a relaxing nervine, has antibacterial and disinfectant properties.

TEA FOR CHICKEN POX AND MEASLES

- 1 part calendula
- 1 part red clover
- 2 parts oats (milky tops)
- 2 parts lemon balm
- 1 part passionflower

1. Mix herbs and store in an airtight container.

2. To make tea, add 1 cup of boiling water to 1 teaspoon of the mixture and steep for 30 minutes. Strain, sweeten with stevia, honey, or maple syrup. Let the child drink as much as desired.

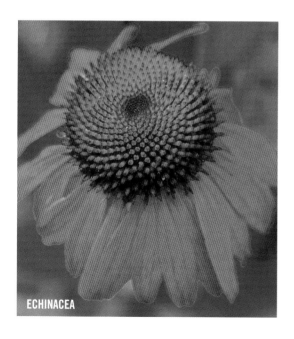

ECHINACEA

VALERIAN–BURDOCK TINCTURE FOR ITCHING AND SKIN RASH

This is my favorite formula to help relieve itching and promote relaxation. You can purchase burdock, echinacea, and valerian tinctures ready-made from most natural foods stores. Mix 2 parts burdock root with 1 part valerian and 1 part echinacea.

- **2 parts burdock root**
- **1 part echinacea root**
- **1 part valerian root**

Make a tincture as instructed on page 384. Give ⅛ teaspoon (or see chart on page 168) every 2 hours.

Note: For some children, valerian acts as a stimulant. If you notice your child becoming more irritated and active after using it, discontinue immediately.

To Prevent Scratching and Scarring

If a sick child is suffering from itching and is scratching frequently, put socks on his or her hands, especially at night, to prevent injury to the skin. A gentle but strong herbal nervine tea or tincture such as skullcap, valerian, or catnip is also recommended.

Vitamin E can be used both topically and internally to prevent scarring. Prick open one end of a 1,000 I.U. capsule and apply the oil directly to the injured area before scars have formed. For internal use, give 50 to 100 I.U. twice daily, depending on the age of the child.

DISINFECTANT POWDER

Mix up this herbal powder and keep it on hand as a disinfectant. It can be sprinkled directly on oozing pox sores, helping dry them as well as preventing infection from setting in. You may also try sprinkling slippery elm powder over the sores. It's so soothing and helps stop the itching.

> 1 ounce green clay (available from natural
>   foods and herb stores)
> 1 tablespoon calendula flower powder
> 1 tablespoon comfrey root powder
> ½ tablespoon cultivated goldenseal or
>   chaparral powder

Combine all the ingredients. Sprinkle on skin sores to stop itching and promote drying. Store the remaining powder in a shaker container or glass bottle with a tight-fitting lid.

> "**Sometimes all it takes** is a warm cup of chamomile tea and a hug to make a miracle."
>
> — Amanda McQuade Crawford

RESCUE REMEDY FLOWER ESSENCE SPRITZER

Try spraying this spritzer in a child's room to relieve the stress and anxiety that accompany the need to resist the urge to scratch that awful itch.

> 3½ ounces distilled water
> 1 tablespoon brandy
> 4 drops Rescue Remedy (Five-Flower Remedy)
> 3 drops lavender essential oil

Combine all the ingredients in a 4-ounce spritzer bottle with a mister top. Shake before using. Use as a room spray as needed.

Colds and Flus

There is probably not a child alive who has escaped childhood without at least a cold or two. Unless this common malady is recurring, there's no need for concern. The various "bugs" and viruses that cause colds and the flu allow the immune system to kick into action and do its job. These illnesses also provide the opportunity for us to observe how quickly our bodies respond to common illness, and they serve as indicators of our overall health.

Lots of fluids, warm soup, a couple of days of rest, and a few specific herbal remedies, along with some immune-strengthening herbs, are generally all that's needed to treat these illnesses.

If your child continues to suffer from colds and flus or is having difficulty recovering from a particularly devastating flu, then seek the guidance of a holistic health care provider or your family doctor.

At the first sign of a cold or flu, start giving your child frequent, higher-than-normal doses of echinacea tincture. For example, a child of four would take ⅛ teaspoon of echinacea tincture every hour until the symptoms subside.

feed a cold?

What and how much a sick child eats will greatly affect the degree of illness. All dairy products, especially milk and ice cream, tend to make the symptoms of a cold worse. Sugar-rich foods should be avoided. So should orange juice, in spite of what the glossy ads say. A large, ice-cold glass of orange juice, no matter how good it tastes, is very acidic and will create more mucus and congestion. Instead, try hot lemonade made with fresh squeezed lemon juice, a pinch of ginger, and a little honey or maple syrup to sweeten. Lemons provide vitamin C, are alkalizing, and will help prevent illness.

Grandma's chicken soup (or, if you're a vegetarian, miso or vegetable broth) is really the best thing to eat when you have a cold or the flu. The mineral-rich broth, the fluid, and the warmth are all beneficial. I often add medicinal herbs directly to the soup base. Astragalus, dandelion root, burdock root, echinacea, and even prince ginseng can be added for extra strength, nourishment, and vitality.

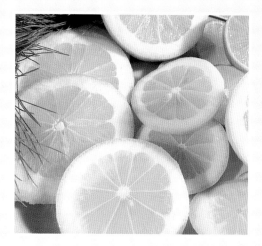

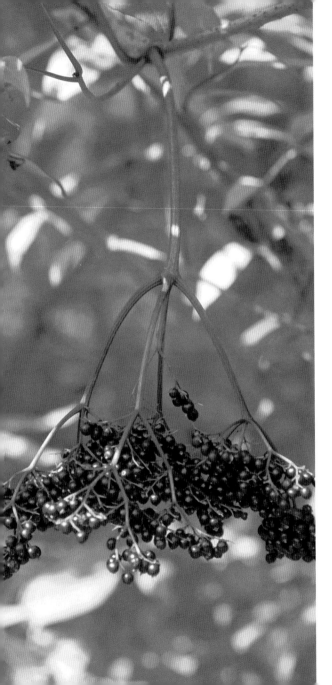

ELDERBERRY SYRUP

This is the most popular herbal cold remedy in Europe, and it's delicious. Every year I try to make two or three batches of Elderberry Syrup, and it's always gone by the end of the season. I've gathered fresh elderberries everywhere from the West Coast to the East Coast and have marked the seasons by the ripening of these dark blue–black berries.

1 cup fresh or ½ cup dried elderberries
3 cups water
1 cup honey

1. Place the berries in a saucepan and cover with water. Bring to a boil, reduce heat, and simmer over low heat for 30 to 45 minutes.
2. Smash the berries. Strain the mixture through a fine-mesh strainer and add 1 cup of honey, or adjust to taste.
3. Bottle the syrup and store in the refrigerator, where it will keep for 2 to 3 months.

Caution: Use only blue elderberries; the red ones are potentially toxic if eaten in large quantities. Never eat elderberries that haven't been cooked first.

FORMULA FOR LUNG AND CHEST CONGESTION

This formula can be made into a tea, syrup, or tincture and is very effective in clearing up bronchial congestion. If making a tea, adjust flavors by adding more licorice, cinnamon, and ginger to the formula. If your child is prone to respiratory infections, make up the formula ahead of time as a tincture.

> 2 parts licorice root
> 1 part cinnamon
> 1 part echinacea
> 1 part elecampane
> ¼ part ginger

1. Combine ingredients and store in an airtight container.

2. To make a tea, see the directions on page 380. To make a tincture, see page 384 for instructions. See the chart on page 168 for dosages.

GINGER–ECHINACEA COLD SYRUP

This is a truly delicious syrup that's very effective. Other herbs can be added, such as wild cherry bark and licorice for cough, valerian for restlessness, and elecampane for respiratory infection.

> 1 part dried echinacea root
> 1 part fresh ginger root, grated
>   or chopped

Follow the directions for making syrup on page 166. Ginger is very warming; if the syrup is too "hot" for your child's taste, serve it diluted in warm water or tea.

warming treatments for lung and chest congestion

A hot-water bottle placed over the back between the shoulder blades helps loosen phlegm and deep-seated congestion in the chest. I use an old-fashioned hot-water bottle wrapped in cotton flannel to keep in the heat. It's even more effective if you rub Bag Balm, Vicks VapoRub, or a homemade vapor type of salve over the back and chest. Because the oils can be irritating to the eyes, don't ever let the child rub these salves on himself. Do it yourself — and be careful not to put too much on that tender young skin.

DECONGESTING HERBAL STEAM

A favorite "instant" remedy for sinus congestion and runny noses is an old-time herbal steam.

Water

Eucalyptus essential oil

1. Heat a large pot of water until it is steaming. Add a drop or two of eucalyptus oil to the water.
2. Set the pot of water on a table. Have the child lean over the pot, being careful not to touch it, and drape a large towel over both the pot and the child's head. Allow the child to inhale the steam for 5 to 10 minutes, or until the sinuses open up. Instruct the child to keep his or her eyes closed tight, as the herbal oil can make them water and cause some discomfort, and encourage him or her to lift up the towel to release some of the steam if it becomes too hot.

Caution: Because you're using a large container of hot water, always stay by the child while she or he breathes the herbal steam and be sure young hands don't touch the hot pot (or pour the water into a heat-resistant bowl before adding the oil). Do not use the steam for children under four years old.

RESPIRATORY TONIC TEA

This blend is an effective and tasty tea for building strong, healthy lungs. It is especially helpful for children who have recurring respiratory problems such as colds, flu, hay fever, asthma, ear

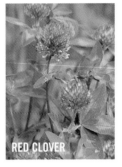

RED CLOVER

infections, and general congestion. This tea is not necessarily the blend you might choose to use in the acute stages of a respiratory infection but, used over a period of time, it will aid in creating a healthy respiratory system.

4 parts fennel

4 parts rose hips

2 parts lemongrass

1 part calendula

1 part coltsfoot

1 part mullein

1 part red clover flowers

1. Combine all ingredients and store in an airtight container.
2. To make a tea, prepare as an infusion, following the instructions on page 380.

HIGH-C TONIC TEA

A wonderfully refreshing blend, High-C Tonic Tea provides bioflavonoids and vitamin C in an organic, naturally biochelated base so that all the nutrients are readily available for absorption. High levels of vitamins supplied in therapeutic dosages, such as commercial vitamins, may be useful to combat illness, but for daily maintenance, a more naturally occurring dose is better for your child.

> 4 parts rose hips
> 3 parts hibiscus
> 2 parts lemongrass
> 1 part cinnamon chips

1. Combine all ingredients and store in an airtight container.

2. To make a tea, prepare as an infusion, following the instructions on page 380. This is a tonic; your child can drink as much of it as he or she wants.

Insect Bites, Cuts, and Scratches

Invariably, all children get bee stings, insect bites, cuts, and scratches. These are perfect opportunities to teach them the art of self-care and make them little "healers." Include your children when you're making homemade remedies. Most children love to participate in these activities and are much keener to use a medicine they've made themselves. What's even more fun is to go out with them to pick the common garden "weeds" that are powerful healing plants: plantain, dandelion, burdock, and other of nature's great gifts.

HEALING CLAY

Clay is composed of mineral-rich deposits accumulated over millions of years. Green clay is particularly rich in minerals and is the one I prefer. You can buy green clay in most natural foods stores or herb shops, and it is a wonderful healing agent when used alone or in combination with herbs for cuts, wounds, and insect bites.

> 4 parts clay
> 1 part dry aloe vera powder
> 1 part comfrey root powder
> 1 part organically grown goldenseal powder or chaparral powder

1. Combine the clay and the powdered herbs. Store in a glass jar.

2. To use, combine a small handful of the mixture with enough water to form a paste. Apply it directly to cuts, wounds, and insect bites.

Alternatively, you can premix the clay and herbal powders into a paste with water. Add a few drops of lavender and tea tree essential oils and store in a glass jar with a tight-fitting lid. If the clay dries out, just remoisten with water.

recipes for baby-care products

Though there is a wonderful variety of natural baby-care products on the market, it's delightful, simple, and far less costly to make your own.

When I first started making my own baby-care products, I was a young, single, working mom. Cost was certainly a factor for me, but not nearly as important as the purity of the product. The only baby products available were the commercial ones, and they were far from natural. So I decided to make my own. Thirty years later, these products are still popular and have been used by hundreds of parents and their children. All are completely natural and easy to make.

BABY'S BATH HERBS

Use the following mixture in the bathwater. These herbs are soothing and relaxing — for Mom and Dad, too.

> 2 parts calendula
> 2 parts chamomile
> 2 parts comfrey leaf
> 1 part lavender
> 1 part roses

Mix all the herbs. Place a small handful of the mixture in a cotton bag and toss it into the baby's bathwater. Use the fragrant herbal bag as a washcloth.

BABY POWDER

This is an excellent daily baby powder. You may wish to lightly scent it, but use only pure essential oil and be certain it is not irritating to the child's sensitive skin. Orange oil is light and refreshing and often used as the scent for baby powders.

> 2 parts arrowroot powder
> 2 parts white clay (available in natural foods stores and ceramic supply stores)
> ¼ part comfrey root powder
> ¼ part slippery elm or marsh mallow root powder

Mix the ingredients together and place in a container with a shaker top, such as a spice jar.

To treat diaper rash, add to this mixture ⅛ part organically grown goldenseal powder, ⅛ part myrrh powder, and ⅛ part echinacea powder. Apply as a powder, or mix into a thin paste and apply as a poultice to the rash.

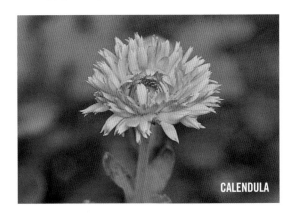

CALENDULA

BOTTOMS-UP SALVE

This is my very favorite salve recipe for diaper rash, cuts and scrapes, and irritated skin. If you don't have the time to steep for 2 weeks or if there's not much sun, let the herbs steep in the olive oil in a double boiler over very low heat for several hours. Check frequently to be sure the oil is not overheating and burning the herbs.

> 1 part calendula flower
> 1 part comfrey leaf
> 1 part comfrey root
> 1 part St.-John's-wort flower
> Olive oil
> Grated beeswax

1. Combine the herbs and store in an airtight container. Make a solar infusion by steeping 2 ounces of the herb mixture in 1 pint of olive oil for 2 weeks. (See page 383 for instructions on making a solar infusion.) This will create about 2 cups of herbal oil.

2. At the end of 2 weeks, place the mixture in a double boiler and warm for 1 hour over very low heat. Strain.

3. To each cup of warm herbal oil, add ¼ cup of grated beeswax. You may need to warm the oil a little longer to melt the beeswax.

4. When the beeswax is melted, check for desired consistency; place 1 tablespoon of the mixture in the refrigerator for a few minutes. If the salve is too hard, add a little more oil; if too soft, add a little more beeswax. Pour it into a glass jar. The salve does not need to be refrigerated and will last for months (or years) if stored in a cool area.

BABY OIL

This is excellent all-purpose oil and is wonderful to rub on baby after baths. It also makes a great massage oil for babies.

> 1 ounce chamomile
> ½ ounce comfrey leaf
> ½ ounce roses
> 1 pint apricot or almond oil

1. Mix herbs and oil and let sit in a glass jar with a tight-fitting lid for 2 weeks in a warm, sunny spot.

2. For a stronger oil, pour the mixture into the top of a double boiler. Slowly warm it over very low heat for 1 hour. Strain and bottle. You may lightly scent it with a few drops of pure essential oil, such as lavender, rose, or chamomile. Use at room temperature.

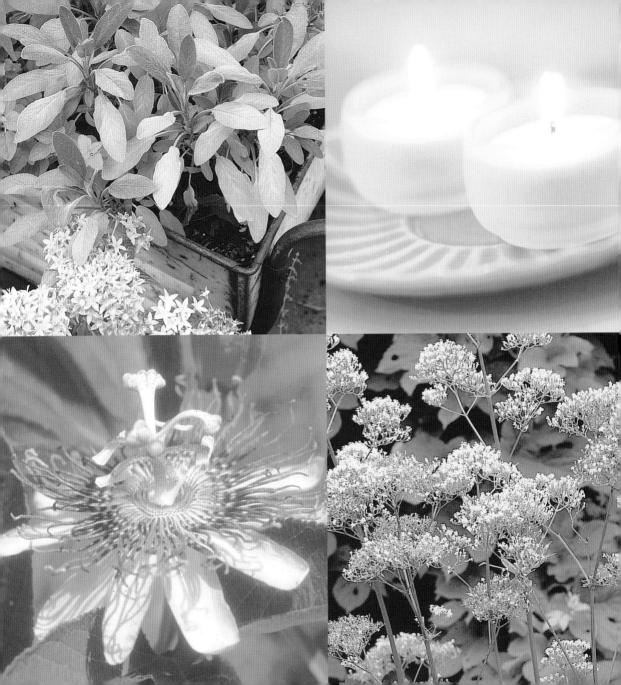

7 For Women

When I first began working as a community herbalist in the 1980s, one of my favorite books was Susun Weed's *Wise Woman Herbal for the Childbearing Year.* It was a favorite reference in my library, and I often lent it to women who were pregnant or trying to conceive. But aside from Susun's, there weren't many books that addressed the subject of herbal medicine for women with any great insight. A handful touched upon menstruation and PMS; even fewer addressed the more challenging health concerns women encounter. I had witnessed firsthand how well herbs and other natural therapies work for problems specific to women, and I felt it was important to alert women to the potential that herbs have for healing. Thus, my first herb book, *Herbal Healing for Women,* was born, and it has proved to be a wonderful help for thousands of women.

As the years have passed since then, I have become increasingly interested in the role of preventive medicine for health and well-being. So much of modern medicine, herbalism included, is about repairing what is unhealthy in the body. But I believe that if we focus our primary attention on ill health, we reduce our opportunity to enjoy the full experience of radiant well-being. If we instead choose to create balance and harmony in our daily lives by emphasizing abundant and sustainable health, we make choices that are good for us and for the earth.

Though I do include effective protocols for the more common imbalances associated with our womanly bodies, I've dedicated the majority of this chapter to those practices that keep our bodies flowing healthfully with the sweet rhythms of life. For many, my words will be a simple reminder of those things that are most important for good health: fresh water, daily exercise, food that supports our life force, work that's meaningful, a spiritual connection, and relationships that are sustaining. There is no better preventive medicine. More than a lack of illness, health is a reflection of inner radiance and vitality. In choosing to live with health, you choose a well-lived, fulfilling, passionate life.

staying healthy

The common health problems that women experience — for example, irregular periods, menstrual cramps, depression, and menopausal disorders — are simply symptoms of imbalances. Often it takes nothing more than "good living practices" to remedy them. Tonic herbs, proper nutrition, adequate rest, connecting with self, and joyful exercise are our primary prescriptions for well-being.

Eat for Health and Vitality

There is no such thing as a diet that is perfect for everyone, so it is important to pay attention to the foods that you eat and how they make you feel, both right after you eat and several hours later. Generally, your body will tell you what is good for it and what isn't.

Dietary principles for women are not much different from those discussed throughout this book:

- Eat food as close to its natural state as possible.
- Eat with the seasons; see what grows in your region in each season and base your diet primarily on those foods.
- Eat foods that make you feel good. Pay particular attention after each meal to how you feel, physically and emotionally, understanding that at different times in our lives and at different times of the month, especially during the menstruating years, women's nutritional requirements change. If a particular food seems to make you feel drowsy, congested, irritable, or sluggish, stop eating it!

- Eat organic whenever possible; it's good for the environment and good for you.
- Eat food that is warming and alkalizing. Many women's disorders thrive in the acidic environment caused by overconsumption of sweets and carbohydrates. Alkalize the system with dark-green leafy vegetables, steamed grains, high-quality protein (fish, tofu, tempeh, organic fowl), and sour fruits such as lemons, grapefruits, and sour cherries.

SEVEN SUPER SUPPLEMENTS FOR THE FEMALE SYSTEM

Supplement	Benefit
Dong quai	A wonder herb for women. Take 2 capsules three times daily, or eat a small piece of the root, about the size of the pink portion of your small fingernail. Do not use dong quai during menstruation or pregnancy.
Spirulina	A complete protein and a good source of energy that's readily absorbed by the body. Take 1 to 2 teaspoons of the powder daily.
Vitamin E	A wonderful nutrient for the reproductive system and a specific remedy for hot flashes, muscle cramps, and vaginal dryness. Also a potent antioxidant. Take 200 to 400 I.U. daily. (However, if you are taking heart medication, do not take more than 50 I.U. of vitamin E without first consulting your health care practitioner.)
Floradix Iron + Herbs	An all-natural liquid vitamin/mineral formula (manufactured by Salus Haus of Germany); rich in iron, in which many women are deficient. Available in most natural foods stores.
Antioxidants	Have a marked beneficial effect on the body and aid in the healthy functioning of women's cycles. They are found in fresh fruits and vegetables and teas made from antioxidant-rich herbs such as bilberry, cayenne, garlic, ginkgo, hawthorn, milk thistle, and green and black tea; they are also available as supplements in most natural foods stores.
Omega-3 fatty acids	Cleanse the arteries, support the heart, boost immune-system function, and nourish the brain. Are often lacking in the Western diet.
Calcium– magnesium	Essential for reproductive health. Supplements are available but should not replace dietary sources, which include seaweeds, seeds (especially sesame), nuts, nettle, watercress, parsley, oatstraw, horsetail, and yellow dock.

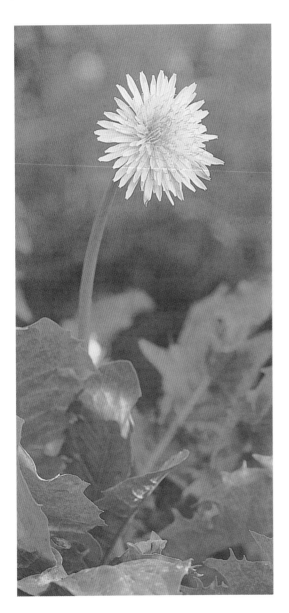

HERBAL IRON SYRUP

This tasty formula abounds in vitamins and minerals, especially iron, in which women are often deficient. Fruit concentrates, available at natural foods stores, are concentrated extracts of fresh fruit; they are a good source of vitamins and minerals and have a delicious fruity flavor.

> 3 parts dandelion leaf
> 3 parts dandelion root
> 3 parts nettle
> 3 parts raspberry leaf
> 2 parts alfalfa leaf
> 2 parts yellow dock root
> 1 part hawthorn berry
> Honey

1. Combine all the herbs. With the honey, prepare as a syrup, following the instructions on page 382.
2. Remove the syrup from the heat. For every 2 cups of syrup, add the following:

> ¼ cup brandy
> ¼ cup fruit concentrate (make sure that it's concentrate, not juice)
> 2 tablespoons blackstrap molasses
> 2 teaspoons nutritional yeast
> 2 teaspoons spirulina powder

3. Stir well, then bottle, seal, and label. Store in the refrigerator, where the syrup will keep for several months. Take 4 to 6 tablespoons daily.

Support Liver Health

When we experience menstrual irregularities, PMS, menopausal problems, fibrocystic conditions, and even erratic mood swings, special attention should be directed to the health of the liver. Our largest and most metabolically diversified organ, the liver performs more functions than any other organ of the body. It is the body's master detoxifier and cleanses the system not only of environmental toxins but also of metabolic wastes. The liver is also a major organ of digestion; every substance that is ingested must be processed by the liver before it can be distributed throughout the body. It manufactures many of the building blocks needed for hormone production and helps regulate hormone activity. The health of the entire body — including our reproductive organs — is directly related to the well-being of the liver.

When an herbal protocol for the reproductive system also addresses the liver, recovery is often faster and more deep-seated. Thankfully — or as part of nature's master plan — many of the herbs recommended for the reproductive system are also beneficial to the liver. And, of course, it's quite easy to add liver-cleansing herbs such as burdock, dandelion, wild yam, yellow dock, milk thistle seed, and garlic to formulas for the reproductive system.

Following are two excellent examples of liver tonic teas that are also specific for the reproductive system. I recommend rotating between them.

LIVER TONIC FORMULA #1

This tonic is excellent for the reproductive system and the liver. If the flavor is too bitter for you, add cinnamon, ginger, lemon peel, or sassafras to taste.

> 2 parts dandelion root
> 1 part chaste tree berry
> 1 part wild yam root
> 1 part yellow dock root
> ½ part Oregon grape root

Prepare as a decoction, following the instructions on page 381, using 4 tablespoons of herb mixture per quart of water, and simmering for 20 minutes. Strain. Drink 3 to 4 cups daily.

LIVER TONIC FORMULA #2

This formula is milder and more pleasant tasting than Formula #1.

> 3 parts nettle leaf
> 2 parts dandelion leaf
> 2 parts lemon balm
> 2 parts red clover flowers
> 1 part alfalfa leaf

Prepare as an infusion, following the instructions on page 380, using 4 tablespoons of herb mixture per quart of water and steeping for 20 minutes. Strain. Drink 3 to 4 cups daily.

Get Rest and Relaxation

A simple prescription for rest and relaxation can be the most important element of a health care program for women. Many women are just plain worn out, whether because of a high-pressure job or the demands of trying to balance work, family, and self. Those of us with recurring health problems often feel chronically tired, but being tired is usually the cause, not the symptom, of the problem.

The best remedy for many health problems is not an assortment of expensive drugs or treatments but simply to slow down, taking time to enjoy the life we live. Granted, this is often the most difficult prescription to fill; rest and relaxation don't fit into a bottle and can't be swallowed twice a day.

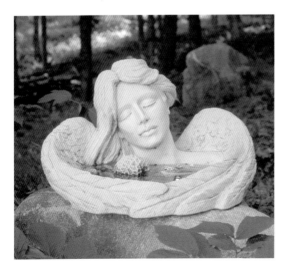

Sleep restores and rejuvenates the body in the deepest sense. If you have trouble sleeping restfully at night, review the suggestions for overcoming insomnia, beginning on page 61. During the day, take a few minutes to rest every afternoon, lying down or relaxing in a comfortable chair, clearing your mind of worries. Allow time for massage, for long soaks in herbal baths, for quiet reflection, and for long walks. For most women, taking time out for rest and relaxation is a quiet act of rebellion. With the heavy weight of responsibilities that each of us carries, it may seem selfish or costly to take time out from our daily performance. But rest and relaxation — even just a few minutes' worth every day — bring peace of mind, and with that comes a renewed sense of vitality and vigor.

Use Herbs Every Day for Well-Being

Following are some of my favorite herbs for women. Though these herbs usually hold great benefit for men, children, and elders as well, they are the ones most often used in blends and formulas designed for women.

Herbs specific for women generally fall into four classifications — uterine tonics, emmenagogues, hormonal balancers, and uterine contractors — depending on their mode of action in the body. Of course, because herbs are composed of a multitude of chemical constituents, they can have several different modes of action. But breaking them down by their major actions, as in the chart on pages 204–205, will help give you a better understanding of how and why the herbs are used in particular combinations and formulas.

Uterine Tonics

These herbs tone and strengthen the entire female reproductive system. They are generally extremely rich in vitamins and minerals. They feed and nourish the reproductive organs and restore vitality and balance to the system. They are generally recommended to take over long periods of time and have few or no known side effects.

Herbal uterine tonics include chaste tree berry, dandelion leaf and root, dong quai root, ginger root, milky tops of oats, nettle leaf, and raspberry leaf.

Emmenagogues

Emmenagogue herbs stimulate and promote normal menstrual flow. They help relieve menstrual cramps and bring on suppressed or delayed menstruation. While many emmenagogues are also uterine tonics, some promote menstruation by irritating or stimulating the uterine muscles; be sure you know which effect an emmenagogue herb has before using it.

Herbal emmenagogues include blue cohosh root, dong quai root, ginger root, motherwort leaf, mugwort leaf, pennyroyal leaf, and yarrow flower and leaf.

Hormonal Balancers and Regulators

Hormonal balancers and regulators normalize the functions of the endocrine glands, thereby aiding the proper functioning of the reproductive system. They balance estrogen and progesterone activity and thus are useful for all aspects of menstrual and menopausal dysfunction. They are rich in phytohormones and provide the hormonal precursors needed by our systems. They often have a strong effect on the liver, which helps explain their effect on the hormonal system.

Herbal hormonal balancers and regulators include black cohosh root, chaste tree berry, licorice root, milk thistle seed, and wild yam root.

Uterine Contractors

These herbs promote uterine contractions. They can be very potent, so learn them well. Some help bring on a late period; others are used to assist in labor. Some of these herbs contain oxytocin, which encourages production of prostaglandins; high levels of prostaglandins cause uterine contractions. Others cause contractions by being directly irritating to the uterine membrane; some are actually poisonous. Though they're potentially very helpful, some can be toxic. You should know these herbs well and do some preliminary work with an experienced herbalist before using them on your own.

Uterine contractors include blue cohosh root, cotton root bark, parsley root and leaf, pennyroyal leaf and flower, rue leaf, and tansy leaf.

HERBS FOR WOMEN

Herb	Effect
Black cohosh (*Cimicifuga racemosa*)	A powerful nervine and muscle relaxant, as well as one of the most useful uterine tonic herbs. Stimulates the estrogen cycle of women and is particularly helpful for menopausal women. Use only organically cultivated supplies.
Black haw (*Viburnum prunifolium*)	Has a long history of "quieting" the uterus and is used for threatened miscarriage, uterine cramps, and dysmenorrhea.
Blue cohosh (*Caulophyllum thalictroides*)	A powerful muscle relaxant and emmenagogue. Used during the later stages of pregnancy (typically the last weeks) to help prepare the mother for childbirth. Of great value in promoting easy labor. Should not be used during the early stages of pregnancy or without the assistance of a qualified herbalist. Use only organically cultivated supplies.
Chaste tree (*Vitex agnus-castus*)	The berries stimulate the pituitary gland, which regulates the menstrual cycle. Used to normalize the menstrual cycle and to increase fertility. Rich in volatile oils, alkaloids, and flavonoids.
Crampbark (*Viburnum opulus*)	An amazing uterine nervine; tremendously helpful for relaxing the uterine muscles. Used to relieve menstrual cramps and in cases of threatened miscarriage due to uterine tension. Its relaxing effects are specific to the reproductive system.
Dong quai (*Angelica sinensis*)	One of the best female tonic herbs. Increases blood flow to the pelvic area. Can be used over time to strengthen the uterus. Excellent for easing the transition of young girls into the menstruating years or of older women into menopause. Should not be used during pregnancy or during the menstrual cycle.
Ginger (*Zingiber officinale*)	Directs blood flow to the pelvic region and helps relieve pelvic congestion and blockages. One of the best herbs for easing menstrual cramps.
Lady's mantle (*Alchemilla vulgaris*)	Helps regulate irregular cycles, relieves cramps, and helps reduce heavy menstrual bleeding. Also used to promote fertility.
Licorice root (*Glycyrrhiza glabra*)	Normalizes hormone production. Useful for treating adrenal exhaustion and hormonal imbalances. Often recommended in cases of infertility.

Herb	Effect
Motherwort *(Leonurus cardiaca)*	Used for promoting delayed menstruation, relieving cramps, and reducing nervous stress. A specific herb for menopausal women.
Mugwort *(Artemisia vulgaris)*	A bitter digestive tonic and liver stimulant. Also functions as a uterine stimulant and aids in bringing on delayed or suppressed menstruation. Helps regulate the cycles of young women just entering their menses.
Nettle *(Urtica dioica)*	One of the best all-around women's tonic herbs. A rich source of iron, calcium, and vitamin A. Used during pregnancy to enrich and increase the flow of mother's milk and to help relieve water retention.
Partridge vine *(Mitchella repens)*	An excellent uterine tonic; often recommended for hormonal disorders. Used by Native Americans to aid in pregnancy and childbirth. Use only organically cultivated supplies.
Pennyroyal leaf *(Mentha pulegium)*	Has a terrible reputation and is, in fact, outlawed in several states. However, it's the oil of pennyroyal, not the leaf, that's the culprit. The leaf is one of the best herbal emmenagogues, promoting menstruation and relieving congestion. Also a good remedy for colds, coughs, and achy muscles.
Raspberry leaf *(Rubus idaeus)*	One of the most famous and widely used female tonic herbs; especially valued as a tonic during pregnancy. Contains fragarine, an alkaloid that tones and nourishes the uterus and pelvic region. A rich source of vitamins and minerals, including calcium, iron, phosphorus, potassium, and vitamins B, C, and E.
Wild yam root *(Dioscorea villosa)*	Contains steroidal saponins that yield diosgenin, an important component of birth control pills. However, wild yam is not a natural birth control agent but is used to regulate hormonal action. It is also a primary tonic for the liver and activates and stimulates liver function.
Yarrow *(Achillea millefolium)*	Used to reduce excessive menstrual bleeding, for easing menstrual cramps, and to stimulate delayed or absent menstrual cycles.

Tonic Herbs & Tasty Teas

There are so many tasty teas one can drink as tonics to nourish and tone the female body. Many of the formulas throughout this book can be used, but the following are two of my favorites.

WOMEN'S TONIC TEA

This is a light, refreshing, nourishing tonic for women.

> 2 parts lemon balm
> 2 parts nettle
> 2 parts peppermint or spearmint
> 2 parts raspberry leaf
> 1 part milky oats
> Stevia

Combine all the ingredients, adding stevia to taste. Prepare as an infusion, following the instructions on page 380. Drink 3 to 4 cups daily.

Roses and blue malva flowers can be added to this formula for beauty and taste. The blue

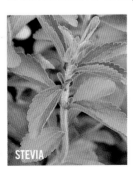

malva makes a gorgeous light blue tea. Though the color is transient, lasting only a few minutes before turning to a dark green, it is lovely while it lasts.

STEVIA

WOMEN'S LIBERTEA

The herbs in this formula stimulate the liver and normalize hormonal function.

> 2 parts chaste tree berry
> 2 parts dandelion root
> 2 parts sassafras bark
> 1 part burdock root
> 1 part ginger root
> 1 part licorice root
> ½ part cinnamon
> ¼ part orange peel

Combine all the ingredients. Prepare as a decoction, following the instructions on page 381. Drink 3 to 4 cups daily.

breast health

Breast health is a major concern for women. And rightfully so — this year, more than 180,000 women in the United States will be diagnosed with breast cancer. Of these, more than 40,000 will die. It is a truly devastating statistic.

Given the prevalence of breast cancer, discovering a lump in your breast is a scary event. It's estimated that more than 70 percent of women have a fibrocystic breast condition, meaning simply that they have nonmalignant lumps — fibrous tissue or cysts — in their breasts. Breast tissue contains fat- and milk-producing glands that are controlled by the hormones estrogen, proges-terone, and prolactin. These hormones are found in the body in fluctuating levels through the course of a month. The hormonal changes that precede menstruation often cause the milk glands to swell and retain fluid. Small cysts may form, especially in the lymph nodes under the armpits. These fibrocystic lumps feel like small sacs filled with fluid. If you press upon one, it may feel something like an eyeball under a closed eyelid. The swollen tissue may be painful. When men-struation begins, the hormone levels in the body change and the cysts disappear or shrink.

Fibrocystic breast lumps are as natural to women as menstruation and menopause. However, they are certainly worrisome, and they can be painful, can make detecting cancerous lumps more difficult, and can be a sign that the hormonal system is unbalanced.

It's vitally important to undertake a weekly breast self-examination. You can find literature with instructions for giving yourself a breast examination in any doctor's office or health clinic. With regular examination, you'll learn to recognize the size and shape of your breasts and to know what lumps are "normal" for you. If a lump appears that you haven't felt before, that feels hard or firm, or that doesn't fluctuate in size over the course of your menstrual cycle, bring it to the attention of your health care provider immediately.

breast milk

Consider this sad fact: Mother's milk, the most sacred of human foods, is now con-sidered to be one of the most toxic of foods. Breast milk is a rung higher on the food chain than the foods adults eat; the toxic residues carried in our bodies — natural by-products of human metabolism overwhelmingly increased by pollution, pesticides, herbicides, fungicides, syn-thetic hormones, and more "miracles" of modern society — are highly concen-trated in the milk our breasts produce. For example, human breast milk contains 10 to 20 times the amount of dioxin that cow's milk has. Even so, mother's milk is still a superior food for babies and provides far more protection and nourish-ment than do infant formulas and other animals' milk.

It's a situation that deserves rage, the kind of healthy rage that incites action. We need to take action against those institutions that allow the poisoning of our environment, making it unfit for our children and other life forms.

The Lymph Nodes

The lymph system is a primary component of our immune system. It contains lymphocytes, white blood cells that destroy bacteria and then help carry infection from the body. The lymph system also plays a major role in maintaining the acid/alkaline balance of the body. If the lymph glands become congested and lymph flow is obstructed, the area surrounding the glands becomes overly acidic, creating a domino effect of cascading pathology.

The breasts have a high concentration of lymphatic tissue and glands. For the health of the body and the health of the breasts, it is important to keep the lymph system flowing freely.

BREAST HEALTH TEA

This mineral-rich tea nourishes the blood and encourages healthy lymphatic flow.

> 2 parts calendula
> 2 parts red clover
> 1 part cleavers
> 1 part lady's mantle
> Spearmint or peppermint (optional; for flavor)

Prepare as an infusion, following the instructions on page 380, using 1 ounce of herbs per quart of water, and letting steep overnight. Drink 3 to 4 cups daily.

LYMPH CONGESTION TEA

The herbs in this formula are renowned for their positive effect on the lymphatic system. Regular consumption of this tea helps ensure proper lymphatic drainage.

> 2 parts calendula
> 2 parts cleavers
> 1 part mullein
> 1 part spearmint (or any flavorful herb of
>   your choice)

Prepare as an infusion, following the instructions on page 380. Drink 2 to 3 cups daily for several weeks.

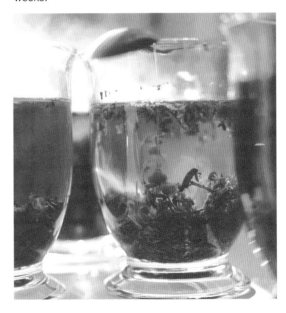

Breast Massage

Breast massage is therapeutically effective and sensuously pleasurable, and it is excellent preventive medicine. It keeps the breasts supple and resilient, enhances proper flow of lymph fluid, helps relieve breast congestion, relaxes the body, and feels great. It also encourages women to know their breasts intimately, which can aid in early detection of cancer. Breast massage takes roughly 5 to 10 minutes a day and should be done at least 5 days a week by women of all ages. I recommend doing the massage while looking at something beautiful — the great outdoors, a painting, yourself in the mirror. Then follow these simple steps:

Step 1. Apply a small amount of massage oil to your breasts. You can use any massage oil, but to enhance lymphatic drainage, try one of the recipes that follow.

Step 2. Cupping your breasts in your hands, move them in a circular motion, rotating outward, away from each other. Use your whole hand, feeling the entire mass of your breast moving beneath it. This motion can be fairly quick or slow and rhythmic, whichever feels better to you. Basically, do what feels good to you and be gentle, as the glands are sensitive. Do this 25 times.

Step 3. Still cupping your breasts in your hands, rotate them inward, toward each other, another 25 times.

Step 4. Repeat step 2, massaging your breasts in an outward motion 25 times.

LOVE-MY-BREASTS MASSAGE OIL

This herbal oil can be used for a stimulating massage. Comfrey is a marvelous herb for the skin, strengthening and healing tissue. Calendula flowers are particularly useful for the lymphatic system and are of tremendous aid in treating fibrocystic conditions. Lavender increases circulation to the breast area and activates the immune system. Pine essential oil also increases blood flow to the breast area and contains compounds that have been proved to destroy cancerous cells. Rosemary is warming and decongesting and stimulates the lymph tissue.

> ½ ounce dried or fresh calendula flowers
> ½ ounce dried or fresh comfrey leaf
> 2 cups almond oil
> 12 drops lavender essential oil
> 6 drops pine essential oil
> 6 drops rosemary essential oil

Infuse the calendula and comfrey in the almond oil, following the instructions on page 383. Add the essential oils to the infused oil.

For fibrocystic breast condition or swollen, sore breasts, add 1 ounce of pokeroot infused oil or 12 drops of pokeroot tincture to the massage oil. Pokeroot can be irritating to the skin, so use only in recommended amount. Do not ingest the berries or the mature stalks and leaves, which are toxic.

YANCE'S POKE OIL PLUS

Donald Yance, author of *Herbal Medicine, Healing and Cancer* and a former Franciscan monk, is beloved in the healing community for his compassionate work with people with cancer and other serious health problems. This is his formula for fibrocystic breasts and tumors. It helps prevent tumors and cysts from forming and can be used as massage oil for fibrocystic breast condition. I like to add a drop or two of lavender essential oil for aromatic pleasure.

> 1 ounce pokeroot *(Phytolacca americana)* infused oil
>
> 2 teaspoons arnica *(Arnica montana)* infused oil
>
> 2 teaspoons mistletoe *(Viscum album)* tincture
>
> 1 teaspoon St.-John's-wort infused oil
>
> 1 teaspoon vitamin E oil

Combine all the ingredients. Bottle and store in a cool, dark location. Use as a massage oil for the breasts.

Caution: Fresh pokeroot is one of the most effective remedies for fibrocystic tissue, but it is also irritating to the skin and can cause a rash, so do not exceed the recommended amount. Do not ingest the berries or the mature stalks and leaves, which are toxic.

Castor Oil Packs

Though the castor bean is extremely toxic, castor oil, which is available at most natural foods stores and pharmacies, is very useful. It is a traditional remedy for constipation and has a long history of use as a poultice for relieving lymphatic congestion and dissolving cysts and tumors. It's a thick and viscous substance that's quite messy to work with, but I've found it very effective; I've used it successfully on fibrocystic lumps in my own breasts.

To make a castor oil pack:

Step 1. Warm a cup of castor oil over very low heat. Remove from heat. You can enhance the effects of the castor oil (and the scent) by now adding a few drops of lavender or pine oil.

Step 2. Thoroughly soak a soft flannel cloth in the warm oil. Place the cloth directly against the skin over the lump. If the oil is too hot or you don't want it directly on your skin, lay it on top of another piece of dry flannel.

Step 3. Cover the compress with another flannel cloth or two, depending on the thickness, and place a hot water bottle or heating pad over the entire pack. Lie back and enjoy the heat and healing power of this simple herbal treatment for at least 35 minutes. This is a good time to practice positive visualization. Make yourself comfortable, close your eyes, and imagine the lump dissolving, becoming smaller and smaller until it has disappeared completely.

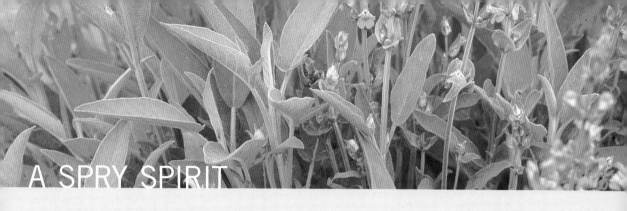

A SPRY SPIRIT

I met Adele Dawson soon after I settled in Vermont. Having barely survived my first winter, I was seriously questioning why any self-respecting herbalist would choose to live in a place where winter ruled for seven months of the year. I might have packed up and gone home to California had Adele not stopped by to visit and bring me some plants from her garden. Watching the way that this tiny spritelike woman walked through the gardens, the way she spoke to the plants, and the way they spoke back, and seeing the sparkle in her eyes, I recognized that I was in the presence of a great herbal elder. That spirit of hers fairly danced around me, drawing me in, forever quelling any doubts about what I was doing in Vermont.

Lucky for me, Adele lived nearby, just over the hill, as the crow flies. Her rambling farmhouse was surrounded by a mostly untamed garden that ran wildly up the hillside. Lush with herbs, wildflowers, and useful weeds, her garden was reflective of the free spirit of its owner.

I was constantly amazed at Adele's accomplishments. I knew her as an herbalist, an extraordinary gardener, and a healer. But others knew her as an artist, a writer, a political activist, and a world traveler. Honestly, I'm not sure there isn't much that is good in this world that Adele wasn't ready to experience, and she filled whatever circle she was in with her stories, laughter, political observations, and endless insights into the many interests she had acquired in her long, rich life.

People often asked her, "Adele, what's your secret for long life?" Perhaps they expected to hear of a secret tonic or special dietary guidance. Little did they know that Adele was a moderation guru. She ate and drank whatever she chose, but, as she would say, "Everything in moderation." She loved her tinctures, which, the way she made them, tasted more like sweet liqueurs than medicine. Her most famous was Sweet Annie's Liqueur. When I'd take my students to visit her, she'd greet us at the door with a small shot glass of liqueur for each of us and a large one for herself. Her other longevity secret, which she repeated often, was quite simple: "One must be very careful whom one chooses as one's parents."

Adele was a very popular lecturer in New England. I got to be Adele's chauffeur, driving her to all of the conferences and events she was invited to. One time she was invited to speak at a conference where all the presenters had a long list of professional-sounding initials after their names. So Adele carefully listed herself as "Adele Dawson, NBEIE." When I asked her what the initials stood for, she answered, "Natural born expert in everything." She said I was the only person who had asked her about it.

No matter where Adele taught, she drew huge crowds. She had a marvelous wit and laughed often. She used to tell all of the older woman, "So long as they think we're crazy, we're safe." She passed on just a few years ago, at the ripe age of 94. I believe she was as surprised as everyone else, not expecting death to knock so quietly. She died at her table having breakfast with friends. I had had lunch with her a couple of days earlier, and she was just as radiant and spry as ever. She was a wonderful, brilliant human being, and she lives on in the hearts of all who knew her.

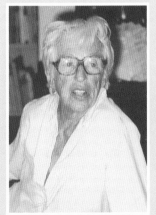

womb and uterine health

Did you know that every woman is born with every egg she will ever have? Tucked deep inside the crevices of our tiny bodies, waiting patiently for our maturity, these eggs form in our ovaries when we are just three months past conception, still living peacefully in the perfect environment of our mother's womb. In essence, when your mother was a babe in your grandmother, you were a seed within her, an egg within her cells, listening to the sound of your grandmother's heartbeat.

Much like the sea embraces the earth, our bodies embrace our wombs. Our wombs are our centers, and they do far more than produce babies — they give birth to the power that is in us. The rhythms of the universe, the ebb and flow of the tides of life, and the energies of the earth and moon are mirrored in our wombs and the cycles of our womanhood.

Uterine Massage

For centuries, healers in Central and South America have treated women with a combination of uterine massage and realignment techniques. My good friend Dr. Rosita Arvigo has been the primary advocate for uterine massage in North America. Having learned this technique in Belize, where she has lived and studied for more than 30 years, Dr. Arvigo finds it to be an amazingly effective therapy for many of the health problems specific to women. She has conducted seminars on uterine massage at many natural health conferences, and she recently began offering training programs for bodyworkers and professional health care providers.

Uterine massage both stimulates and relaxes the uterine muscles and helps restore balance to the reproductive system. For a variety of reasons, including childbirth, back injury, traumatic sexual experiences, lifting and straining, and the chronic stressful effects of a modern lifestyle, a woman's uterus may prolapse, becoming misaligned in the pelvis. Prolapse of the uterus leads to inadequate circulation, poor lymphatic drainage, and general congestion in the pelvic region. Uterine massage helps realign the womb and the muscles. After just a few massage treatments, many women have experienced complete reversal of symptoms ranging from irregular menstruation and painful PMS to backache and numerous other complaints. As Dr. Arvigo states, "These Mayan uterine massage techniques eliminate the primary cause of female complaints, the congested uterus, thereby preventing the progression of symptoms to chronic disease."

Uterine massage can be practiced at home by you and your partner, though I recommend that you see a person trained in the technique for initial treatment and instruction. For more information or to find someone in your area trained in uterine massage, contact Dr. Arvigo's North American organization: The Arvigo Technique, care of Coletta Abergale, 43 Beacon Street, Northampton, MA 01062.

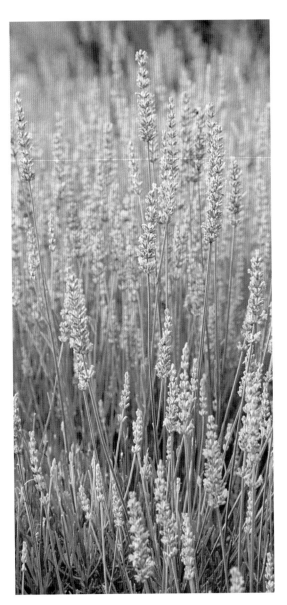

WOMB TEA

This simple tea tones the pelvic region and is highly recommended for womb health. It can be used in conjunction with uterine massage.

> 2 parts nettle
> 2 parts white oak bark
> 1 part lady's mantle
> 1 part oats
> 1 part raspberry leaf
> Spearmint or peppermint (optional; for flavor)

Prepare as an infusion, following the instructions on page 380. Drink 2 to 3 cups daily.

WOMB & BELLY RUB

To bring warmth and energy to the womb and pelvic area, use this gentle, soothing, aromatic oil during massage of the belly.

> 1 cup coconut oil
> ½ cup cocoa butter
> ½ cup sesame seed oil
> 1 tablespoon castor oil
> Vanilla or lavender essential oil

1. Warm the oils until they are thoroughly mixed, then remove from heat and add essential oil to scent.

2. Rub your hands together vigorously, until there is heat dancing between them. Imagine your hands as being full of radiant healing energy. When they feel warm and tingling, alive with their own fire, hold your hands just over your pelvic region, without touching the skin. Let the warm healing fire from your hands penetrate your womb. Imagine healing rays of light sweeping your womb, removing any obstructions, congestion, or painful memories.

3. Take a generous fingerful of the oil and begin gently massaging the area in a circular motion from right to left, spiraling in and then out. Continue for 5 to 10 minutes.

Warming Ginger Poultices

The area surrounding our uterus, that soft area above and between our pelvic bones, should feel warm, juicy, and alive, but it often feels cold or damp. This "stagnation" can result from uterine prolaps, poor circulation, congestion caused by food allergies, or injuries and abuse. In these cases, a warming ginger compress can help restore warmth and heat to the womb.

To make the poultice, grate fresh ginger and pour ¼ cup or so of hot water over it, or combine powdered ginger with enough hot water to make a paste. Place the hot ginger mixture on a soft cotton cloth and fold it several times. Place the poultice directly over your womb area, that space in the soft crevice above and between your pelvic bones. Cover the poultice with a thick towel and place a hot water bottle or heating pad over the pack. Lie back comfortably, close your eyes, and relax for 20 to 30 minutes. This is a perfect time to enjoy a clay facial or a relaxing eye bath.

Sitz Baths

Though this old-fashioned therapy may sound torturous, sitz baths are a wonderful and very effective method for restoring the health and vitality of the reproductive system. They can be employed monthly as a tonic treatment or used more frequently as part of a specific health program. The application of hot and cold water draws fresh blood to the pelvic region, helping remove stagnation and blockages of energy. Sitz baths have been effectively used to treat menstrual irregularities, pelvic congestion, and infertility and to restore tone to the pelvic region.

Step 1. Place two large basins in the bathtub. Fill one with very cold or ice water. Fill the other with a hot herbal tea (raspberry, comfrey, and chamomile are good choices).

Step 2. Lower your buttocks into the hot tea. It's important that it be hot, but not so hot that it's really uncomfortable. Stay in the hot water for about 5 minutes. Then quickly immerse your buttocks in the basin of cold water. Stay in the cold water for 3 to 4 minutes.

Step 3. Continue moving back and forth for at least four rotations.

Kegel Exercises

Kegel exercises are among the most important exercises for strengthening the pelvic region. The pubococcygeus (PC) is a large muscle that stretches from the tailbone to the pelvic bone and supports the entire pelvic area. If not exercised on a regular basis, the PC will, like any other muscle, weaken and eventually atrophy. Lack of PC muscle tone can contribute to urinary incontinence, prolapsed uterus, lack of sensitivity in the vagina, and vaginal dryness. With regular PC exercise, the entire pelvic region will become stronger and healthier (and your sex life will get better). Exercise draws fresh blood to the vaginal tissue, creating thicker walls and more moisture; the supporting muscles become stronger, and there is an overall improvement in the health of the vagina.

Exercising the PC is fun. It is naturally stimulated by any activity for which you must squeeze and release the pubococcygeus, such as in sexual intercourse and urination. Kegels, developed by Dr. Arnold Kegel in 1940 as a nonsurgical alternative for urinary incontinence, are excellent for the PC, and they can be done spontaneously anywhere, anytime. Do them when you're driving, standing in line at the grocery store, watching television, or working at your computer. No one will ever suspect what you're up to.

First, identify the PC muscle. It's the muscle you feel when you squeeze your anus or when you stop urinating midstream. A well-toned pubococcygeus works like a faucet, turning on and off quickly. To perform a kegel exercise, simply squeeze and then release that muscle. For best results, do 100 kegel squeezes a day (this takes only about 10 minutes). Alternate between fast and slow contractions. If you're just getting started, spread the exercises over the course of a day, starting with 25 in the morning, 50 in the afternoon, and 25 again in the evening. As with any form of exercise, it is important to increase only gradually and to be consistent. Find a time of day or activity that works for you and go for it! It's certainly worth the effort.

healthy menstruation

The menstrual cycle can be broken down into two phases: the follicular phase and the luteal phase. The follicular phase is marked by a gradual buildup of estrogen, a hormone produced by the ovaries. Estrogen affects the body as well as the emotions. It stimulates protein synthesis and cell division. Vital capacity of the lungs and sweat gland production are highest during this phase of the cycle. At the end of the follicular phase, estrogen levels peak and ovulation occurs.

After ovulation, the luteal phase begins. Estrogen levels decline and progesterone levels increase. During this stage, body weight increases and bowel transit time becomes slower or sluggish. Levels of the hormone aldosterone rise,

which can encourage water retention. The luteal physiological processes are slower, weightier, and damper than those of the follicular phase.

The entire cycle fluctuates between yang and yin, the outward and inner movements of our bodies. The stimulatory, outward-directed effect of estrogen is balanced by the depressive, more inward-directed effects of progesterone.

Yin menstrual ailments are characterized by dull, achy cramps and a listless, tired feeling. Yin imbalances can result from external cold and chills or immediate stress. In these situations, blood tends to pool in the inner core of the body to preserve warmth, often resulting in circulatory congestion in the pelvic region. Symptoms are relieved by warmth and pressure. Common herbal treatments employ diaphoretics to open up peripheral circulation and direct blood away from the body's central core. Alternating hot and cool footbaths will also improve circulation and relieve congestion in the pelvis.

To prevent yin menstrual distress, dress very warmly and make sure your feet are very warm and dry. In addition, make sure that your diet is not too rich in yin foods, especially refined sugar, fruit, and raw vegetables. The recommended diet for yin ailments emphasizes protein, grains, and beans.

Yang menstrual imbalances are characterized by restlessness, thirst, swollen or painful breasts, and sharp cramps with abdominal pain. Pain is worse with heat and touch. Yang imbalances often result from excess protein in the diet. To prevent yang menstrual distress, eat more vegetables, fruit, raw food, and whole grains and less animal protein. Be sure that you're getting adequate calcium and magnesium. Supplement your diet with

treat the liver first

A central problem in many types of menstrual disorders is an imbalance in the levels of estrogen and progesterone. The imbalance can have many sources, sometimes involving serious physiological disorders. Many times, however, an imbalance arises because the hormones are not properly eliminated from the system. Normally, estrogen and progesterone are broken down in the liver and sent as waste products to the kidneys for excretion. If the liver is not functioning well, hormones are not processed effectively, and disorders result. Most hormonal imbalances respond to a diet that supports the healthy function of the liver. You'll see this idea reflected in the treatment protocols for menstrual disorders that follow.

cooling, liver-cleansing herbs such as dandelion root, burdock root, and red clover.

I offer many thanks to fellow herbalists Ellen Greenlaw and Bhavani Worden, who contributed greatly to the discussion of the physiology of the menstrual cycle in my home study course, The Science and Art of Herbalism. Ellen, a brilliant student who attended my herb school many years ago, became a practicing herbalist and worked for many years in a women's health collective. Bhavani Worden was a friend and herbalist I worked with in my early days on the Russian River. Bhavani died of uterine cancer in the early 1980s but left a rich body of information in her wake. Her small booklets, long since out of print, are still sources of information and inspiration.

Painful or Cramping Menstruation (Dysmenorrhea)

About 10 days before menstruation begins, calcium levels in the blood begin to drop, and they continue to drop until about 3 days into the cycle. Blood calcium deficiency is responsible for many of the symptoms of painful menstruation: muscle cramps, headaches, water retention, achiness, depression, and insomnia.

Following are suggestions for preventing and relieving menstrual cramps. If you follow this program diligently, within 3 to 4 moon cycles you should begin to note a significant difference in your menstrual symptoms.

Preventing Cramps

To prevent cramps from happening:

- Increase your calcium intake 10 days prior to your period. See page 199 for a list of calcium-rich foods and herbs to include in your diet.
- Support liver health with a tonic formula such as the one below.

LIVER TONIC FORMULA FOR MENSTRUATION

If you're preparing this formula as a tea, you may wish to add a pinch of stevia to improve its flavor.

2 parts burdock root
2 parts dandelion root
2 parts sassafras (for flavor)
1 part chaste tree berry
1 part licorice root
¼ part ginger

To prepare as a tea, decoct the herbs following the instructions on page 381, using 1 teaspoon of herbs per cup of water and letting steep for 5 to 10 minutes. Drink 3 to 4 cups daily.

To prepare as a tincture, follow the instructions on page 384. Take ½ to 1 teaspoon of the tincture two or three times daily.

HIGH-CALCIUM TEA FOR MENSTRUATION

This variation of High-Calcium Tea is designed especially for preventing menstrual cramps. Pennyroyal leaf is an excellent emmenagogue, relieving uterine congestion and helping promote menstruation. Raspberry is a wonderful tonic for the reproductive system, and peppermint gives the tea a refreshing flavor. I like to add a handful of organic rose petals to the tea for flavor and beauty.

2 parts nettle
2 parts oatstraw
2 parts pennyroyal leaf
1 part horsetail
1 part peppermint
1 part raspberry leaf

Combine the ingredients. Prepare as an infusion, following the instructions on page 380, using 1 teaspoon of herbs per cup of water, and steeping for 15 to 20 minutes. Drink 3 to 4 cups a day for 10 days prior to your period.

Caution: Never use the oil of pennyroyal for internal purposes; it is highly toxic.

Relieving Cramps

If you're suffering from menstrual cramps, try the following:

- Don't eat or drink anything cold, as cold foods exasperate the cramps.
- Place a warm ginger poultice (see page 213) or a heating pad over the pelvic area.
- Drink Cramp-Relief Formula tea or tincture every few minutes until the cramps cease.

CRAMP-RELIEF FORMULA

1 part crampbark

1 part pennyroyal leaf

1 part yarrow

Peppermint (optional; for flavoring the tea)

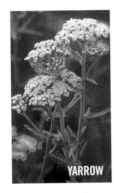

YARROW

To prepare as a tea, decoct the crampbark, following the instructions on page 381. Remove from heat and add the pennyroyal, yarrow, and peppermint. Cover, let steep for 15 to 20 minutes, and strain. Drink ¼ to ½ cup every 15 minutes until the cramps subside.

To prepare as a tincture, follow the instructions on page 384. Drink ½ to 1 teaspoon every hour until the cramps subside.

Excessive Bleeding During Menstruation (Menorrhagia)

In cases of menorrhagia, it's important to focus on building and strengthening the liver and the endocrine system, specifically the thyroid, which is often implicated in excessive menstruation. However, do not expect to see dramatic change in the first month or two. Give the body a chance to progress slowly and steadily. The results will be long-lasting.

The following protocol has been helpful for many women who bleed excessively during their menstrual cycles.

- **Seaweed.** Each day include seaweeds in your diet. They are incredibly rich in trace minerals, vitamins, and calcium and are highly recommended for endocrine gland imbalances, specifically those of the thyroid. You can take seaweed capsules, but a better choice is to incorporate seaweed into your meals. If you're not crazy about the taste of seaweed, try hizike, which is quite mild in flavor. Dulse is also good. Try mixing them with grains, soups, casseroles, and salads.
- **Iron.** If you're bleeding heavily during your period, you're losing a lot of iron. Restore your body's iron levels by taking liquid Floradix Iron + Herbs (available in most natural foods stores) or Herbal Iron Syrup (see recipe on page 200) daily.
- **Reproductive tonics.** To tone, strengthen, and improve the general health of your reproductive organs, take a reproductive-system tonic daily.

WOMEN'S REPRODUCTIVE TONIC

This tea is a strong tonic for both the liver and the reproductive organs. For flavor, try adding sassafras, birch bark, and orange peel to the blend.

- **3 parts licorice root**
- **1 part burdock root**
- **1 part chaste tree berry**
- **1 part dandelion root**
- **½ part cinnamon**
- **½ part ginger root**

Prepare as a decoction, following the instructions on page 381. Drink 3 to 4 cups daily for at least 4 months.

BALANCING BLEND

This blend should be used throughout the month to help create a balanced hormonal system.

- **2 parts chaste tree berry powder**
- **2 parts dandelion root powder**
- **1 part dong quai powder**
- **1 part milk thistle seed powder**
- **1 part yellow dock root powder**

Combine the herb powders and encapsulate in size 00 capsules. Take 2 capsules three times daily on a rotational cycle, that is, 5 days on, two days off, for up to 6 months. Discontinue during menses.

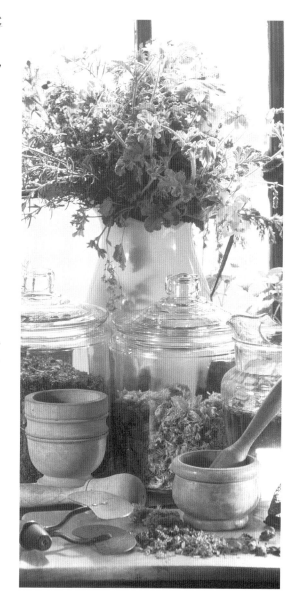

yeast and nonspecific vaginal infections

The vagina is the perfect petri dish for bacteria. Warm, moist, and sweet, it is home to many lively species of bacteria. Most live in symbiotic relationship with one another and are necessary for the overall health of the vaginal area. Some bacteria help keep the vagina in its normal state of acidity (with a pH between 4.0 and 5.0), which helps control the growth of fungus, yeast, and other harmful organisms. When the pH of the vagina changes even slightly, however, one or more of the bacteria can grow out of control, reproducing rapidly and generating copious amounts of metabolic waste that causes inflammation and irritation to the vaginal membranes.

The common treatment for vaginal infections is antibiotics or sulfa drugs, which, though very effective in killing the infection-causing bacteria, also indiscriminately kill all the other bacteria. In fact, in the long run, they often make matters worse. The symptoms of the infection may disappear for a few weeks, but the problem that first created the imbalance is not corrected, and the infection-causing bacteria often begin to thrive again. They multiply much more quickly now, because the antibiotics destroyed the other bacteria that were part of the natural system of checks and balances. A cycle of infection and antibiotic treatment ensues, leaving your body exhausted and your psyche irritable.

A CAUTION FOR PARTNERS

When you have a yeast or other vaginal infection, avoid intercourse. Sexual activity can irritate the already inflamed tissue and force the infecting organisms up into the uterus and fallopian tubes. Also, infections are easily passed back and forth between partners. If you are fighting a vaginal infection, it is important that your partner follow a treatment program as well.

Identifying a Yeast Infection

There is a broad spectrum of triggers for yeast infections. The most common are emotional stress, general physical weakness, poor diet, hormonal changes (such as those occurring during menopause or pregnancy), vaginal irritations, excessive douching, birth control pills, hormone pills, stressful sex, and antibiotics, sulfa drugs, and other medications.

Common symptoms of yeast infections are:
- Itching, irritation, and a thick white discharge that may smell like baking yeast
- Inflammation and redness of the external vaginal area (the vulva), sometimes with a rash or sores

- Inflammation and redness, sometimes with a discharge, of the internal vaginal mucous membranes, which can be examined with the use of a speculum

Treating a Vaginal Infection

The only way to successfully cure a yeast or other vaginal infection is to correct the underlying cause. In holistic therapy, the major considerations are reestablishing the normal vaginal flora, restoring pH, and promoting healing from within.

Natural therapies have as high or higher a success rate as do drug therapies for "curing" yeast and vaginal infections. However, a holistic treatment program requires dedication. Drinking herb teas, douching, swallowing homemade pills, and eating a light and nourishing diet is more complex than taking prescription drugs three times a day, but considering the results, it's certainly worth the effort.

Keeping Dry

A moist environment encourages the growth of yeast bacteria, so it's important to keep the area around the vulva dry. Wear cotton underpants and avoid panty hose. Panty hose do not permit the vaginal area to "breathe," which further irritates and inflames a yeast infection. Use a hair dryer on its cool setting after you bathe to dry your vaginal area. For added dryness, apply Yoni Powder as a medicinal talc.

YONI POWDER

1 cup fine white clay

½ cup cornstarch

2 tablespoons black walnut hull powder

2 tablespoons myrrh powder

1 tablespoon goldenseal root powder (organically cultivated)

A drop or two of tea tree essential oil (optional)

Combine all the ingredients and mix together using a wire whisk. Spoon some into a jar with a shaker top for easy application. Store the remainder in a glass jar with a tight-fitting lid.

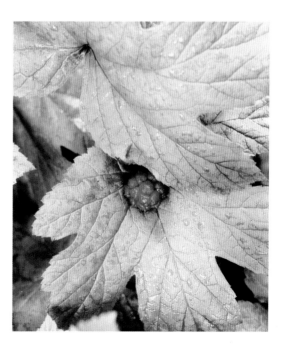

Dietary Therapy

Often, simply attending to diet is enough to cure a yeast infection. Emphasis should be placed on light, wholesome meals that are healing to the body and help restore a normal, slightly acidic pH to the vagina.

Meals should center on whole grains such as brown rice, millet, buckwheat; nourishing soups such as miso and chicken and vegetable broths; and steamed vegetables, especially the dark-green leafy types. Avoid red meat. Eat plenty of lemons and grapefruit, but avoid sweet citrus fruits such as oranges. Cranberries and unsweetened cranberry juice are highly recommended.

Yogurt and acidophilus help replenish the normal flora of a healthy vagina and are important elements of a dietary program to combat a yeast infection. If you have allergies to dairy foods, goat yogurt and nondairy acidophilus are available.

With each meal, drink 1 teaspoon of apple cider vinegar mixed with 1 teaspoon of honey in ¼ cup warm water. This old-fashioned tonic helps restore the body's acid/alkaline balance.

Avoid alcohol and sweets (except for your honey/vinegar water) during the course of a yeast infection. What do you do when you're baking bread and you want your yeast to activate? You drop the yeast in some warm water and add a little sugar or honey. Likewise, a raging yeast infection can be encouraged to grow by eating sugary foods. Oftentimes a yeast infection can be cleared completely just by eliminating all sweets from the diet.

ANTI-YEAST TEA

This tea is quite bitter, so you may wish to mix it with cranberry juice.

> 2 parts mullein
> 2 parts raspberry leaf
> 2 parts sage
> ¼ part goldenseal root (organically cultivated)

Combine all the ingredients. Use 4 to 6 tablespoons of the herb mixture per quart of water. Add the herbs to cold water and bring to a simmer, keeping the pot covered. Remove from heat immediately and let steep 20 minutes. Strain. Each day drink 3 cups of the tea between meals or 30 minutes before eating.

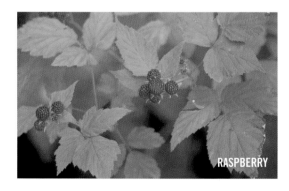

RASPBERRY

ANTI-YEAST CAPSULES

This formula contains powerful antifungal, anti-yeast herbs.

- 1 part black walnut hull powder
- 1 part chaparral powder
- 1 part echinacea root powder
- 1 part goldenseal root powder (organically cultivated)
- 1 part marsh mallow root
- 1 part pau-d'arco powder

Mix the powders thoroughly and encapsulate in size 00 capsules. Take 2 capsules three times daily for 5 days, then take 2 days off. Continue this cycle for 4 weeks, or until symptoms subside.

Garlic Suppositories

Quick to make and easy to apply, garlic suppositories are especially effective for trichomoniasis, a more persistent type of yeast infection. Follow these simple steps.

Step 1. Carefully peel a clove of garlic. Most women nick or bruise the clove to release its oil, but if your vaginal tissue is particularly sensitive, you may want to be cautious about this.

Step 2. Place the clove (nicked or not) in the center of a piece of thin gauze. Fold the gauze over the clove and twist its corners into a tail. It will look vaguely like a homemade tampon with a tail.

Step 3. Insert the garlic suppository deep inside the vaginal cavity. You may want to rub a small amount of oil onto the end of the suppository for easier insertion.

Remove the suppository and insert a fresh one every 3 to 5 hours. Repeat for 3 to 5 days, or until the infection is gone.

Douching

Gentle douching with Anti-Yeast Douche formula every few days can be very helpful for clearing a vaginal infection. If the infection is severe, douche every day.

ANTI-YEAST DOUCHE

- 1 quart water
- ½ ounce Anti-Yeast Tea herb mix (see the recipe at left)
- 2 tablespoons apple cider vinegar
- 1 tablespoon acidophilus culture or ¼ cup yogurt
- 1 tiny drop of tea tree essential oil

1. Bring the water to a boil. Remove from heat, stir in the herbs, and let steep 1 hour. Strain.
2. Add the rest of the ingredients and mix well. Let cool slightly (it should be warm, but not hot).
3. Pour the herbal liquid into a douche bag and use it to very gently douche the vaginal area.

healthy menopause

Women have been experiencing menopause for eons, so it amazes me that in our era menopause is so often designated as a medical condition, an anomaly that requires medical intervention. Menopause is a state of being, not a disease. Medical intervention should be the exception, not the norm.

As a woman approaches menopause, she experiences a great hormonal change that may last for several years. This change begins some years before menstruation ceases and menopause begins. The ovaries stop producing a monthly egg and secrete a smaller supply of estrogen. At the same time, there is a decline in the production of the hormone progesterone, which each month has been stimulating the buildup of the uterine lining in preparation for a fertilized egg. This is a tremendous amount of physiological change to adjust to. The last time we experienced such dramatic hormonal changes was in our puberty — and we all remember what that was like!

Many of the symptoms of menopause are similar to those of adrenal stress: nervous disorders, severe depression, irritability, fatigue, and unpredictable mood swings. The adrenal glands take over the biological function of the ovaries by producing small amounts of estrogen once menopause begins and continuing to do so until about the age of 70. But because of stress and poor eating habits, the adrenals of many women are prematurely worn out by the time they reach the age of menopause. Exhausted and depleted, the adrenals are unable to function in optimum capacity, and adrenal stress — and/or the symptoms of menopause — results.

Most women begin to experience menopause sometime between the ages of 40 and 55, and they experience some type of noticeable change for a period of 6 months to 2 years. Some of the signs of menopause can be attributed to the dramatic hormonal changes that take place during this time. Generally, however, physical health and attitude are primary factors in our well-being and contribute to our ability to adjust to the changes. Many of the disagreeable signs associated with menopause are a reflection of "ungraceful" aging, a direct result of poor eating habits, stressful living, and lack of exercise. Men in this age range experience many of these same symptoms. (Yes, men really do go through a male form of menopause; just ask any woman who has lived with a man over 40!) For both men and women, these symptoms are often corrected with good nutrition, exercise, and lifestyle changes.

Six Essential Supplements for Menopause

The chart at right offers suggestions for foods that provide the vitamins and minerals especially needed during the menopause years. Prepare a checklist of these foods and see how many are included on a regular basis in your diet. If they are lacking, you may wish to begin to include them daily.

ESSENTIAL SUPPLEMENTS FOR MENOPAUSE

Supplement	Benefit and Best Food Sources
Calcium	**Benefit:** Helps prevent osteoporosis and other bone problems, as well as hot flashes. **Sources:** Almonds, amaranth, chickweed, comfrey, dandelion greens, dark-green leafy vegetables (broccoli, chard, kale, mustard greens, spinach, and turnip greens), High-Calcium Tea (page 51), horsetail, nettle, oatstraw, seaweed (hizike, kelp, and wakame), sesame seeds and sesame products, watercress, and yogurt and other cultured milk products.
Dong quai	**Benefit:** A wonderful herb for the female system; used in the treatment of almost every gynecological ailment. A powerful uterine tonic and hormonal regulator. Excellent for the circulatory system and also high in minerals, especially iron. **Sources:** Eat ⅛ inch of the root or take ¼ teaspoon of the tincture two or three times daily.
Ginseng	**Benefit:** An excellent tonic herb. Slowly and surely builds life force; is excellent for long-term deficiencies and imbalances. Produces a steady flow of grounded, well-balanced energy and aids in the elimination of mood swings and depression. **Sources:** Eat ⅛ inch of the root daily or take ¼ teaspoon of the tincture two times daily.
Iron	**Benefit:** Essential for robust health and high energy. Keeps the blood oxygen-rich. Iron deficiency leads to exhaustion, fatigue, and stress. **Sources:** Alfalfa, apricots, beets and beet greens, blackstrap molasses, bran, cereal grains (especially oats), comfrey, eggs, Floradix Iron + Herbs (available at most natural foods stores), Herbal Iron Syrup (page 200), horsetail, nettle, parsley, raisins, seaweeds, spinach, sunflower seeds, tofu, watercress, wheat germ, whole grains, and yellow dock root.
Spirulina	**Benefit:** By weight, 55 to 70 percent protein. Also contains concentrated amounts of B vitamins (helpful for strengthening the nervous system) and gamma-linolenic acid (helpful for preventing degenerative diseases such as osteoporosis and arthritis). **Sources:** Take 1 to 2 tablespoons of the powder or 6 tablets daily.
Vitamin E	**Benefit:** A wonderful nutrient for the reproductive system and a specific remedy for hot flashes, muscle cramps, and vaginal dryness. **Sources:** Whole grains, cold-pressed oils, dark-green leafy vegetables, bee pollen, and some nuts. Supplements are often recommended during menopause. Suggested dosage is 400 to 600 I.U. daily. *Caution:* Those with diabetes, rheumatic heart, or high blood pressure should not exceed 50 I.U. of vitamin E daily without consulting a health care practitioner.

Focusing on the Adrenals

Adrenal stress can play a role in exacerbating the symptoms of menopause. To minimize mood swings and depression, work on strengthening the entire glandular system, especially the adrenals. The following formulas are adrenal strengtheners.

ADRENAL TONIC TEA

3 parts sassafras

1 part ginger

1 part licorice

1 part wild yam

½ part chaste tree berry

½ part cinnamon

¼ part dong quai

⅛ part orange peel

Prepare as a decoction, following the instructions on page 381. Drink 3 cups daily.

ADRENAL TONIC CAPSULES

2 parts kelp

2 parts licorice

1 part black cohosh

1 part ginger

1 part ginseng

½ part dong quai

Powder the herbs and encapsulate in size 00 capsules. Take 2 or 3 capsules daily.

Hot Flashes

About 75 percent of menopausal women experience hot flashes. Every woman's experience of hot flashes is different. They can be absolutely unpredictable or occur like clockwork; they can last but a second or two or for several minutes.

Ginseng and sage are excellent herbs for hot flashes. Ginseng normalizes the body's response to hot and cold; take as directed in the chart on page 227. Sage is a yang, or grounding, herb, and many women have found it helpful in relieving hot flashes. Try drinking several cups of sage tea daily.

In addition, try the following herbal formulas.

HEAT RELIEF

2 parts black cohosh

2 parts motherwort

2 parts sage

1 part blue vervain

1 part chaste tree berry

Mint to taste

Combine all the ingredients. Prepare as an infusion, following the instructions on page 380, using 1 teaspoon of herbs per cup of water, and letting steep for 30 minutes. Strain. Drink in ¼-cup doses throughout the day as needed, up to 3 cups.

If the tea tastes too strong for you, powder and encapsulate the herbs in size 00 capsules. Take 1 or 2 capsules three or four times a day.

HOT-FLASH RELIEF TINCTURE

2 parts black cohosh

1 part ginseng

1 part licorice

1 parts wild yam

Prepare as a tincture, following the instructions on page 384. Take ¼ teaspoon diluted in warm water or tea three times daily, or as often as needed.

Thinning Vaginal Walls (Atrophic Vaginitis)

The thinning of the mucous membranes along with the decreased elasticity of the walls of the vagina cause an uncomfortable dryness in many women during the menopause cycle. This thinning of the vaginal lining, known as atrophic vaginitis, is caused by the decreased production of estrogen. It does not always cause problems, but it can be painful if the lining of the vagina becomes inflamed, dry, or rough. Estrogen creams and pills are the common allopathic solution for this problem, but these products have serious health risks and should be used, with caution, only when necessary.

Natural therapies for atrophic vaginitis include:

- **Vitamin E.** Take 200 to 400 I.U. daily. You can also use the gel from a vitamin E capsule to lubricate the vagina before sex.

- **Herbal salves.** Homemade or commercial salves made from comfrey and aloe or from calendula, comfrey, and St.-John's-wort are very effective when applied inside the vulva.

- **Water.** Lubrication increases in proportion to water intake. Drink 3 to 4 quarts of water daily.

- **Aloe–slippery elm paste.** To soothe and lubricate the inflamed, dry vagina, mix enough slippery elm powder with aloe vera gel to form a thick paste. Apply inside the lips and up into the vagina. It will feel very cool and soothing. This paste also makes an effective lubricant for the vagina before sex.

- **Kegels.** Exercising the PC muscle (see page 216 for instructions) strengthens and tones the vaginal area. Kegels also stimulate circulation, encouraging fresh blood flow to the area, which helps keep it moist.

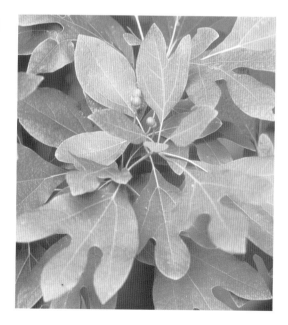

Osteoporosis

A crippling degenerative disease that affects about 25 percent of American women, osteoporosis is marked by a gradual loss of bone mass, which can lead to skeletal deformities and fractures, especially of the hips. It is more prominent in women than in men, due to the hormonal changes of menopause, dietary differences, and general lack of exercise. Though osteoporosis is most noticeable in older women, bone loss begins in our early to mid-30s.

Contrary to former reports, synthetic sources of estrogen (estrogen-replacement therapy) do not significantly increase bone density. Nature's answer — a healthy diet, adequate exercise, and concentrated nutrients found in herbs and natural supplements — is still our best bet for strong bones.

The Question of Calcium

Calcium has long been regarded as essential for healthy bones. In North America, we look to dairy products as our major source of calcium. The American Dairy Council advises drinking 4 glasses of milk a day to ensure that we receive adequate calcium. We're the only country in the world that drinks that much milk; we're also the country with the highest rate of osteoporosis. What's going on?

Phosphorus enhances the body's absorption of calcium; foods with a calcium/phosphorus ratio of 2:1 maximize calcium absorption. Milk has only a 1:1 calcium/phosphorus ratio. The best sources of calcium are, instead, dark-green leafy vegetables, some nuts and seeds, and seaweeds, which generally have a 2:1 ratio. Sadly, these foods are missing from the typical American diet.

Though calcium is essential for healthy bones, lack of calcium alone does not cause osteoporosis. Even in countries where calcium intake is low, the rate of osteoporosis does not match that of the United States. I believe that the prevalence of osteoporosis in this country is due, in part, to the typical Western high-protein, high-fat diet. Biochemists have known for years that a high-protein diet causes bones to lose calcium. The medical community largely ignores this information. The rapid bone development that occurs in many American children due to high-protein diets contributes to a weak and porous skeletal structure. The remainder of the diet can't support this rapid bone growth, and bone density never becomes substantial, leading to bone loss in later years.

The Exercise Connection

Lack of proper exercise is probably the number one cause of osteoporosis. We've become a sedentary society. Our bones, which long to run and jump and dance in graceful movement, are bound by the times we live in. We're restricted in the clothing we wear, the shoes we walk in, and the jobs we tend. Without the exercise our bodies yearn for, our bones become stiff and brittle.

Exercise has proved not only to prevent osteoporosis but also to alleviate symptoms of it. A recent study showed that menopausal women who exercised vigorously for 1 hour each day for a year increased bone calcium levels by one-third. Exercise ensures adequate bone density and improves circulation. It is one of the surest ways to keep bone calcium where it belongs — in the bones. It is also an excellent antidote to the hormonal and metabolic changes of menopause.

Preventing and Reversing Osteoporosis

Though the medical establishment generally advises that osteoporosis is not reversible, Dr. John Lee of Sebastopol, California, feels otherwise. He conducted a study of 100 women with varying degrees of osteoporosis in his family practice. With a combination of a low-protein and low-fat diet, exercise, vitamin and mineral supplements, and low doses of estrogen and transdermal progesterone, the symptoms of osteoporosis were reversed in each of these women.

Osteoporosis is predominantly a disease of modern society. Lack of exercise, diets rich in protein and fat, overemphasis on dairy products as our primary calcium source, high intake of citrus, and hormonal imbalances are all contributing factors. To prevent osteoporosis from becoming even more widespread, cultural as well as personal lifestyle changes need to be implemented.

- **Dairy.** Reduce the amount of dairy you consume. Do not rely heavily on dairy products for calcium.

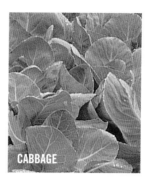

CABBAGE

- **Diet.** Eat a low-protein, low-fat diet. Include plenty of dark-green leafy vegetables, nuts, seeds (especially sesame seeds), soy products, and seaweeds. Avoid those substances that deplete the body of calcium, including coffee, carbonated beverages, salt, and sugar.

- **Exercise.** Find an exercise routine that you enjoy, and stick to it. Strength-building exercises such as weight lifting are most effective for building bone density. However, any type of exercise is beneficial, including low-impact exercises such as yoga and walking. Remember, exercise is the surest way to slow down the advances of osteoporosis.

- **Calcium supplements.** Though calcium supplements will neither prevent nor correct osteoporosis, they may be taken as extra insurance against the disease. A high-quality biochelated supplement (such as that manufactured by Rainbow Light, available in most natural foods stores) in the amount of 1,000 to 1,500 mg is recommended daily for women susceptible to osteoporosis.

- **Adrenal balance.** Hormonal imbalances definitely contribute to osteoporosis. It is imperative, therefore, to nourish and build the endocrine glands and the liver. Make the adrenal tonics on page 228 a part of your daily supplement routine.

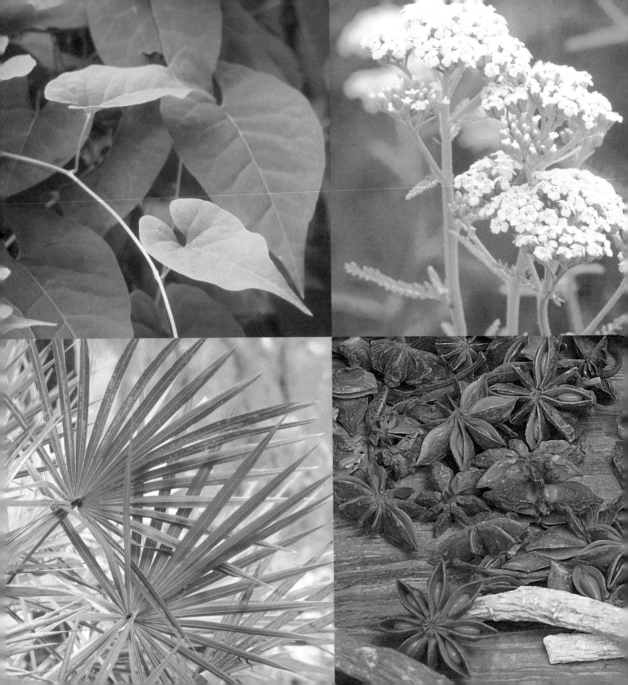

8

For Men

The section of my library labeled "Women's Health" is getting rather crowded and books are beginning to topple one another. Not surprisingly, there's been a plethora of books published on women's herbs, health, and healing in the past few years. Written by caring practitioners, both men and women, many of the topics are excellent. They focus their attention on women's health issues and offer the reader a rich tapestry of views and information.

Unfortunately, the same cannot be said for men's health. There are few published articles, fewer books, and very little information circulating. My library of men's health titles is dismally empty except for one brave classic, *The Male Herbal: Health Care for Men & Boys*, by James Green. Published in 1991, this book was groundbreaking not only because it was the first book of its kind on the subject, but also because it presented Green's revolutionary and rather unique views on male health.

So why isn't there more information available on natural health for men? Different approaches, different views to draw upon? Aren't men interested? Don't they get sick? They may tell you they don't, but statistics of male health in the United States present an entirely different picture. Forty percent of sexually active men are infertile; in its first year on the market, more than one million prescriptions for Viagra were written solely for impotence. Heart disease is the number one killer of men in America, and hypertension is rampant. More than 70 percent of men over the age of 60 will have prostate problems requiring medication of some kind, and men continue to die on the average eight years before women.

These data don't present a very healthy picture of the American male. Information is sorely lacking, books are not available, and men seldom, if ever, talk about their needs. Sadly, the holistic healing community has little to offer men for their health problems or for maintaining well-being (except for anabolic protein powders to build mass). Something's wrong with this picture.

herbalism for men

When I opened an herb store in 1972 in the midst of a lively alternative community in Sonoma County, California, most of my customers were women. They came to buy herbs for themselves, their children, and sometimes their partners. I can remember the occasional male customer who ventured into the store. He would generally wait until no one else was in the shop, slowly wind his way to the front counter, and begin talking about everything under the sun but the specific problem that had brought him there. I'd find some quiet way to create a space for him to talk about his prostate problems, or herpes, or impotence, or even heartbreak. Sometimes, it was something as simple as a cold or a bad case of poison oak that he was so hesitant to ask for help with.

Being young, I figured that men weren't comfortable talking to me about their health problems simply because I was a woman. I hadn't yet discovered that men seldom talk about these things with other men, either. I also erroneously thought, as many people do, that men don't have the same degree of complexity of physiological function as women. After all, where are the breasts, the womb, the ability to give birth? I find this rather limited perspective amusing now, and I apologize for it, having discovered how complex, marvelous, and cyclic the male system is.

It's a "Guy Thing"

What is finally being acknowledged is that men's bodies are just as complex as women's, and that men have many concerns about their health — they just deal with them differently. Women talk about their problems. They seek help. They turn to other women. Women spend a great deal of time talking together about their feelings, their desires and dreams, their health, and men. These are not topics that come up often in men's circles. Jobs, sports, and women are often the talk. It's not considered "manly" to be ill or, worse, to be emotional. It's the "get tough and stay tough" mentality.

My former husband, Karl, likes to tell the story of an exciting football game he played in college. He was the quarterback, had the ball, and was racing toward the end zone when he was tackled hard; he injured his shoulder badly. Nevertheless, he played out the game, in severe pain and with a shoulder practically pulled out of the socket. His teammates admired him for his tenacity, and to this day, many years later, he tells the story with a mixture of pride and sheepishness, because that shoulder still gives him a lot of pain. For me, this story demonstrates the way we train males to get the job done no matter what — often at great cost to their bodies, and certainly to their feelings. It's what we admire them for, and what they take pride in.

Women foster this attitude in men as much as men do, and we may have a greater interest in doing so than we like to admit. It's easy to see the stupidity of sacrificing your body to carry a ball across a mown field. It's easy to get outraged about the ludicrousness and horrors of war. But who benefits when you translate that same attitude to mean "women and children first" at any cost?

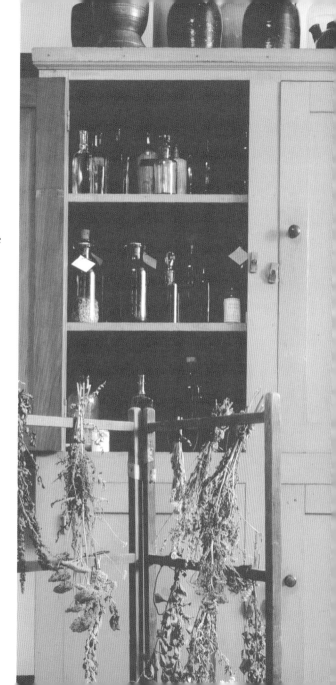

teaching men's herbal health

At the apprenticeship programs I offer at my home, Sage Mountain, we always devote a few days to discussing herbal protocols for the reproductive systems of women and men. I will be honest in saying that we generally devote a full two days to women's health, while the topic of men's health is given, at most, a mere half day. Is this discrimination? We could argue that it's because there are more women in the class and a greater percentage of women will seek out herbal health care. Up to this time, that's been true.

Rather than teach the workshop on men's health, I spend some time sharing information on the herbs most often used for men's health problems and highlight some of the major health concerns men have. Then I invite all the men in the class to participate on a panel. The women are invited to ask men questions about health and healing.

In the early years of this course, the women would ask their questions, and before the men had a chance to answer, another woman would answer. There were always lively discussions — usually among the women. The men generally added a comment or two, when they could be squeezed in, but, on the whole, they listened politely. The outcome was that we never did learn much other than what we already knew, and certainly learned nothing from a male perspective.

After a couple of tries with this failed format, we changed the rules. The women were still invited to ask the questions, but they couldn't answer them, nor could they offer their perspectives. I learned a lot about men's health listening to the heartfelt responses of these men as they struggled to answer deep and sensitive questions about health, communication, safety, and healing.

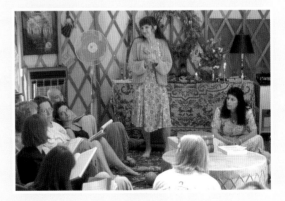

Where Are All the Men?

It has often been said that modern medicine, the Western allopathic model so familiar to us today, is a heroic system of medicine. It is the medical model of choice for emergency situations, for the "cut and stitch" care needed in accidents and life-threatening situations. The healer is often the hero. Allopathic medicine offers quick fixes and crisis intervention but does not support a person's natural process of healing and does not encourage preventive health care.

Does this help explain the paucity of information about men's health in herbal medicine, or why herbalism seems to be overwhelmingly dominated by women? Do the self-care and preventive medicine emphasized by herbalism contradict the "tough it out," "get the job done no matter what" attitude Western society seems to foster in men? Are men more comfortable working in the "healer as hero" allopathic system because we expect them all to be heroes? Author James Green speculates that "today's Western, technological, crisis medicine is the male's folkloric tradition in the making."

Striking the Perfect Balance

Allopathic and herbal medicine together form a perfect balance for the many health problems facing both men and women today. Men are just discovering the same potential for their own herbal health care that women have been taking advantage of for years. Herbs such as saw palmetto,

St.-John's-wort, nettle, and ginseng are finding their way into health care products for men, not as a crisis type of medicine but as preventives. Perhaps as men find ways to explore their own health and healing, they'll have less need for crisis intervention, because they will focus on prevention and well-being. Perhaps we'll find more information readily available on men's herbal health. And perhaps we'll experience a boom in the population of male herbalists.

Sharing Different Perspectives

I want to thank you for your patience with my obviously feminine perspective of men's health. I hope it will provide insight and balance, but I must admit that I feel a bit like one of the women in my classes on men's health, asking the men their thoughts, then proceeding, without a pause, with my own ideas and opinions.

So it is my hope that this chapter will offer a unique and valuable perspective. I am venturing into a subject that I know well through the men in my life, my male clients, fellow herbal practitioners, and the place of maleness in myself. But I am a guest here, so please excuse me if I'm sometimes clumsy and don't always know the proper protocol. Somewhere, I think, there exists a silent agreement between men and women that we are all venturing into new territory, exploring different ways to be and feel together, and creating a healthier threshold of understanding.

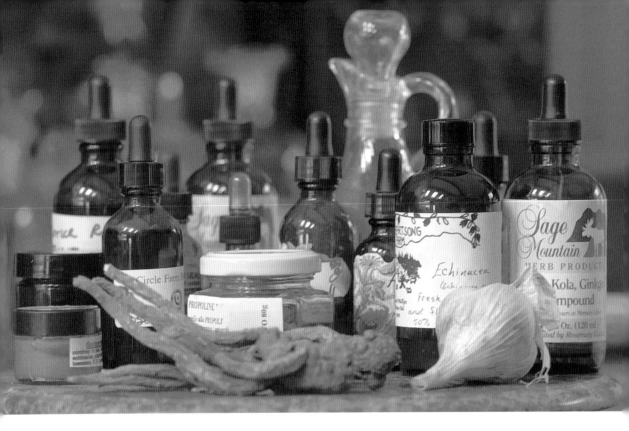

invigorating formulas especially for men

Good health is not a complicated matter. Being in good health doesn't mean you are never sick, or tired, or sore, or depressed. But it does mean that you feel hardy most of the time; your body is invigorated and your spirits are high. In the words of that wonderful singer Taj Mahal, "You wake up and morning smiles back at you." Maintaining good health requires excellent daily habits and practices. Preventing, rather than treating, problems is the key to living a long, high-quality life.

These are some of my favorite tonic formulas. They are strong, invigorating, and flavorful. Most are best used on a daily basis, but each of them can be used as a medicinal and incorporated into health programs. I've provided recipes here for you to try, but you need not follow them to a tee. Be creative and have fun with the recipes; you can alter the formulas and flavors to suit yourself. Experimentation might lead to an even better formula!

FERTILITY & POTENCY SYRUP

This formula has a reputation for increasing virility in men and helping with fertility (if not due to structural causes). It is a tonic formula and needs to be used over a period of 3 to 6 months.

1 ginseng root

2 ounces muira puama

1 ounce ashwagandha

½ ounce saw palmetto berries

½ ounce wild yam root

2 quarts water

2 ounces oats (milky green tops)

½ ounce raspberry leaf

1 ounce damiana

1 ounce nettles

1 to 2 cups honey (or to taste)

1 cup fruit concentrate (available in
    natural foods stores)

½ cup brandy (optional, but will help
    preserve syrup)

1. Combine the ginseng, muira puama, ashwagandha, saw palmetto berries, and wild yam with the water. Decoct slowly, as instructed on page 381, over low heat until the liquid has been reduced to 1 quart. Keep the lid slightly ajar so that some of the steam can evaporate.

2. Turn off the heat and immediately add the oats, raspberry leaf, damiana, and nettles. Cover tightly and let the herbs sit overnight.

3. The next day, strain the herbs through a fine-mesh strainer lined with muslin or cheesecloth. Add honey to taste, the fruit concentrate, and the brandy. Store in the refrigerator. Take 2 to 4 tablespoons daily for 3 to 6 months.

10 SUPERFOODS FOR THE MALE SYSTEM

Food	Benefit
Chicken	Contains high-quality proteins
Cultured milks, such as buttermilk	Aids digestion; supports the immune system
Dark-green leafy vegetables	Excellent sources of minerals, vitamins, and fiber
Fish	Contains high-quality proteins
Fresh fruit	Excellent source of vitamins, minerals, and fiber
Pumpkin seeds	Rich in zinc; excellent for the prostate
Sesame seeds	Calcium-rich; support the nervous system
Sesame or tahini butter	Calcium-rich
Squash seeds	High in zinc; good for the prostate and male glandular system
Yogurt	Aids digestion; supports the immune system

"elixir for the gods"

The first time I made this recipe, I stored it in an antique glass bottle that had engraved upon it the Tree of Life and the words "long life," so I named it Long-Life Elixir. The name seemed fitting and has stuck. That first jar, brewed so many years ago, went to James Green, author of *The Male Herbal,* who said upon first tasting it, "Its flavor and culinary presence brings to mind words such as 'exquisite' and 'elixir for the gods.'"

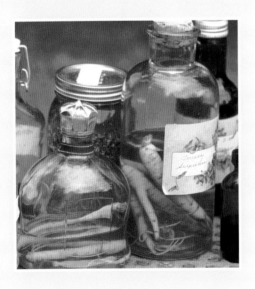

MEN'S LONG-LIFE ELIXIR

This is one of my all-time favorite recipes. It's a variation of the Long-Life Elixir in chapter 2; this formula is predominantly a masculine yang type of tonic that builds strength and vitality.

> 2 parts damiana leaf
> 2 parts fo-ti
> 2 parts ginger root
> 2 parts licorice
> 2 parts sassafras root bark
> 2 parts wild yam root
> 1 part Chinese star anise
> 1 part sarsaparilla root
> ½ part saw palmetto berries
> Asian ginseng roots (2 good-sized, quality
>   roots for each quart of tincture)
> Brandy
> Black cherry concentrate (available at
>   most health food stores)

1. Prepare a tincture with the herbs and brandy, as instructed on page 384. Let the mixture sit for 6 to 8 weeks; the longer, the better.

2. Strain. To each cup of liquid, add ½ cup of black cherry concentrate. Be sure this is a fruit concentrate, not a fruit juice. Shake well and rebottle. I often put the ginseng roots back into the rebottled tincture. A standard daily dose is about ⅛ cup — just enough for an evening aperitif. Try sipping it with your sweetie before a sensuous night.

ENERGY BALLS

This special, high-powered food supplement is delicious and easy to make. Though there are many "superfood bars" on the market, they are expensive and generally not as good as what you can make at home. Try these; they contain nutrients essential to the yang male energy system. They are energizing, restorative, and formulated to build and renew the male reproductive system when used over time. Be sure the herbs are finely powdered, or else you'll be picking out little chunks of nonchewable roots.

> 3 parts pumpkin seeds, powdered
> 2 parts Siberian ginseng powder
> 1 part ginkgo or gotu kola powder
> 1 part ginseng powder
> ½ part spirulina or Super Blue Green Algae
> 1 cup sesame butter (tahini)
> ½ cup honey
> ½ cup crushed almonds
> Coconut, cocoa powder, raisins, chocolate
>   or carob chips, and granola for flavor
> Carob powder or powdered milk

1. Combine the powdered herbs and spirulina and mix well.

2. Combine the sesame butter and honey, mixing to form a paste. If you want your Energy Balls to be sweeter, add more honey.

3. Add enough of the powdered herbs to thicken, then add the almonds and the flavoring additions. Thicken to the desired consistency with the carob powder or powdered milk. Roll into walnut-sized balls. Eat two Energy Balls daily.

energy balls and then some

One year, I wanted to make something special for several of my older neighbors who were going on a holiday cruise. In the midst of making my Energy Balls, some devious little creature took over and they became Aphrodite's Super-Aphrodisiac Balls. I added passion-promoting flavors such as black cherry liqueur, then a host of aphrodisiac herbs, plus a tablespoon or two of guarana, just to keep things moving. The final touch was coating them each with organic bittersweet dipping chocolate. My neighbors loved them! They came back and said, "What in the world did you put in those balls?" To this day, people I don't even know sometimes accost me on the streets of my little Vermont town and ask, "Are you the woman who made those chocolate herb balls for my friends on that cruise?" This is always followed by, "Will you make some for me?"

ONCE-A-DAY MALE TONIC

This is my version of "one a day"; that is, 1 tablespoon a day. I love to use herbs in food and cooking, rather than always taking them in a medicinal preparation such as tinctures or capsules. Herbal pastes can be spread on toast, licked from the spoon, or added to boiling water for instant tea. Stored in the refrigerator, the paste will last indefinitely. Here's one version of the recipe.

> 2 parts fo-ti powder
> 1 part astragalus powder
> 1 part ashwagandha powder
> 1 part cardamom powder
> 1 part cinnamon powder
> 1 part licorice root powder
> 1 part Siberian ginseng powder
> ½ part echinacea powder
> ¼ part ginger powder
> Honey
> Fruit concentrate

Mix all the herbs in a bowl. Add enough honey and fruit concentrate (blended according to your taste) to form a paste. Pure rose water also can be added for an exotic flavor. Be sure that the paste is moist enough. It will dry out a bit in the refrigerator, even when tightly closed. If it becomes too dry, moisten it with a little more fruit concentrate and honey.

GOOD-LIFE WINE

This aromatic herbal wine should be served as a tonic. It can be taken in small dosages of ¼ cup daily to promote health and well-being.

> 4 astragalus roots
> 1 good-quality medium-sized ginseng root
> 1 ounce ashwagandha root
> 1 ounce damiana leaf
> 1 ounce fo-ti
> 2 tablespoons cardamom seeds, crushed
> 2 tablespoons Chinese star anise
> A couple of cloves (for flavor)
> A pinch of ginger root (for flavor)
> 1 quart good-quality wine

1. Place the herbs in a widemouthed canning jar and pour the wine over the mixture. Cover and let sit for 3 to 4 weeks in a warm location.

2. Strain and rebottle the liquid into the original wine bottle. The ginseng root can be sliced and added back to the wine.

GINSENG TONIC TEA

When I met Nam Singh many years ago, I knew that I was in the presence of a master. Of African-American descent, Nam was raised in a Taiwan monastery by his elderly grandfather and was instructed early in the arts of tai chi, Chinese herbal medicine, and acupuncture. Now in his late 40s, Nam still looks 25. I think he's on his way to becoming one of those ageless sages.

Nam taught me most of what I know about Asian ginseng and also instructed me on how to prepare it using a ceramic ginseng cooker, which can be found in most Chinese herb stores. A regular double boiler will do as well.

> 1 large, well-aged ginseng root
> Water

1. Place the root in the cooker and cover with water. Tie the cooker shut, then place it in another pan filled with water. Cook over low heat for 6 to 8 hours.
2. Strain, and drink all of the resulting liquid. It is very potent, to say the least.

the ginseng fast

Nam Singh recommends fasting for 3 days prior to and after drinking the ginseng tea. This is the traditional Chinese practice for drinking this tea; it is undertaken once or twice a year.

MALE TONER TEA

A flavorful, well-balanced tea especially formulated for the male system, this used to be my personal favorite and was one of the best-selling blends of the early Traditional Medicinal line. However, the F.D.A. ordered us to remove the sassafras due to questions about its safety (see appendix 1). I never felt it was quite as good after that. You get to choose: Sassafras or no? Adjust the flavors as you please.

> 3 parts sarsaparilla
> 3 parts sassafras
> 1 part burdock root
> 1 part cinnamon
> 1 part Siberian ginseng
> 1 part Asian or American ginseng
> 1 part licorice
> 1 part muira puama
> 1 part wild yam
> ¼ part ginger
> ⅛ part orange peel

Prepare a decoction as directed on page 381. Drink 3 to 4 cups daily.

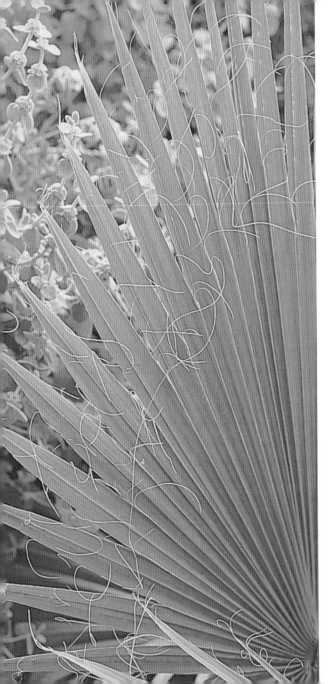

CHAI HOMBRE

There are literally thousands of recipes for chai, a robust, spicy herbal blend originating in India, Nepal, and Tibet. Following is a chai blend especially formulated for men. It has some of the traditional chai herbs, but added are a number of herbs for male health. Serve it hot or chilled with frothy steamed milk.

> 6 slices fresh ginger root, grated
> 5 tablespoons black tea leaves
> 3 tablespoons cinnamon chips (or 1 stick broken into small pieces)
> 1 tablespoon sliced fo-ti
> 1 tablespoon sliced ginseng root
> 1 tablespoon sliced licorice root
> 2 teaspoons crushed cardamom
> 6 black peppercorns
> 4 whole cloves
> 6 cups water
> Honey
> Steamed milk (cow's, soy, or rice)
> Nutmeg or cinnamon

1. Gently warm the herbs and the water in a covered saucepan for 10 to 15 minutes. Do not boil.
2. Strain the mixture into a warmed teapot and add honey to taste. Pour into a large cup, add a generous heap of steamed milk, and sprinkle with nutmeg or cinnamon.

DAMIANA CHOCOLATE LOVE LIQUEUR

When you need that something extra on that oh-so-special night, try this blend from the love goddess herself, Diana DeLuca. This stuff is dangerously lip-smacking good — and daringly easy to prepare. Prepare it ahead of time and serve it at the beginning of a hot date.

> 1 ounce damiana leaves (dried)
> 2 cups vodka or brandy
> 1½ cups spring-water
> 1 cup honey
> Vanilla extract
> Rose water
> Chocolate syrup
> Almond extract

1. Soak the damiana leaves in the vodka or brandy for 5 days. Strain; reserve the liquid in a bottle.
2. Soak the alcohol-drenched leaves in the spring-water for 3 days. Strain and reserve the liquid.
3. Over low heat, gently warm the water extract and dissolve the honey in it. Remove the pan from the heat, then add the alcohol extract and stir well. Pour into a clean bottle and add a dash of vanilla and a touch of rose water for flavor. Let it mellow for 1 month or longer; it gets smoother with age.
4. To each cup of damiana liqueur, add ½ cup of chocolate syrup, 2 or 3 drops of almond extract, and a touch more of rose water.

There are many herbs that can be used in the bath. They should be **aromatic**, filling the steamy bathroom with a delicate scent. They should be **relaxing**, bringing peace to body and mind. And they should be pretty, intoxicating the soul with nature's **beauty**. Get a big bathtub — one of those deep, old claw foots or even a modern Jacuzzi-style one will do — and fill it with water, herbs, and essential oils. Light incense and candles. Serve up that **Damiana Chocolate Love Liqueur** that you made weeks ago, along with some **chocolate-covered strawberries.** And in Diana style, sprinkle a path of fresh rose petals leading to the tub that your heart's desire can't refuse to follow. Your heart will be nourished — and perhaps other parts of your body as well.

bath blends

These three wonderful bath blends are formulated especially for men. To use them, first combine the herbs, then mix in the essential oil. Place a handful of the mixture in a cotton bag, nylon sock, or muslin bag and tie it onto the nozzle of the tub. Run very hot water into the tub for a few minutes, letting the water run over the herb bundle. Then release the bundle into the tub and adjust the temperature of the water to your liking.

As an alternative, you can prepare an extra-strong herbal tea, strain it, and add it directly to the bathwater.

Good health is not a complicated matter. Being in good health doesn't mean you never are sick, or tired, or sore, or depressed. But it does mean that you **feel hardy** most of the time; your body is invigorated and your spirits are high. In the words of that wonderful singer Taj Mahal, "You wake up and morning smiles back at you."

REFRESHING/STIMULATING BATH BLEND

If you need to energize, use this invigorating blend.

> 2 parts peppermint
> 2 parts rosemary
> 6 to 8 drops pine essential oil

DEEP RELAXATION BATH

Try this bath whenever you need to unwind. The recipe makes enough for four to six baths.

> 2 parts chamomile
> 2 parts sage
> 1 part hops
> 1 part lavender
> 6 to 8 drops clary sage or lavender essential oil

BATH BLEND FOR SORE MUSCLES

Sore muscles will benefit from soaking in this eucalyptus, sage, and pine blend. The recipe makes enough for two to four baths.

> 2 parts eucalyptus leaf
> 2 parts sage
> 6 to 8 drops pine or sage essential oil

good health for the prostate

The prostate is getting a lot of press these days. It may even be the most talked-about male organ; it's certainly in the running for second place. Even so, many men are still not sure what the prostate does, why it's important, or even where it's located, until it starts aching or creating health problems.

A chestnut-shaped organ no larger than a walnut, the prostate is a part-muscular, part-glandular organ that is located below the bladder and next to the rectum. It surrounds the urethra, the tube that runs from the bladder to the tip of the penis. If the prostate becomes inflamed or engorged, it squeezes the urethra, and bladder infections, urinary incontinence, and kidney problems ensue. The prostate is also directly related to fertility, because it produces and secretes into the semen an alkaline, proteinlike fluid that is critical for sperm motility.

The prostate is an inconspicuous little organ, but it can cause a lot of problems. Nearly 60 percent of the North American male population between the ages of 40 and 60 suffers from benign prostatic hyperplasia (BPH), also called noncancerous prostate enlargement, a condition that occurs when the prostate becomes enlarged or engorged.

The causes of prostatitis (inflammation of the prostate) are varied, but most are directly related to stress. Often, though not always, the stress may be of a sexual nature. Irregular sexual patterns, that is, intense sexual activity after a long period of inactivity or a period of inactivity after intense sexual play, can also be a precursor of prostatitis. It seems the prostate prefers regularity. Other factors that can contribute to prostatitis include an unhealthy diet, consumption of alcohol, consumption of caffeine-rich products, lack of physical exercise, too much sitting, infections of the gums and tonsils, and venereal disease.

The symptoms of prostatitis and BPH are similar. They include:

- Painful urination
- Difficulty in emptying the bladder completely
- Having to get up at night to urinate
- Reduced force when urinating
- Pain upon sitting
- Unexplained chills and fever
- Blood in the urine (sometimes)

Prostate problems generally respond incredibly well to home treatment, which includes lifestyle changes, dietary changes, and herbal remedies. However, if your symptoms don't improve within a few days of beginning treatment, you'll want to consult your holistic health care practitioner or physician for further examination and advice.

Dietary Treatments for the Prostate

Eat simple, nourishing foods to enhance prostate health, as well as overall health. Diet should consist primarily of steamed vegetables, grains, and miso or chicken soup. Add medicinal herbs such as echinacea, astragalus, fo-ti, and ginseng to the soup base.

Include lemon juice and unsweetened cranberry juice in your daily diet. Don't eat foods that you know will further irritate the prostate gland. Caffeine-rich foods, alcohol, and sugar seem to be particularly irritating.

Several foods, vitamins, and minerals are excellent in helping alleviate prostate enlargement and inflammation, including:

- Pumpkin seeds (¼ to ½ cup or more daily)
- Cucumbers (2 to 3 daily)
- Calcium/magnesium (600 mg combined daily)
- Vitamin E (400 I.U. daily)
- Zinc (20 to 50 mg daily)

Watermelon Cooling Tonic

Watermelon seeds are a wonderful remedy for prostate imbalances. If watermelon is in season, you're in luck. Put as much watermelon and seeds as you can drink in one serving into a blender (cut off the rind). Add a handful of unsalted pumpkin seeds. Blend until creamy. Drink 1 quart daily. Fresh watermelon is wonderful for the kidneys and the prostate, providing a mineral-rich flush. If there is a lot of congestion in the gland, this is an excellent cooling tonic.

If watermelon is not in season, you can still make this remedy by using the seeds of the watermelon. Watermelon seeds can be purchased at some herb stores, but why not collect and dry your own in the warm summer months? Place the watermelon seeds and the pumpkin seeds in the blender with unsweetened cranberry juice. Blend until creamy. Drink 3 to 4 cups daily.

preventing and treating prostate cancer

Though saw palmetto isn't a cure for prostate cancer, it may be a preventive. And it's certainly wise to use it as part of a holistic treatment program for prostate cancer. Many allopathic doctors now recommend it as part of their treatment protocol. Prostate cancer is generally very slow growing and easily monitored, and the latest findings suggest that men live the same length of time with or without the surgery, but have much greater discomfort with the surgery. Often the recommendation is managing the cancer through the use of herbs and diet, rather than surgery.

Medicinal Teas for Prostatitis

The following two medicinal formulas are excellent remedies for swollen, inflamed prostate. Drink 3 to 4 cups daily of one or both formulas. For greater effect, add 10 drops of saw palmetto tincture and 10 drops of pygeum tincture to the tea.

PROSTATE FORMULA #1

This formula aids in better urinary flow.

- 3 parts corn silk
- 3 parts watermelon seeds
- 2 parts nettle
- 1 part cleavers
- 1 part uva-ursi

Infuse the herbs as instructed on page 380.

PROSTATE FORMULA #2

This formula is designed to ease inflammation and congestion of the prostate.

- 2 parts marsh mallow root
- 1 part echinacea
- 1 part gravel root
- 1 part organically cultivated pygeum
- 1 part saw palmetto

Prepare as a tincture as instructed on page 384.

Making an Herbal Poultice

Though messy, poultices are very helpful for relieving congestion of the prostate. Mix equal amounts of clay, comfrey leaf, and slippery elm powder in a bowl with warm water. Place the mixture on gauze or muslin fabric and apply

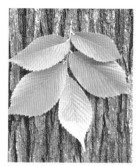

directly to the skin covering the gland twice a day for 20 minutes. Use a jockstrap or underwear to hold the poultice in place.

You can also mix fresh comfrey leaves in a blender with a little water to make a paste, place the mixture on gauze or muslin fabric, and use this as a poultice. If nothing else is available, try an oatmeal poultice.

Hot and Cold Compresses

Hot and cold compresses are also very effective for relieving congestion of the prostate. This treatment requires a bit of willpower. Wrap an ice pack in a towel and place it directly on the skin covering the prostate. Leave it on for a minute or two. Remove the cold pack and place a hot compress on the skin for a few minutes. Repeat this process three or four times at least once a day.

A variation of this is sitz baths, alternating between hot and cold tubs. Drs. Michael T.

Murray and Joseph E. Pizzorno, in their excellent book *Encyclopedia of Natural Medicine,* highly recommend these "contrast baths," stating that they're extremely beneficial for prostatitis and BPH, but also difficult to employ. They are very effective for increasing circulation to and improving muscle tone of the prostate and other reproductive organs.

Malignant Prostatic Enlargement (Prostate Cancer)

Until recently, the only accepted treatment for prostate cancer was surgical removal and/or chemotherapy and radiation. Many men who underwent the procedure considered the side effects worse than the cancer. Incontinence, impotence, and depression are just a few of the many possible side effects. Recently, however, conventional medicine has changed its tune about its procedure for prostate cancer and often will recommend a "management program."

Most cancers of the prostate are very slow growing. They can be managed and often slowed down even further, and they sometimes go into complete remission. It's easy to monitor prostate enlargement and to know if the cancer is increasing or decreasing in size.

Follow the suggestions listed on the preceding pages for BPH and prostatitis. In addition, add to your diet herbs, foods, and supplements that are known to have cancer-inhibiting properties:

Essiac is a somewhat notorious herbal formula that was known as an old Native American cancer cure. A dedicated nurse, Rene Caisse (essiac spelled backward), was given the formula to treat cancer patients. She had great success with it until the Canadian government forced her to stop using the formula. It went underground for several years and has now surfaced, at outrageous prices, in a flurry of marketing madness. Though not, as marketed, a "cancer cure," essiac has been known to reduce the size of tumors. It is also highly effective in lessening the painful side effects of conventional cancer therapies. The best sources for high-quality essiac at reasonable prices are Jean's Greens and Healing Spirits (see Resources).

Pau d'arco is an herb native to South America that has excellent anticarcinogenic properties. It can be taken as capsules, tincture, or tea. I generally blend it in tea, as it has a robust, tasty flavor.

Shiitake and **reishi mushrooms** have demonstrated antitumor activity. Though they can be obtained as tinctures and are often found combined in anticancer formulas, shiitake mushrooms are delicious and should be incorporated into the diet. You can grow them on mushroom logs in your basement, join a shiitake mushroom club and get them delivered to your door, or buy them at most grocery and natural foods stores. Shiitake mushrooms also significantly lower blood cholesterol.

TREE MEDICINE

When I first met Grandpa Roberts, back when I lived in California, he was living up the coast in an old trailer parked on a windswept hill, a lonely old guy whose family was scattered far and wide. He used to drive the 30 or so miles to my herb shop in his beat-up old jeep to pick up his herbs and whatever new herb book had been recently released, and we'd talk for a while. I could tell he was quite knowledgeable about plants, but mostly I knew he was just lonely and lost without a life calling.

We were hosting a small herbal event at Orr Hot Springs, a lovely little spot nestled in the California coastal hills, and I thought Grandpa Roberts might enjoy coming. I also figured folks would enjoy meeting him. He was a ripe old character who knew his herbs and had a barrel of good stories to tell. So along Grandpa Roberts came, and that trip changed his life forever. Grandpa had found his clan!

Shortly afterward, I invited him to move to the California School of Herbal Medicine. He was getting elderly and I feared for him living all alone.

Besides, he needed a family, and we, like every community, needed an elder. He moved into this small earthen podlike structure, barely bigger than 20 feet across and set down a steep path in the heart of the woodlands, and there he set up house. He found that people loved to listen to his stories — and he loved to talk — and soon people were traveling from all over the country to hear him. He often had two or three people camped out on his cramped floor. His favorite thing was to take people out, get them to put their arms around a tree and listen, listen to the heartbeat of the tree and their own heartbeat as it merged with that of the tree. He taught them about tree medicine and heart medicine and how to walk gently on the earth. He taught us to go into the forest as healers, to take our hands and touch the trees and plants and rocks. He would take us on "medicine walks" through the woodlands. We'd enter the forest to heal and be healed, to care and be cared for. He'd instruct us to find large strong trees that naturally lent themselves to our leaning up against, and we'd stretch out bodies to meet theirs, embracing them with our arms and letting their life force move into us. Then he had us look for trees that were injured — and there were plenty. Large old redwoods that had been struck by lightening but were still surviving after 500 years. Douglas firs that had huge gashes carved out by passing logging trucks. Trees crippled by disease. Our job would be to go to these trees and place our hands on them and to let our energy and light force move into them. And there truly was an energy force moving between the life form of the plants and ourselves. No one missed it; it was big.

Grandpa soon learned that within the herbal community, older folks are honored. So he quickly upped his years. We knew he was over 70, but we're not sure that he was the 85 he quickly claimed to be. We decided it didn't matter. You're only as young — or old — as you think you are. And Grandpa had become ageless. He was a big man with a large belly and a long white beard; he looked amazingly like a real-life Santa Claus. He had the energy of a bear, who legend had it taught the skills of herbalism to the people. So Grandpa was our Santa, our Bear Medicine, and our ceremonialist, as well as a teacher and tree hugger.

What I realized in watching Grandpa blossom is that there are so many elderly people, so full of stories and the rich experiences of life, who are never invited into the circle where they belong. Often it's just a simple matter of asking them to share, providing opportunities for them to teach and pass on their knowledge. Everyone becomes the richer for it.

Grandpa lived at the herb school for many years. In the last few years, his bones began to ache and breathing became labored. When it became difficult for him to maneuver up the path from his tiny pod to the road, we helped him move to Harbin, his favorite hot springs community. He spent his last days there. Jane Bothwell, one of my dear friends, was visiting him on the day he died. She sat with him while he took his last breaths and was with him to help him on his journey into the spirit world.

I think often of the lessons that Grandpa taught us. How to heal and be healed by trees. How to walk in the forest and listen. But mostly he taught people about love and kindness and gratitude. I'm teaching my grandson about this medicine now so that when he grows up he will remember and believe in it.

glandular imbalances

Lack of energy, depression, impotence, and lack of vitality characterize glandular imbalances. The usual route to resolve these problems is to seek quick-fix stimulants such as caffeine to maintain energy, but these will only further exhaust already depleted energy levels. Instead, try some of the following suggestions to build and stabilize inner chi and vitality:

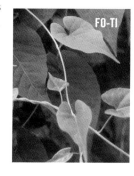
FO-TI

- Take Men's Long-Life Elixir daily (see the recipe on page 240).
- Eat two Energy Balls daily (see the recipe on page 241).
- Snack on organic pumpkin seeds; eat ¼ to ½ cup daily.
- Drink 3 to 4 cups of Male Toner Tea daily (see the recipe on page 243).
- Eat a small piece of ginseng root daily, drink ginseng tea, or take 2 ginseng capsules three times daily.
- Take a cold shower at least every other day. I'm a great advocate of cold showers and have found them to be wonderfully restorative. Take a quick warm shower and follow with a cold burst from the faucet. Cold water strengthens the overall constitution of the body and creates greater energy levels. It also stimulates immune function by improving circulation and regulating body temperature. You may need to work up your nerve to try it, but believe me, it's well worth it!

impotence and infertility

Infertility is the inability to conceive after a period of adequate effort (a one-year period, by clinical standards). The latest statistics show that men's systems are the root of at least 40 percent of couples' infertility problems. Most cases of male infertility are due to low sperm count and/or weak or inactive sperm. Stress and lack of activity can be contributing factors. Some less common causes are obstructions in the reproductive system, liver problems, and glandular imbalances in the thyroid (hypothyroidism) or the pituitary gland.

Impotence, or erectile dysfunction, afflicts more than 30 million men. A comprehensive men's health study performed in Massachusetts reported that 52 percent of men between the ages of 40 and 70 experience some degree of impotence.

The Viagra Phenomenon

With the advent of Viagra, the first pharmaceutical drug found to be effective in treating impotence, one of men's best-kept secrets may have

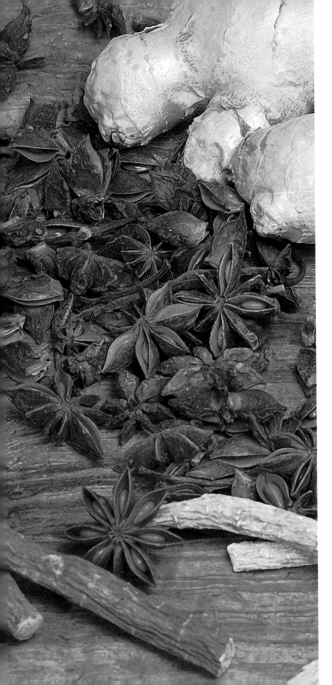

been revealed. Viagra was introduced in the early spring of 1998, and more than a million prescriptions for it were filled by the end of that year. However, there have been many side effects reported, several deaths have been related to its use, and no studies have been conducted to determine what its long-term effects on the human body are.

Viagra works by causing the muscles surrounding the penis to relax, thereby increasing blood flow into the spongy tissue of the shaft of the penis. While Viagra is effective 60 to 90 percent of the time in producing the desired outcome, it does nothing to correct underlying causes of impotence. And it's far more important to address the causes, I believe, than the symptoms that they produce

Factors such as stress, poor eating habits, high or low blood pressure, mental exhaustion, and possible prostate infection are overlooked. Aging is also considered a cause of impotence in men in their middle years and onward, though I believe it's the unhealthy habits we acquire as we age that create many of the problems, including impotence, associated with the elderly years. Lack of exercise, sleep and dreaming, mineral-rich foods, and good relationships, plus many stress factors, lead to unhealthy physical changes. Men as well as women have the opportunity to continually recharge their sexual health by creating good living habits.

How Can Impotence and Infertility Be Treated?

I prefer to use herbs, exercise, and diet to help correct the underlying problems and restore balance to the overall system. The *penis erectis* isn't a solo performer, nor does it function independently of the rest of the body; it is an indictor of overall well-being. When it refuses to respond, listen to it. Generally its message is that something is awry — and it's not always about sex.

● Emphasize the following herbs in your formulas: Siberian ginseng, muira puama, saw palmetto, astragalus, ashwagandha, nettles, oats, dandelion, sarsaparilla, licorice, wild yam, and fo-ti, or ho shou wu.

● Follow the suggestions listed for prostate health, including use of saw palmetto.

● Take 400 I.U. of vitamin E daily.

● Take zinc supplements (30 ml) daily.

● Take 1 teaspoon of bee pollen daily.

● Establish a nonstressful but vigorous daily physical exercise program.

● Eat plenty of fresh raw vegetables, high-quality protein sources, fresh fruit, and grains. Avoid all processed refined foods, alcohol, sugar, and caffeine-rich foods.

● Every day, take 2 Energy Balls (see the recipe on page 241), ¼ cup of Men's Long-Life Elixir (see the recipe on page 240), and 1 to 2 teaspoons of Once-a-Day Male Tonic (see the recipe on page 242).

genitourinary infections

Though women tend to be more susceptible than men to urinary tract infections, men do experience many systemic imbalances as infections in their genitourinary system.

Inflamed Penis or Foreskin Infection

Though inflammation of the foreskin and penis shaft is fairly uncommon in most circumcised men, I have seen and treated foreskin infections in babies and young boys. An infected foreskin can be painfully disruptive.

There are several external applications that will cure an inflamed penis or infected foreskin.

● **Herbal powder.** The quickest and most effective action is to make a powder of 3 parts slippery elm powder or marsh mallow root powder to 1 part organically grown goldenseal powder. Sprinkle this powder over the head and shaft of the penis.

● **Herbal soak.** In *The Male Herbal,* James Green describes how to do penis soaks, the equivalent of an herbal douche, and thoughtfully instructs on choosing a proper-sized container. Make a strong tea of comfrey and organic goldenseal. Pour the warm tea into a small glass and place the penis in it for as long as possible. (For children, this may be only a few minutes, considering the activity level of most small boys.) As an alternative method, soak a soft cotton cloth in the tea and place it directly on the infected area.

● **Herbal wash.** I've also had success clearing up foreskin infections with a wash made of a decoction of witch hazel bark (not the extract), white oak bark, and raspberry leaf. Gently wash the infected area two or three times daily with this astringent, disinfectant tea.

If the infection persists, treat it internally with a mixture of organically grown goldenseal or chaparral, echinacea, marsh mallow root, and myrrh. These herbs can be powdered and encapsulated in size 0 caps and taken at regular intervals throughout the day. Give small children 1 capsule three times daily. For infants, mix a pinch of the powder with warm milk or juice. Adults may take 2 capsules three times daily.

This mixture, useful for many types of infections, can also be tinctured. For a small child or an infant, mix 3 to 10 drops of the tincture in warm water, milk, or tea and administer three times daily. For adults, take ¼ teaspoon of the tincture three to six times daily.

Urinary Tract Infections

Weak bladders and urinary tract infections often plague men, most probably due to the placement of that male organ, the prostate. Follow the advice for prostatitis and enlarged prostate glands beginning on page 247. In addition, try the suggestions listed here.

Drink cranberry juice. Drink 2 to 4 glasses of cranberry juice daily. Cranberries are the natural treatment of choice for the bladder and the kidneys, since they contain a chemical that prevents bacteria from adhering to the urethra wall, thus helping prevent urinary tract infection. If you're prone to bladder infections, keep on hand unsweetened cranberry juice. Dilute the tart juice with apple juice or tea. You also can use fresh or frozen cranberries and cranberry tablets for urinary tract infections.

Use herbs to support the system. There are a host of wonderful herbs used to support urinary health, including:

● Buchu
● Corn silk
● Couch grass
● Dandelion leaves
● Goldenseal (organically grown)
● Marsh mallow root
● Oregon grape root
● Saw palmetto
● Uva-ursi

Practice kegel exercises. Kegel exercises are the best strengthening tool we have for toning and conditioning the bladder and the entire genito-urinary tract. They were designed by a doctor to treat urinary incontinence. If you're prone to bladder infections, the caliber and force of your urine is steadily getting weaker, and you are beginning to "dribble," get on with those kegels immediately.

I've yet to meet anyone knowledgeable about reproductive health who doesn't advocate doing kegels on a regular basis for the health of the entire genitourinary system. It's a simple little exercise that was developed in the 1940s by Dr. Arnold Kegel, a gynecologist, to help women with urinary problems and bladder control.

Quite by accident, it was discovered that exercising the pubococcygeal muscle on a daily basis not only helped with bladder control but also enhanced sexual performance, increased circulation to the pelvis, and increased overall health of the reproductive area. Kegels are beneficial for both men and women; they are especially recommended for men with prostate problems, low sexual energy, lack of bladder control, and poor circulation. The wonder of this exercise is that you can do it anywhere, anytime, anyplace: while driving in the car, while sitting reading or watching TV, or while standing in line at the grocery store.

The pubococcygeal muscle is a large, bandlike muscle that runs from the pubic bone to the coccyx. It's the muscle you feel when you squeeze your anus. One way to test its strength is to get up a good flow of urine, then try stopping it midstream. A well-toned pubococcygeal works like a faucet, turning on and off quickly.

To do kegels, first identify the muscles by pulling inward and upward while tightening the anus at the same time. Pull up as hard as you can, hold, relax, and release. It's suggested to start off by doing 10, then 20, 30, and slowly working up to 100 a day. It's guaranteed to make your sex life better (especially if your partner is exercising, too).

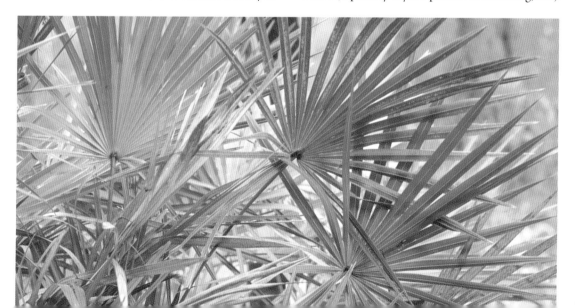

> "The art of medicine consists of amusing the patient while nature cures the disease."
>
> — **Voltaire**

Yeast Infections

Men, if your partner has a vaginal infection of any kind, chances are you have it, too. The problem is that men are often asymptomatic, and partners unwittingly pass the infection back and forth. Women's reproductive organs are like warm petri dishes; living organisms thrive in the warm, deep, moist recesses of the vaginal cave. Yeast and other bacteria tend to grow more quickly and produce more intense symptoms in women than in men with the same infection. No matter how careful a woman is and how committed she is to following a treatment program, it will be futile unless you follow through, too.

Traditional allopathic medicine isn't always necessary in treating yeast-related infections and, in fact, will often make the condition worse. Follow these simple guidelines to prevent and treat your yeast infections:

Herbal soaks. Penis soaks should be done both before and after lovemaking. These are the equivalent of vaginal douches. Follow the instructions on page 255. Enjoy the experience; it's not often that one gets an excuse to hang out in a cup of tea.

Cut back on sugar consumption. All yeast and yeast-related infections thrive on a sugar-rich diet. Sugars — whether from candy bars, white cane sugar, raisins, dates, mangoes, oranges, or a chocolate-covered granola bar — create an acidic condition and a perfect medium for bacteria to grow in.

Alkalize your body. Eat an alkalizing diet consisting of dark-green leafy vegetables, miso, fish, organically raised chicken, soy protein, seitan, salads, root vegetables, and cultured milk products such as yogurt, buttermilk, and kefir.

Support your immune system with herbs. Use herbs that build immunity, such as echinacea and astragalus; herbs that fight infection, such as organically grown goldenseal or chaparral; and herbs that soothe irritated reproductive tissue, such as marsh mallow root. These herbs can be powdered and taken daily in capsules, made into tinctures, or served as tea.

Minimize your dairy intake. Dairy products (except for cultured milk products) such as milk and cheeses are acidic and will promote infection.

treating inguinal hernia

Though not normally classified as a male health problem, far more men than women get hernias. Hernias often result from heavy lifting or straining or because the tissue or muscle at the lower end of the abdominal cavity is either congenitally weak or becomes weak and loosens, leaving an opening through which a loop of the intestines protrudes. Inguinal hernias are most often noticed as a lump protruding from the lower abdomen and sometimes a pain that radiates from the groin. The pain can become quite severe. Chronic constipation can exacerbate inguinal hernias, since the straining will create extra pressure.

To treat a hernia, apply clay packs to the affected area twice daily. Any clay will do, but my preference for medicinal purposes is green volcanic clay. Mix the clay with enough water to form a paste and apply it directly to the hernia. Cover with a cotton cloth and hold in place with a bandage. Hernia supports can be obtained at most medical supply stores. The clay poultice can be wrapped in gauze and placed inside the support belt. Wear this for at least an hour a day, and longer if it's not too uncomfortable.

If you suffer from a hernia, avoid all lifting and straining. Take care to avoid constipation:

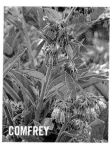

COMFREY

Drink plenty of water and supplement with gentle herbal bowel tonics, such as psyllium, yellow dock root, and licorice root. If you develop constipation, take small amounts of senna or cascara sagrada blended with fennel and licorice root. In addition, take 2,000 mg of vitamin C daily and drink herb teas that are astringent and healing.

OATSTRAW AND HORSETAIL HERNIA REMEDY

- 4 parts comfrey leaf (optional)
- 3 parts raspberry
- 2 parts lemon balm
- 2 parts nettle
- 2 parts white oak bark
- 1 part horsetail
- 1 part oatstraw

Make an infusion of the herbs by following the directions on page 380. Drink 3 to 4 cups daily.

comfrey controversy

There is a current, as yet unresolved controversy surrounding the use of comfrey for internal purposes. Generally, I no longer recommend comfrey internally for others, though I continue to use it myself abundantly. In the case of hernias, because of its extreme usefulness in healing torn or damaged tissue, I am braving the wrath of the herbal community and including it in the formula. Please educate yourself as to the controversy, and make up your own mind. For further information, you can send a SASE to Sage Mountain or write to the Herb Research Foundation (see Resources).

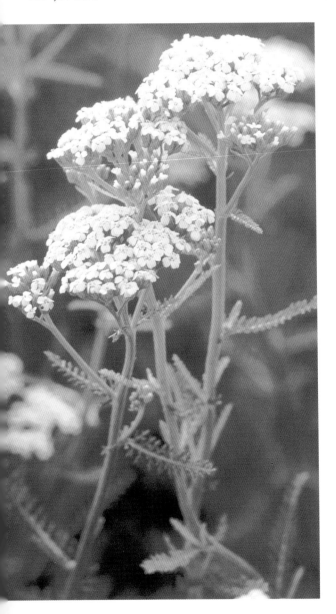

heart health

I find it so sad that the heart, that great throbbing center of emotions and feelings, is the number one killer of men today. I know that this is in part because of "heart unfriendly" dietary patterns established in this century and because most men no longer work as hard physically or get the exercise they did a hundred years ago. We know that stress levels are incredibly high as we begin this new millennium and contemplate enormous changes on this planet that will affect life for centuries hereafter. That's a lot of weight on a man's heart.

But the real reason for this rash of heart disease and troubled hearts may be less obvious, or less talked about. A poignant line from the novel *The English Patient* has always stayed with me: "The heart is an organ of fire." The heart is fed and nourished by love, touch, and feeling, sensory experiences that many men are lacking. Love, touch, bonding — feelings so enormously important to the human heart — are often lacking in the workplace of most men. Oftentimes, home doesn't provide that intimate heart energy, either.

Sadly, most men don't even recognize this as a problem. But heart disease continues to rise. Dr. Dean Ornish, in his outstanding book *Dr. Dean Ornish's Program for Reversing Heart Disease,* offers excellent counsel. His advice goes far beyond dietary and exercise measures and explores the realms of "maleness" in our society and its effect on heart disease. Sam Keene and Robert Bly are other authors whose insights into men's hearts are worth exploring.

Herbs for Heart Health

Hawthorn, in its many delicious forms, is an absolute must. Include it as a food, tea, and medicine (tinctures and capsules) daily. Studies in Europe have verified its ability to reduce angina attacks as well as lower blood pressure and serum cholesterol levels. Hawthorn is a food herb and can be used safely with heart medication.

Other tonic herbs that are specific for heart health are motherwort, garlic, valerian, cayenne, and yarrow. Each of these herbs has a specific toning effect on the heart. Use herbal reference guides to explore each of them in more detail.

SAFETY PRECAUTIONS

If you are taking heart medication, be very cautious about which herbs and supplements you use. Though I've recommended only benevolent and safe herbs, it is wise when dealing with heart problems to work in conjunction with a holistic health care practitioner, who can provide insights on the best formulas for your particular constitution and condition.

Dietary Factors and Supplements

Diet is critical to the health of the heart. There are so many good publications and books about the effects of diet on the heart that I'll only remind you of its importance here and steer you toward the works of Dr. Ornish and others. Evaluate your diet thoroughly and throw out those things you know are destroying your heart. While you're at it, you might evaluate the rest of your life and begin to clear out or change whatever else may be causing you pain and heartache.

Supplement with 20 to 30 mg of coenzyme Q10. This natural substance found in most foods assists in oxidative metabolism and seems to improve the utilization of oxygen at a cellular level. People with poor circulation and heart problems seem to benefit most from it.

Exercise!

One of the most important factors in building and maintaining a healthy heart is exercise. James Green states that "exercise alone may be the most effective nondrug method for normalizing blood pressure." Lack of exercise and a diet high in rich, fatty foods that packs on extra poundage (take a look at the "normal" American male's diet) is a deadly combination.

Take your heart out for a walk today. Keep lean and trim as you grow older, if your heart is at stake. Exercise comes in many forms, from simple stretches to vigorous workouts at the gym, to yoga and sports. All are good. Never forget the importance of life exercise where you exchange energy with the natural world as you're hiking, biking, running, or stretching fully in response to your own body's need to move.

While visiting with my longtime friend and farmer extraordinaire Tim Blakley, we were reminiscing about the "good old days at herb school," which ultimately led to dreaming about future plans. I've known Tim since he was in his early 20s; he's now in his mid-40s. He still looks 20, really. He's trim and fit, with a radiant sparkle in his eyes. His dreams for the near future? To spend a summer hiking the Pacific Crest Trail with his wife, Heather. And they're already planning it. It's a good way to stay fit and trim, as well as the best way to commune with nature. Good heart medicine all the way around.

hypertension

Hypertension, or high blood pressure, is one of the major medical problems of the 21st century. It is directly related to cardiovascular disease, angina, and heart attacks. Although 92 percent of all diagnosed cases of hypertension are termed essential (i.e., the underlying mechanism is unknown), the primary cause is almost always directly related to diet, stress, and lifestyle choices. Hypertension is almost unknown in undeveloped regions of the world where people still enjoy a diet untainted by fast food and other overprocessed culinary wonders of modern civilization. In these regions, hypertension is not a common, accepted aspect of aging, as it is in more developed countries.

Excess body weight, caffeine, alcohol, stress, smoking, and lack of exercise are major factors contributing to hypertension. Given the wide range of side effects — including impotence and exhaustion — attributed to antihypertensive medication, it seems exceptionally worthwhile to consider lifestyle changes related to the above factors as your primary "treatment." In fact, according to long-term clinical studies reported by the American Medical Association and *The American Journal of Cardiology,* people taking medication for high blood pressure actually fared worse than those with hypertension who didn't take medication.

For dietary suggestions and lifestyle modifications for hypertension, consult *Dr. Dean Ornish's Program for Reversing Heart Disease.*

To treat hypertension, consider the following:

Coenzyme Q10 plays a significant role in metabolic processes involved with energy production. Individuals with cardiovascular disease and hypertension show decreased levels of coenzyme Q10. Supplements are available.

Essential fatty acids, especially those found in black currant seeds, flaxseed, and evening primrose, have a profound effect on hypertension. Flaxseed can be ground and added to food. (Store it in the refrigerator to reduce rancidity.)

Garlic is very effective for normalizing blood pressure levels. I like to chop up raw cloves and add them to salad dressings. Encapsulated garlic, which is mostly odorless, also works well. Other helpful herbs are hawthorn, motherwort, onion, shiitake mushroom, Siberian ginseng, vervain, and yarrow.

High-potassium herbs, such as dandelion leaf have a mild diuretic action and work as a kidney tonic as well. The health of the heart is directly connected to the health of the kidneys.

Mistletoe is one of the most widely used herbs for hypertension in Europe, where it is frequently combined with hawthorn. However, mistletoe can be very toxic, even in moderate doses. Use only under the supervision of a competent herbalist or naturopathic doctor.

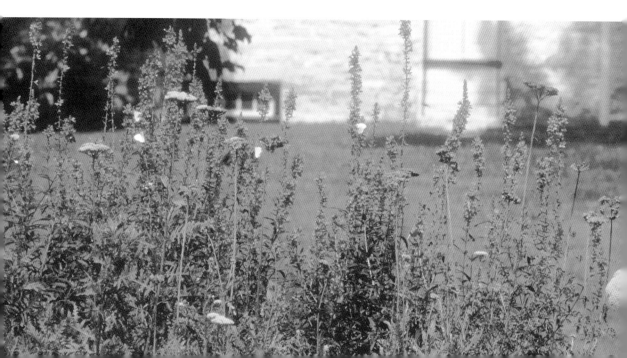

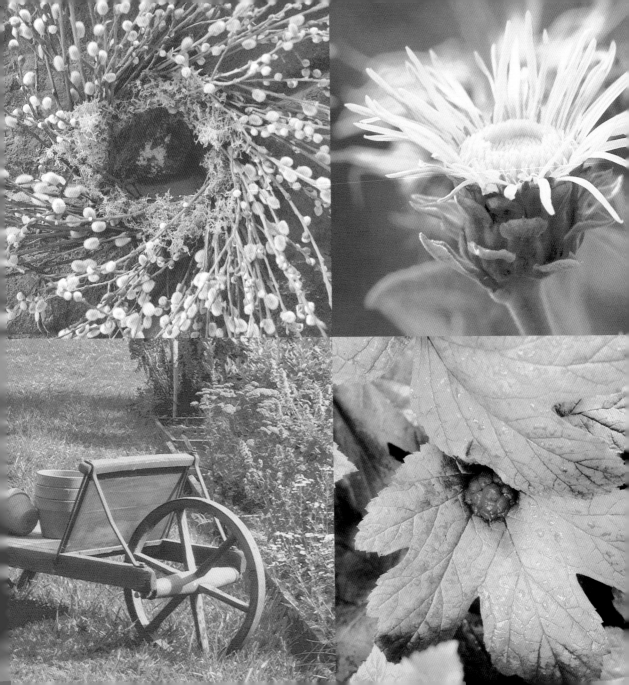

9

For Elders

For the past few years, I have been compiling and giving a slide presentation about my favorite elders in the field of herbal medicine. Much to my surprise, "Voices of Our Herbal Elders" has been such a hit that I have been asked to present it as the keynote address at several large herbal conferences and events throughout the country. The audience often arrives expecting to see a slide show of herbal remedies and treatments for the elderly or perhaps an educational slide show of ancient plants. Instead, they're treated to photographs and stories of my teachers, the herbalists I studied with 20 and 30 years ago. Some of them I knew well; others I met only in passing. The presentation also features elders whom I never had the privilege to meet but who belong in the slide show by virtue of their contributions to herbalism and the examples they share of good living.

Though several of these wise elders have passed on, most are still very much alive and full of the spice and élan of life. The slide presentation brings their stories and teachings to life, especially for those of the younger generation who never had the opportunity to meet such greats as Dr. John Christopher, Adele Dawson, Dr. Bernard Jensen, Keweydinaoquah, Don Jose

Matsua, Norma Meyers, Adelma Simmons, and Ann Wigmore, among many others. It keeps those who are still living in our thoughts and prayers, ensuring them a respectful place in the great circle of life.

remembering our elders

The reason I began to collect the photos and stories of our herbal elders was simple. Aside from the fact that these were extraordinary individuals whose words and lives espoused the world of the green with vigor and passion, I wanted to preserve their memory for future generations of herbalists. When I taught, I noticed that few of my younger students recognized the names of these elders when I mentioned them, as I often did. For me, this was sorely amiss; these individuals were each great characters in their own right, and they had kept alive the teachings of the plants during a time when herbalism was not mainstream, was not popular, and was, in fact, illegal to practice.

Of course, when I began this photo project, I had no idea where it would lead. Like any journey, it had its own agenda, which soon took over. Shortly into the project, I began to question not only where our herbal elders were but where *all* our elders were, in our communities and our families. They were missing from our dialogues, our education, our lives. Had they all gone south to warmer climes? To special homes designated for those over 65? If so, I wondered, how does a community function without its elders? Is it possible to have a healthy community without their teachings and stories? Obviously, we can, because we do. But I feel strongly that the absence of elders creates a large gap in the integrity of community life.

I remember the excitement I first felt when I moved to the Northeast and discovered the great northern hardwood forests. But as beautiful as these woodlands were, I sensed something was amiss. The northeastern forests have been continuously logged for more than 400 years. Though clear-cutting is rare these days, taking "the best timber" — cutting the largest, strongest trees, the elders of the forest — is not. When the first European settlers arrived on the North American continent, they discovered an ancient hardwood forest interspersed with great stands of white pine that were commonly several feet in diameter or larger. One would be wont to find even one tree of such grandeur in all of New England these days.

Our forests are in constant recovery from endless cycles of timbering, yet they hold a beauty born of genetic tenacity that is awesome to behold. Most of the trees are still young, however, and will never have the opportunity to reach the status of elder. Though I honor the youthful energy and clamoring vitality in these new forests, I dearly miss the elder trees. Those trees that live to be hundreds of years old hold the ancient stories and memories of the forest in their rings of growth, in their roots, in the sap that flows thickly in the riotous spring.

In researching the stories of the herbal elders, I began to observe a tender lack in the world around me, not only in the forests but also in our communities and families. Where are our elders? What place in our communities have we created for them? Who listens to their stories, hungering for the rich experiences they store in a lifetime of memories? What is a community without its wizened elders?

For centuries, in cultures around the world, elders were honored by their communities. They were entrusted with teaching traditions and ceremonies to the children. They were the respected healers, herbalists, shamans, and midwives; they took care of the spiritual and physical needs of the community. In council, the elders held the sacred space while the younger members listened with due respect. Often, the final decisions rested with them. These were the sages, the honored ones.

How things have changed.

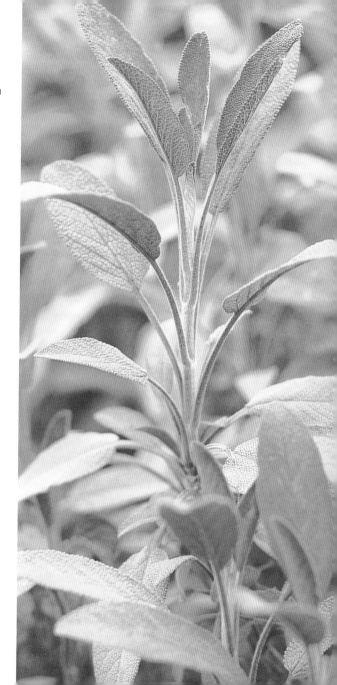

We live in a culture that worships the young for their unbounded potential but devalues the elderly and their rich store of experience. Worse yet, our culture treats aging as an illness, a "terminal illness" at that. A large and profitable industry has grown up around keeping our elders out of sight, out of mind, segregated from the rest of society. Our parents and grandparents are bundled off to homes for the elderly, often against their wishes; once they are safely "stored," many are largely ignored. Though this is not true of every family or community, it is a growing trend. Just look at current statistics or, better yet, look in the community around you to see how visible seniors are in community events, school programs, and family affairs. Sadly, the important role of elders in community life has been largely forgotten.

Even in the herbal community, where elders have long been honored for their sage advice and contributions, our aging parents and grandparents are overlooked to some degree. Though there have been many herb books written in the past couple of decades, there is only one that specifically addresses the needs of our elder population: *An Elder's Herbal*, by David Hoffman, which provides great recipes and remedies specific for the elderly population. Given that people over the age of 65 make up 13 percent of the overall population in the United States, consume the greatest amount of medication, and require

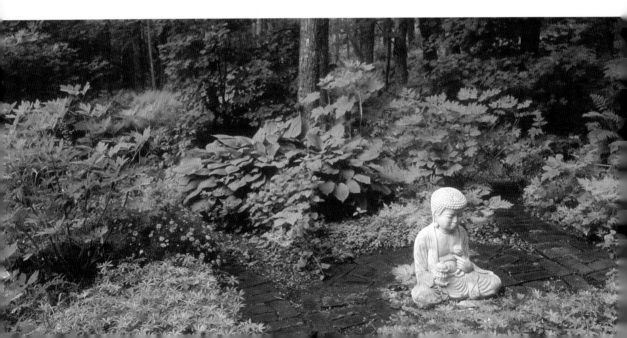

the most medical assistance, wouldn't you think that we would see a predominance of books and articles on natural health and healing for that age group? But we don't — though there are certainly enough television commercials and magazine advertisements, articles, and pharmaceutical medications that specifically target this age group. Aren't the elderly interested in natural remedies, preventive medicine, and self-care?

It is true that the needs of the elders are different from those of a younger person. Much like the plants in the garden at different seasons of their lives, our bodies and spirits reflect the needs of our cycles of life. When we are children, the herbs and herbal remedies we use focus on growth, childhood illnesses, and foundational health. When we become childbearing adults, our needs change. Herbal remedies often focus on reproductive health, remedies for stress and anxiety, and digestive and liver problems. Health concerns for the elderly change as well. Though there is a rich body of information available on herbs and natural therapies for the elderly, it is often overlooked and underutilized. Herbs that maintain life force and contribute to a keen mind, healthy heart, and good digestion have been supplanted by synthetic medications and pharmaceuticals. Rather than use diet and natural therapies to promote and maintain well-being, this "modern" medicine focuses on disease detection and intervention. Used not as preventives but as

> "Elderhood offers us the **wonderful opportunity** to complete our lives triumphantly."
>
> — **Zalman Schachter-Shalomi,**
> *From Age-ing to Sage-ing*

palliatives, many prescriptions in Western allopathic geriatric medicine create a cycle of dependency, as more and ever stronger drugs are needed to keep the system intact. Much of what is prescribed for even the most common health problems can have grave side effects for an elder's more sensitive system. Often elderly people face institutionalization, hospitalization, or becoming burdens on their loved ones with little hope of recovering self-sufficiency or dignity. No wonder many of our elders fear for their quality of life, rather than enjoying, as they should, the harvest of a life well lived.

the "sage-ing" years

Elderhood is often a time for introspection. This stage of our life initiates, far more than any other, a deepening of our relationship with our Creator, our belief system, and our own mortality. In *Longer Life, More Joy,* psychologist Gay Luce states that elderhood "is the time to discover inner richness for self-development and spiritual growth. It is also a time of transition and preparation for

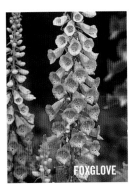

FOXGLOVE

dying, which is at least as important as preparation for a career or family. Out of this time of inner growth come our sages, healers, prophets, and models for generations to follow." Elderhood marks the time when we distill a life full of experiences into wisdom and pass on this synthesized wisdom as our legacy to future generations.

Perhaps one of the most important issues facing us at this "sage-ing" time in our lives is the growing awareness of what impact our life will have on future lives — and the future of the planet. The question we begin to ponder is not what we get from life but what we can give back. What are we leaving as our legacy to future generations on this beautiful planet? David Hoffman, one of the sages of the herbal community, wisely says of elderhood, "The fundamental importance of vision and spirituality is qualitative, not quantitative. By bringing such qualities into our lives we heal and transform ourselves and the world around us. Living for a longer chronological span is beside the point."

Our health is inextricably linked to that of the earth. Modern allopathic medicine has need for a big improvement in this area. In 1994, the United States Environmental Protection Agency (EPA) reported that medical waste incinerators were the biggest source of dioxin air pollution in the United States. Mercury thermometers are still marketed and are widely available, though it's been proved that mercury is a deadly neurotoxin. Pharmaceutical pollution from birth control pills, antibiotics, estrogen, painkillers, and other drugs fills our landfills and permeates our water supplies, affecting every form of life.

Allopathic medications have a negative impact not only on the health of the environment but also often on the health of the individual they are intended to cure. Prescription and over-the-counter drugs kill more than 100,000 people every year; they are the fourth leading cause of death in the United States today. Although allopathic medicine has much to offer to the health of the world, these numbers indicate a dire need to address the toxic nature of prescription drugs.

Modern medicine gives little thought to the connection between human health and planetary health. However, individual health can be possible only when the entire community — people and planet — is healthy. Part of the reasoning behind choosing herbal medicine as your primary health care modality, then, is that it is nature's ultimate ecological medicine.

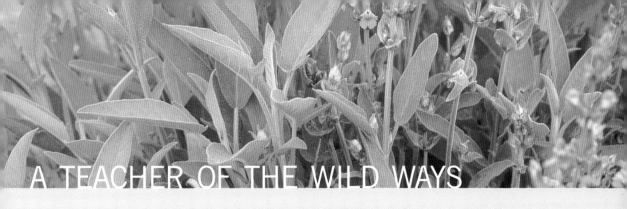

A TEACHER OF THE WILD WAYS

Though Norma Meyers left no books in her wake, she is well remembered by all who knew her. An eccentric and passionate human being, Norma influenced an entire community of fledging herbalists, including James Green, Michael Tierra, Sun Bear, and myself. She was a teacher of the green and wild ways, being a free spirit herself and just about as unconventional as they come.

Norma was married to a Native American fisherman, and they lived in a small house on a reservation on Alert Bay, a remote island off the furthermost tip of northern Vancouver Island. It was one of the most out-of-the-way places imaginable, but Norma's house was always overflowing with people. Whether they were there to attend her classes or because they were ill and needed help, people found their way to her doorstep. And Norma never turned anyone away; no matter how ill or how poor, every person was welcomed warmly into her generous heart and her tiny home.

Many years ago, I invited Norma to teach at the California School of Herbal Studies, because I thought my students would benefit from the teachings of this wise elder. But as radical and "New Age" as the young students were, they weren't ready for Norma. She made them look like conservatives! Norma had lost her front teeth and never had the funds necessary to fix them — whatever money she earned she gave back to her clinic and healing work, never thinking of her own needs. So there was Norma in front of the class, in khakis, no front teeth, a bit frumpy, and her dark hair trimmed in one of those bowl cuts to just above her ears, getting ready to teach about energy and dowsing. But she couldn't find her favorite dowsing pendulum. So off she ran to the kitchen, a bundle of energy, and returned triumphantly a couple of minutes later with a used tea bag dangling from a string. Though soggy, it worked! But when the tea bag fell apart after a few minutes of successful dowsing, Norma disappeared into the kitchen once more and returned with the kitchen sink plug swinging from a thin chain. If only I could have taken a picture of my students' surprised faces!

Oh, Norma, it's been twenty years now, and you are still rememberd by those students. But I remember you for much more

— for your generosity, your greatness of spirit, your kindness and love, the sharing of your teachings, the way you opened your heart and house to us, your garden, how you gave the little that you had so willingly. And I remember you for saving lives; you were a great healer. And when it came time for you to lay down your bones, your Give Away back to the earth that fed and nourished you, you did so quietly, surely, and reverently. Norma, your book is written in our hearts.

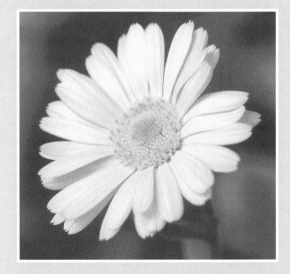

putting herbs to work for elders

Aside from its environmental impact, modern allopathic medicine offers little for our elder population in the way of preventive medicine, the type of honest prevention that works to maintain well-being and radiance rather than to avert medical crisis through all-out "heroic" warfare. Though herbs certainly won't cure all the problems experienced by the elderly, they can, depending on the situation, be as effective as modern medicine at treating ailments, without the long list of side effects, and they can serve as a wonderful system of preventive medicine. For most of the non-life-threatening disorders experienced by our elderly population, herbs offer a safe, gentle alternative to the harsher actions of synthetic drugs.

Herbal therapies for an elder in good health are not much different from herbal therapies for any other stage of adulthood. You must, however, be mindful that elders' systems are generally more sensitive than those of younger adults. In general:

- Digestion and absorption are slower or not as effective.
- Herbs circulate in the system longer, creating different effects than otherwise noted.
- Food sensitivities are higher.
- Eliminative organs — the skin, colon, and kidneys — are less effective.

Be particularly careful when suggesting herbs to elderly people who are already taking prescription drugs. Combining prescription drugs and herbs can have unforeseen effects. However, when used consciously and wisely, herbal medicine can be combined with many other systems of healing, including allopathic treatments, to offer a highly effective health care program.

WHEN TO ASK FOR HELP

Elders in poor health, with a complicated health condition, or who are taking prescription drugs should seek guidance from their doctor before beginning an herbal therapy. If your doctor hasn't been trained in herbal medicine, find a good holistic, naturopathic, or homeopathic practitioner to work with. Many Western-trained doctors are unfamiliar with herbs and their actions other than the warnings and scare stories — most resulting from inappropriate use of high-potency extracts of herbs — that are well publicized in popular media. Thankfully, increasing numbers of doctors are studying herbs and natural remedies so that they can combine the best of allopathic and herbal medicine in their practice.

Determining Dosage

The dosages suggested here are appropriate for an elderly person of average size (140–175 pounds) and in fairly good health. When determining dosage, always consider the individual's sensitivities, allergies, body weight, and constitutional health. These play a bigger role in a person's reaction to medication, herbs or otherwise, than is generally accounted for.

For all individuals, but especially for seniors, always start with smaller doses and work up only as necessary.

If you are uncertain how much of an herbal formula to use, a general rule is that people over 60 should take half of the recommended adult dosage.

For Chronic Problems and Tonic Therapy

Chronic problems are long-term imbalances such as hay fever, arthritis, back pain, insomnia, and long-standing bronchial problems. Chronic problems can, however, flare up with acute symptoms.

Tonic therapies are designed to nourish, tone, rehabilitate, and strengthen the body or particular body systems. They are preventive medicine: incorporating herbs into daily life as a means of building health, energy, and vitality.

For chronic conditions and tonic therapy, the following dosages are appropriate.

Tea: Take ½ to 1 cup two times daily for several weeks.

Tinctures and Syrups: Take ¼ to ½ teaspoon two times daily.

Capsules/Tablets: Take 1 to 2 capsules two times daily.

Herb Powders: Take ¼ to ½ teaspoon two times daily.

For Acute Problems

Acute problems are sudden, reaching a crisis and needing quick attention. Examples of acute problems include toothaches, migraines, bleeding, burns, and sudden onset of cold or flu. You must be keenly observant and apply common sense when administering herbs to elders suffering from acute illness. Though herbs can be particularly helpful in these situations, the sensitive nature of an elderly person's system can elicit unusual and reactionary responses. Start with low dosages and increase as necessary only after observing the individual's response to initial treatment.

For acute conditions, the following dosages are appropriate.

Tea: Take ⅛ to ¼ cup every hour or two throughout the day, up to 3 cups.

Tinctures and Syrups: Take ⅛ to ¼ teaspoon every 2 hours until symptoms subside.

Capsules/Tablets : Take 1 capsule every 3 to 4 hours until symptoms subside.

Herb Powders: Take ⅛ teaspoon every 3 to 4 hours until symptoms subside.

rosemary's rules for living well in our elder years

1. Eat sagely. Several small meals are better than one or two large ones. Eat foods as close to their natural state as possible; the fewer preservatives, the better.

2. Exercise wisely. Every day, move that body as though you're a dancer moving to the smooth rhythm of time.

3. Sleep serenely. Nothing restores the body and the brain like a night of good sleep. Although the body is usually ready to go after only 4 to 5 hours of sleep, the brain requires at least 8 hours of sleep to be restored and revitalized.

4. Drink deeply. Americans are a nation of "underdrinkers" — at least when it comes to water. Drink at least a quart of clean, pure water every day. Remember, 80 percent of the human body is water; we need it inside and outside to survive. So drink up!

5. Breathe fully. The "secret of long life" of the sages of Tibet and India is breathing exercises, elaborate and complex patterns of breathing that exercise the internal organs, soothe the smooth muscles, relax the mind, and encourage wellness. It seems to work — many of these sages are well over 100 and still going strong. I've found that just being conscious of breath — breathing in slowly, filling my lungs, expanding down into my stomach, out to my arms and legs, holding the breath all the while, holding until I can feel my blood being oxygenated, then breathing out slowly, slowly — helps me feel both relaxed and energized.

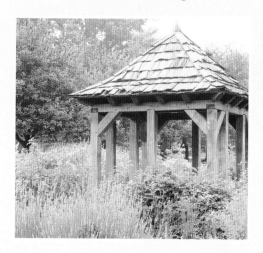

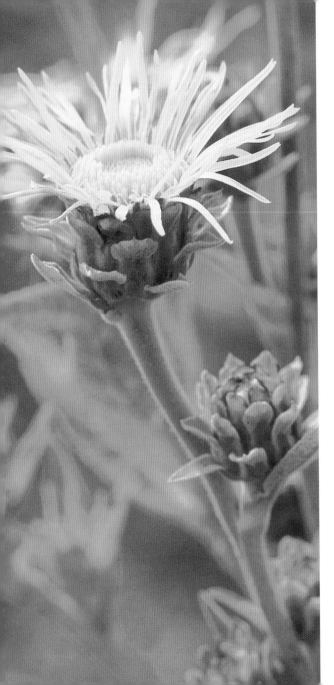

Building Energy, Health, and Vitality

Energy, health, and vitality — the three faces of well-being — are a function of everyday awareness of our body's strengths and weaknesses. It's not often difficult to realize that we don't feel vibrant, but it is sometimes hard to figure out what to do about it.

The chart at right offers a wide range of herbs to choose from for addressing the most common detriments to well-being. The best advice for selecting which herbs and herbal therapies are right for you is the same bit of common sense and simple wisdom I have advocated throughout these pages:

- Know your herbs well, and know why you're using them in each given situation. You don't have to know or use hundreds of herbs to keep healthy, especially in your elder years, but make friends with those you do use.
- Always use the gentlest and safest herb that will get the job done.
- Begin with simples, not compounds, so that you can identify the effects of each herb.
- Start with small doses and work up.
- If side effects are noted or suspected, suspend use for a day or two, or until the symptoms clear up. Then, if you're unsure whether the herb was the cause of any unusual symptoms, commence taking it again. If the herb was the culprit, the symptom will appear again. If this happens, discontinue use or decrease the dosage.

USING HERBS TO BUILD WELL-BEING

Desired Effect	Appropriate Herbal Aids
Improve digestion	Burdock, chamomile, cinnamon, dandelion root, fennel, ginger, marsh mallow root, peppermint, spearmint, yellow dock
Aid with fading memory or memory loss	Ginkgo, gotu kola, rosemary, Siberian ginseng
Improve circulation	Cayenne, garlic, ginger, ginkgo, hawthorn, prickly ash
Improve immune system	Astragalus, boneset, calendula, echinacea, lemon balm, maitake mushroom, milk thistle, pau-d'arco, reishi mushroom, schisandra berries, shiitake mushroom, Siberian ginseng
Lessen joint pain	Black cohosh, boneset, cayenne, comfrey, crampbark, meadowsweet, turmeric, valerian, willow
Enhance sleep and restfulness	Hops, passionflower, skullcap, valerian, wild lettuce
Lessen anxiety and depression	Chamomile, damiana, lavender, lemon balm, oats, rose, St.-John's-wort, Siberian ginseng
Strengthen respiratory system	Calendula flowers, coltsfoot, elderberries, elecampane, garlic, horehound, licorice, lungwort, mullein, sage, thyme
Improve eyesight	Bilberry, blueberry, ginkgo, lycium
Help regulate blood pressure	Buckwheat, garlic, ginkgo, hawthorn
Improve energy levels	Ginseng (any kind), guarana (contains caffeine), yerba maté (contains caffeine), and my Elder Energy Balls (see page 298)

aging eyes, deteriorating eyesight

It seems that almost everyone over 45 notices a change in eyesight. I chuckle at myself and my older friends when we're out to dinner and the menus arrive. There are always a few long seconds of shifting menus back and forth as we attempt to find our best range of vision. When did they start making the type so small? Have we just seen too much? Stretched our vision past its point of focus? I know my own eyesight started deteriorating shortly after I turned 50. The earliest indication was when the road signs whizzed past before I had had a chance to read them. I knew it was time for glasses as much for others' sake as for my own. But when my near vision began to fade as well, it was time to take action. With the help of a few faithful herbs and my own persistence, I noticed a general improvement in my sight. Though I still use my driving glasses, my close-up vision is nearly perfect again.

Though relatively small compared with our other organs, our eyes are very complex. Described as windows to the soul, they also serve as windows to the outer world and fill our life with vibrant colors and visual stimuli. But our eyes can become overused and worn, especially in a world filled with so much visual stimuli. Our eyes need to rest, to exercise, and to be properly nourished in order to function well. Oddly, as visible as they are and as dependent as we are on our vision, we seldom consider the health of our eyes unless they are functioning poorly. I believe that we should be taught routine eye care just as we're taught to brush and floss our teeth daily. The eyes respond so quickly to just a bit of simple care.

Rest Your Eyes

Eyestrain is a common cause of deteriorating eyesight. Without rest, the eyes become tired and don't function at optimal levels. Working on computers, watching television, reading in poor light, and stress can all cause eyestrain.

It's important to use good lighting when reading or doing handiwork. Remember what your parents told you about reading in bad light? They were right. Poor lighting results in poor eyesight. But it's not just dim light that affects the eyes; glaring light can also be a problem. Soft, warm light is best.

If your eyes need a break during the day, try eyecupping. This is a marvelous technique that is fun to do. Simply rub your palms together vigorously, then place them against your eyes. Press firmly and count to 50, enjoying the light show all the while.

In the evening, refresh your tired eyes with a warm chamomile poultice. Infuse 2 chamomile tea bags or 2 tablespoons of loose chamomile in ½ cup of hot water. Soak a couple of cotton balls or squares of cotton flannel in the tea. Cool to an acceptable temperature, wring gently so they won't drip, and place them over your eyes. Turn the lights down, turn on some relaxing music, and lie back and enjoy this soothing ritual for 20 to 30 minutes. Ah. . . .

Exercise Your Eyes

Like all the muscles of the body, the eye muscles can be strengthened by proper exercise, which improves circulation and muscle coordination. My dear friend Andrea Reisen was fitted with

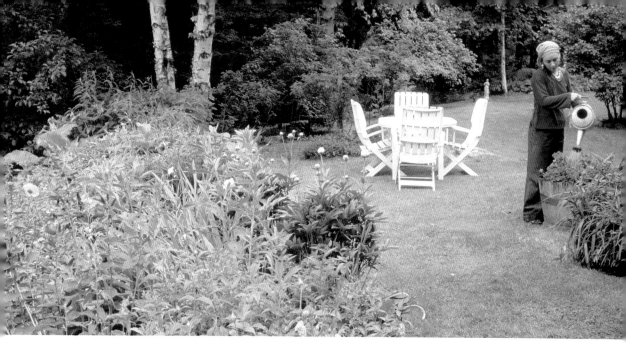

thick glasses when a child and wore them most of her life. When she was in her 40s, a time when statistics say that her vision should have worsened, she began practicing a series of simple eye exercises every day. In time, she was able to discard her glasses altogether.

Eye exercises take just a few minutes of daily practice and will make your eyes feel and see significantly better. Here's what to do:

Start by turning your eyes to the right as far as you can, stretching the muscles. Pause. Roll your eyes slowly up to the center top. Roll them back as far as you can, as if you were trying to see into the top of your head. Pause. Continue slowly rolling your eyes to the left, stretching them as far

as you can. Pause. Slowly roll your eyes down to the center, stretching the muscles downward. Then move your eyes together, peering toward the tip of your nose.

Repeat this exercise four times. Then reverse directions. When you're finished, your eyes will feel rejuvenated, your eye muscles will feel relaxed, and the tiny capillaries that surround the eyes will be filled with fresh, nourishing blood.

Feed Your Eyes

Our eyes need the full spectrum of nutrients to maintain optimum health. A healthy diet filled with dark-green leafy vegetables, fresh fruits, and high-quality protein will supply your eyes with most of the nutrients they need. But when you are focusing on improving eye health, concentrate on foods that are particularly rich in vitamin A, zinc, protein, antioxidants, and lutein. Many yellow and orange fruits and vegetables, such as carrots, pumpkin, winter squashes, and apricots, are rich in beta-carotene and other carotenoids, the precursors to vitamin A, and so are particularly good for the eyes. Fruits that are dark blue or red in color, such as bilberries, blueberries, cranberries, raspberries, and huckleberries, tend to be rich in lutein and in anthocyanosides, compounds that are especially beneficial to the eyes.

Though direct sunlight is detrimental to eye health, natural lighting nourishes the eyes. It's

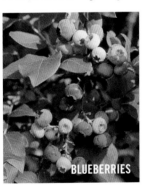

BLUEBERRIES

important to expose your eyes to sunlight every day. Dark tinted sunglasses are helpful for protecting your eyes from the full glare of the sun, but they should be worn only when necessary.

Vision Food

What better medicine than delicious food? Make these recipes a regular part of your diet, and your eyes will stay fit and functional for years to come.

VEGETABLE JUICE FOR THE EYES

1 part beets
1 part carrots
1 part cucumbers

Combine the vegetables in a juicer, process, and drink.

BERRY GOOD TEA

2 parts elderberries
2 parts dried hawthorn berries
2 parts lycium berries
1 part huckleberries or bilberries
1 part raspberry leaf
Honey (optional)

Mix together all the ingredients. Brew as an infusion, following the instructions on page 380, using 1 tablespoon of the herb mixture per cup of water, and steeping for 30 to 60 minutes. Sweeten with honey, if desired. Drink 1 cup daily.

GOOD-VISION
NO-COOK HERBAL JAM

It's a long name for a simple concoction, but you'll find this recipe helpful, delicious, and easy to make.

1 part blueberries
1 part elderberries
1 part dried seedless hawthorn berries
1 part dried seedless rose hips
Freshly grated ginger
Honey

1. Mix the berries together in a saucepan. Add a pinch or two of ginger. Add enough water to cover the fruit completely, then add another 2 cups of water.

2. Place a lid slightly ajar on the saucepan. Bring the mixture to a boil, then turn the heat to low and simmer until the water level again just covers the fruit.

3. Remove from heat and let cool. Place the mixture in a blender and puree.

4. Return the mixture to the saucepan and add honey to taste. Warm it just until you can mix in the honey thoroughly.

5. Pour or scoop the jam into glass jars and store in the refrigerator, where it will keep for up to 2 weeks. If you make a big batch, you can pour some of the jam into freezer bags and freeze it for later use. Eat a dollop or two of the jam every day, spread on toast, crackers, bagels, or whatever suits you.

blueberry heaven

When I first noticed my eyesight changing, I began supplementing with lutein and a special dietary supplement for the eyes. If there was improvement, it was slight. Two years ago, we had a record blueberry season. I enjoyed handfuls daily throughout the summer months. When fall came, I filled my freezer with the large, succulent berries. I ate them daily throughout the winter in morning shakes, in hot cereal, and sprinkled liberally in yogurt. I was in blueberry heaven. When spring rolled around the following year, I can quite honestly say that I noticed a definite improvement in my eyesight. Once again, nature in all her infinite finesse put together the proper formula. Blueberries, rich in lutein, vitamin C, anthocyanosides, and other bioflavonoids necessary for capillary health, are a perfect supplement for the eyes.

Good-Sight Supplements

It's important to make eye care — rest and exercise — a daily habit. In addition, nourish, support, and protect your eyes with good-quality supplements, including the following:

- **Antioxidant formulas.** A daily antioxidant supplement will help protect the eyes from free radical damage
- **Commercial supplements.** OcuGuard (Twinlab) and Ocu-Care (Nature's Plus) contain a full spectrum of nutrients that nourish the eyes.
- **Spirulina.** This blue-green algae, a descendant of the oldest living plant life on the earth, is rich in antioxidants and proteins that protect and nourish the eyes. A tablespoon a day will supply your eyes with the best of green nutrients
- **Vitamin A.** Vitamin A is essential to healthy vision. Retinal, which in combination with proteins forms the visual pigments of the retinal rods and cones, is derived from vitamin A and is continuously used up as images are formed in the eye. Fortunately, vitamin A is readily available in a diet of natural foods, but assimilation by the body may be less than perfect, especially as we age. If vision is failing, then supplementing with vitamin A is recommended. Take 25,000 I.U. daily.
- **Zinc.** Though too much can be just as harmful as too little, zinc is considered to be one of the most important mineral supplements, both because of its importance to physical function and because it is deficient in the standard American diet. Zinc supports the health of the immune system and is essential for our enzyme system. Because of its importance to the vascular coating of the eye, it is thought to improve vision and help protect the eyes.

Though zinc is found in many common foods, such as eggs, whole grains, nuts, seeds (especially pumpkin and squash seeds), and shellfish (particularly oysters), it is often deficient in the diets of elderly people. The recommended supplemental dosage for those over 65 is 10 to 20 mg daily. Do not exceed the recommended dosage, as too much zinc can cause nausea and vomiting. Try taking zinc lozenges, available in most natural foods stores, which are easier for the body to absorb than capsules or tablets.

Cataracts and Macular Degeneration

Cataracts and Age-Related Macular Degeneration (ARMD) afflict as many as 13 million people in the United States. They are generally curable if caught in the early stages, but their symptomatic progressions are very slow, making them sometimes difficult to detect; they are the leading causes of blindness in the world.

Cataracts are characterized by the thickening and clouding of the lens of the eye; macular degeneration is the slow disintegration of the macula, the area of the retina responsible for fine vision. Most prevalent in those 65 or older, cataracts and ARMD are frequently the result of free radical damage.

However, free radicals themselves are not the problem. As an element of our immune system, free radicals respond to stress. A system that is overly stressed, whether from internal or external stimuli, produces an excess of free radicals.

According to *Science* magazine, the body's inability to deal with high dietary sugar is the single highest cause of cataracts. Lactose (milk sugar) and refined white sugar are at the top of the list of offenders. Other factors that weaken the eyes and make them susceptible to cataracts and ARMD include excess dietary fat, diabetes, poor digestion and assimilation, environmental pollutants, UV rays, and protein deficiency.

Prevention is the best remedy for these twin afflictions. Rest, exercise, and nourish the eyes as outlined above. In addition:

- Take ginkgo and hawthorn extracts to improve microcapillary circulation to the eyes; they also are excellent antioxidants, protecting against free radical damage.

- Eat bilberries and blueberries, or supplement with their extracts; these berries are exceptionally rich in antioxidants.

- Supplement with 75,000 I.U. of beta-carotene daily. Studies show that the higher the intake of carotenoids, the lower the risk of ARMD.

- Increase your consumption of sea vegetables and blue-green algae. A tablespoon of spirulina and an ounce of seaweed every day will help keep your vision clear.

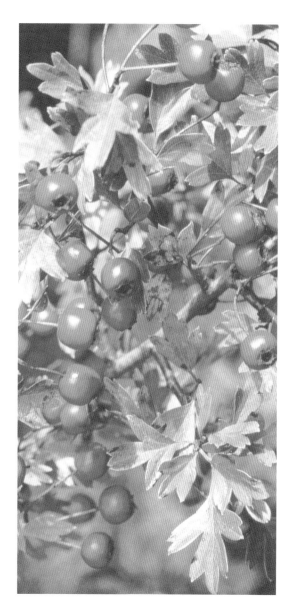

Glaucoma

Another age-related eye illness, glaucoma is characterized by a slow buildup of pressure in the eyeball. It is often asymptomatic in the early stages and thus goes unnoticed. If unrelieved, the building pressure can cause considerable damage to the retina and optic nerve. Blindness can result.

Glaucoma affects two to three million people in the United States, most over the age of 65. It has no single cause, though there are several contributing factors, including nutritional imbalance, stress, high blood pressure, excess glutamic acid and glutamate, and faulty collagen metabolism. Prevention is the best treatment. Follow the suggestions outlined above for healthy eyes and for treating cataracts and ARMD. In addition, consider supplementing with the following:

● Lecithin, a good source of choline and inositol, B vitamins that are important for the health of the eyes and brain. Follow the dosage instructions on the label.

● Jaborandi, an herb of the rain forest that has been used for more than a hundred years to treat intraocular pressure specific to glaucoma. Its active ingredient is pilocarpine.

● *Coleus forskohlii,* an East Indian herb used in Ayurvedic medicine that has shown promise in studies for treating glaucoma.

In addition, every evening apply to your eyes a poultice of chickweed, which is tremendously soothing and relieves inflammation. To make the poultice, place 2 tablespoons of finely chopped chickweed in a bowl. Mix in enough hot water to form a mash. Place on a small square of soft cotton cloth. Lay this poultice over the eyes, relax, and let chickweed work its wonders for about 20 minutes.

maintaining brainpower and memory

It is natural at any age to forget names, where the car keys are, or where we left the grocery list. Even the occasional anniversary or birthday slipping by unnoticed should give no cause for alarm. But it is not natural for us to become disoriented and/or to experience memory lapses so frequently that they affect the quality of our lives. What we have come to accept as a normal characteristic of elderhood is more an issue of health than of age. Extensive research from around the world shows that elders normally have bright, inquisitive minds and cognitive abilities that match those of the rest of the members of their community, no matter the age. What we assume to be the natural order of aging in our society is due largely to huge amounts of stress and poor nutrition. Our brains are simply tired and malnourished; as a result, they short-circuit. This is extremely unfortunate; at a time when we most need thoughtful, concerned elders to guide the younger generation, we are experiencing cultural brain fatigue. But there is much we can do to awaken the full potential of the brain.

The following tips and recipes will help sharpen the mind, improve memory, and boost brainpower. It may take from 4 to 6 weeks to notice an improvement in your cognitive abilities, but it's certainly worth the time it takes.

● Follow the suggestions outlined in chapter 2 (see Improving Your Mental Acuity, page 28).

● Supplement with lecithin, a rich source of choline, which is necessary for brain function. You can take lecithin capsules or sprinkle lecithin granules on your food.

● Supplement with omega-3 fatty acids; omega-3 is vitally important to brain function and is often lacking in the Western diet.

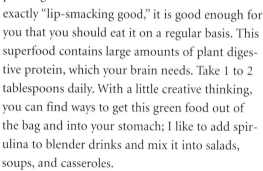
AMERICAN GINSENG

● Add spirulina to your daily diet. Though this potent green food isn't exactly "lip-smacking good," it is good enough for you that you should eat it on a regular basis. This superfood contains large amounts of plant digestive protein, which your brain needs. Take 1 to 2 tablespoons daily. With a little creative thinking, you can find ways to get this green food out of the bag and into your stomach; I like to add spirulina to blender drinks and mix it into salads, soups, and casseroles.

● Make herbal brainpower formulas a regular supplement to your diet. Following are three of my favorite recipes.

BRAIN BALLS

A delicious treat that you *will* remember to take each day!

> Tahini or other nut butter
> Honey
> 2 parts powdered ginkgo
> 1 part powdered gotu kola
> 1 part powdered Siberian ginseng
> ½ part powdered lycium berries
> ¼ part powdered rosemary
> Carob or chocolate chips (optional)
> Coconut (optional)
> Lycium berries or raisins (optional)
> Slivered almonds (optional)
> Carob powder

1. Mix together equal parts of tahini and honey, or mix to taste (you may prefer less honey and more sesame butter, for example).

2. Combine the powdered herbs. Add enough of them to the tahini–honey mixture to make a thick batter or paste.

3. Mix in whatever goodies you prefer — carob or chocolate chips, coconut, lycium berries, or slivered almonds.

4. Add enough carob powder to thicken into a dough. Roll into small balls. Store in the refrigerator, where they will keep for 2 to 3 months. Eat one ball a day.

BRAINPOWER SEASONING SPRINKLE

Use this seasoning sprinkle on salads, popcorn, in soups, and in any main course dish.

> 3 parts sesame seeds
> 4 parts nutritional yeast
> 2 parts powdered kelp
> 1 part powdered ginkgo
> 1 part powdered gotu kola
> 1 part lecithin granules
> 1 part spirulina
> ¼ part powdered rosemary
> Kitchen herbs of choice, powdered (I like to use thyme and garlic)

1. Toast the sesame seeds in a heavy skillet, then grind them in a seed or nut mill.

2. Combine the sesame seeds with the remaining ingredients, adding kitchen herbs of choice to taste.

> "**I would rather know** what sort of a person has a disease than what sort of disease a person has."
>
> — Hippocrates

BRAIN ALERT FORMULA

You can make this brain-boosting formula as capsules or a tincture.

> 2 parts ginkgo
> 2 parts gotu kola
> 1 part blueberries or bilberries (dried)
> 1 part reishi mushroom
> ¼ part rosemary

To make capsules, powder the herbs in a small grinder or blender and use them to fill size 00 capsules. Take 2 capsules three times daily.

To make a tincture, follow the instructions on page 384, using this formula. Take 1 to 2 teaspoons three times daily.

Alzheimer's

The biggest fear that most elderly people face is not cancer or heart disease but Alzheimer's. And it's no wonder — a shocking four million Americans, most over the age of 50, are affected by this haunting disease. The idea of losing not only your cognitive abilities but also your memories and personality is a frightening prospect. But advancing age and elderhood are not a sure dance to dementia. Alzheimer's was relatively unknown until the early part of the past century and rare enough that most people didn't even worry about contracting it; so there must be some factor or factors, as yet unidentified, in the environment that explains its epidemic growth in this country. Is there a brain-weakening contaminant prevalent in our daily living? What effects do food colorings, preservatives, and genetically engineered food have on our bodies? These substances were introduced into the food chain only in the past 60 or 70 years. What does the human body do with food that it has no way of assimilating or eliminating? Does the increase of synthetic hormones in the food chain affect the health of our bodies? Given that it has so adversely affected the health of the animals, we can only imagine what it's doing to us. Of course, it may not be food additives and synthetic hormones that are causing the incredible increase of Alzheimer's, but there certainly is something introduced to our environment in the past 100 years that is causing the brain to decay.

Scientist David Snowdon has been conducting a 15-year research program with 678 nuns at the School Sisters of Notre Dame. This groundbreaking study, aptly called the Nun Study, indicates that, in addition to genetic predisposition, diet, lifestyle, and mental stimulation play a bigger role in Alzheimer's than was previously thought. In addition, Snowdon found that nuns who had suffered strokes were twice as likely to develop Alzheimer's as those who hadn't. In his recently published book, *Aging with Grace,* Snowdon gives a moving personal account of his research and sheds some new light on this dark subject.

According to the Nun Study and other research, there are many possible risk factors for Alzheimer's. Nutritional deficiencies have been identified as a possible factor; many patients with Alzheimer's have abnormally low levels of folic acid, zinc, and vitamin B_{12}. In addition, mercury, a toxic metal, has been found in higher than normal concentrations in people with Alzheimer's.

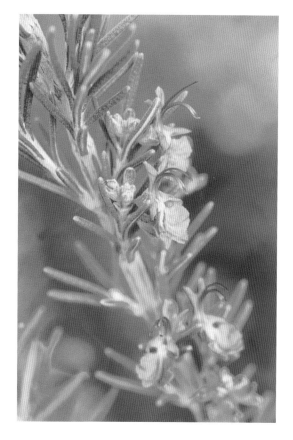

There is also a possible link between Alzheimer's and aluminum. Many of the symptoms of aluminum poisoning are the same as those of Alzheimer's: memory loss, reduced mental capacity, seizure disorders, headaches, anxiety, slurred speech, and gastrointestinal disturbances. Though potentially toxic in even small amounts, aluminum is widely found in a variety of products from common cookware to deodorants. Even more disturbing is the relationship among Alzheimer's, aluminum, and fluoridated water. It has been found that drinking fluoridated water increases the body's absorption of aluminum by 600 percent — and just think how many municipal water supplies are fluoridated!

As for many other of our modern "plagues," all the factors that contribute to Alzheimer's have not been positively identified, though health practitioners tend to agree that there are many of them. But even though we may never know the exact cause, there are things we can do to prevent it from happening. First, follow the suggestions for improving memory and brainpower given above. Second, avoid aluminum in all its many guises: canned foods, aluminum cookware, deodorants, antacids, aspirin, aluminum foil. And, by all means, avoid mercury; even the small amount of mercury found in the old-fashioned thermometers is highly toxic. Then consider the following supplements as further preventive medicine.

- **Antioxidants.** Eat a diet rich in antioxidants. Ginkgo, bilberry, garlic, blueberry, spinach, hawthorn, green tea, and milk thistle seed extract, among many, many other fruits, herbs, and vegetables, are all rich in antioxidants. The quest is not so much to find antioxidants but to make a variety of fresh greens, fruits, and herbs a regular part of your diet. Nature provides the medicine; we just have to remember to eat it.

- **Carnitine.** Acetyl-L-carntine (ALC) is a natural substance found throughout the body. It helps transform fats into mitochondria and improves the activity of important brain neurotransmitters such as dopamine and acetylcholine. Research has shown some promising results using ALC with Alzheimer's patients. In a placebo-controlled clinical study on 279 patients with mild to moderate cognitive decline, those taking ALC showed significant improvement in their cognitive function tests, while those taking the placebo showed little improvement. Dietary sources of ALC are milk, fish, and other animal protein. However, in the treatment of Alzheimer's, ALC is recommended as a regular supplement; take two 500 mg tablets for 5 days, discontinue for 2 days, and repeat. Continue for 3 months, discontinue for 1 month, then repeat the cycle again. The biggest drawback to ALC is its cost; a month's supply can cost as much as $100.

- **Exercise.** Exercise daily. Exercise moves energy throughout the body, stimulates circulation, and invigorates the mind. There is a definite link between cardiovascular health and Alzheimer's prevention. In fact, yoga for elders is one of the best remedies for a variety of health issues associated with aging.

• **Folic acid and vitamin B$_{12}$.** Older people (as many as 30 percent, according to a report in *The American Journal of Clinical Nutrition*) are often deficient in folic acid and vitamin B$_{12}$, nutrients important to the healthy functioning of the brain. Take a daily supplement that contains folic acid and B$_{12}$, and include in your diet foods that are high in these nutrients, such as nutritional yeast, spirulina, and whole grains.

• **Ginkgo.** Several studies reported in *The Journal of the American Medical Association* have shown standardized extract of ginkgo to have a measurable beneficial effect on people with Alzheimer's. Ginkgo improves blood flow to the brain and slows down the brain's aging process. The recommended dosage is 100 to 200 mg two or three times daily, or follow the dosage recommended on the package. Though I generally don't feel that it is necessary to use standardized herbal products, the studies that showed success with slowing the progression of Alzheimer's all used standardized extracts of ginkgo.

• **Herbs for the heart.** Include herbs and foods that build and maintain cardiovascular integrity, such as ginger, cayenne, ginkgo, gotu kola, blueberries, raspberries, and bilberries.

> Speaking of hawthorn, Dr. Ellingwood, a prominent late-19th-century physician, said, **"It is superior** to any of the well-known and tried remedies at present in use for treatment of heart disease, because **it seems to cure** while other remedies are only palliative at best."

And don't forget hawthorn, the supreme cardiovascular tonic.

• **Omega-3.** Include foods rich in omega-3 fatty acids; sea vegetables, spirulina, flax and evening primrose, black current seed, borage seeds, eggs, and whole grains all provide these brain-nourishing essential fatty acids.

heart health

The heart has long been associated with our emotions and our sense of vitality. It is the source of all life for us, a river coursing through the internal landscape of our being, nourishing every cell, supporting the entire system. A large muscular organ, it tracks our time on earth, beating steadily every day of our life, whether we're awake or asleep. When it stops beating, life ends.

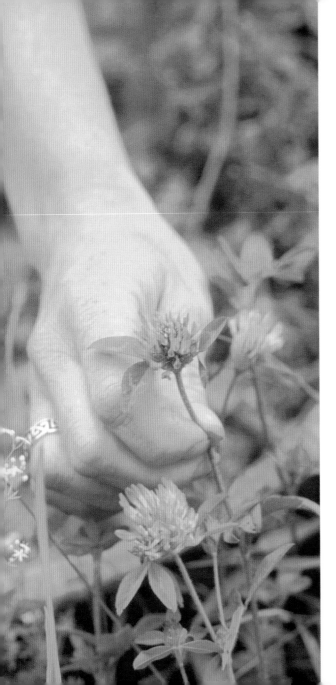

A healthy heart, like a healthy mind, is essential to vibrant well-being. It's common sense. For us to feel energized and vibrantly alive, our blood, our personal river of life, must flow swiftly and undisturbed through its waterways, the vernacular system of the body, feeding, cleansing, and nourishing the entire system. Even more sensible is acknowledging that diet and lifestyle have a dramatic effect on the health of the heart. But interestingly, throughout most of the 20th century, the medical profession denied the link between diet and heart disease, preferring heroic measures over preventive medicine. Bypass surgery, angioplasty, and laser endarterectomy became more popular than the simple and often more effective measures offered by nature. Though each of these medical procedures has inarguably saved countless lives, my father's included, many lives have been lost as well. Cardiovascular disease is the leading cause of death in the United States; more than a million deaths are attributed to various forms of it each year.

Given the importance of diet and lifestyle in the health of the heart, it's insane not to emphasize them as essential aspects of health care for every person at risk of heart disease. In fact, studies show that people live longer with fewer complications by following standard medical treatment and incorporating dietary and lifestyle changes than by having bypass surgery and/or angioplasty.

There are many factors involved in heart disease. Elevated cholesterol levels, arteriosclerosis (hardening of the arteries), and hypertension are among the most commonly known causes of cardiovascular problems. I think broken hearts, loneliness, and depression play a bigger factor than we suppose. How can we deny the importance of the emotional body, our sense of feeling and our ability to heartfully relate to the world around us, in heart health or as a potential cause of heart disease? Both men and women are often isolated from their feelings, spending their days away from family and friends, working in situations that are less than supportive. People often live far from family and childhood friends, often in communities that are not emotionally gratifying or stimulating. Like my friend James Green, I believe that heartbreak — not the classic heartbreak of breaking up with your first sweetheart, but the loneliness of spirit so many people experience today — is the underlying cause of most heart disease.

"The heart is an **organ of fire**."

— *The English Patient,*
by Michael Ondaatje

We need community to have a healthy heart. We need one another. Having close friends and family nourishes and fills the heart. We also need wholesome food, fresh air, exercise, and work that is satisfying and life supporting. It's not too much to expect, is it?

Four Steps to a Happy, Healthy Heart

Health care for the heart should be based on preventive medicine, which encompasses lifestyle, diet, and natural supplements. By following four simple rules for daily living, you'll keep your heart healthy and happy for a lifetime.

1. Exercise Daily.

The human body was engineered for movement, so a sedentary lifestyle almost always leads to heart problems. Exercise should be a normal part of every day. "Too busy to exercise" is an oxymoron. Being busy should be exercise! Even when you're working long hours at a desk, stay aware of your body's needs. Take frequent stretch breaks, wiggle in your seat, get up and move. If you exercise as you work, you'll find that your mind stays focused, your body relaxed, and your productivity optimal.

Exercising doesn't have to mean long hours at the gym, treadmills, and stationary bikes. Healthy exercise is simply getting up and moving — walking, gardening, stretching, chasing a baby around the house. It matters less *what* you do than that you get out and *do* it. While I was working on the manuscript for this book, my good friend and fellow herbalist Christopher Hobbs was teaching at the advanced herbal training program at Sage Mountain. The author of more than twenty books, he understands deadlines. But between classes, he'd come and fetch me and we'd head off for a short walk, twenty minutes or so, into the woodlands. We'd look for new spring flowers, stand under an elder tree raining spring blossoms, or just talk as we passed among the trees. It was fun and invigorating, and when I returned to my desk, my heart was full and happy. How can we be too busy for a daily walk in the world around us? Without it, the heart becomes lonely.

As you grow older, your body may begin to be less flexible, less strong, and less capable of exercise. But it is still vitally important that you move as much as possible. Be physically challenged. Move more slowly and more surely, but move a lot. Walk more. Wiggle more. Laugh more. It's all good exercise, for both body and soul.

In every city and town across the country, there are exercise programs for the elderly. Offered at YMCAs, senior citizen centers, hospitals, and health spas, these programs are often free for people over 60. If you don't like to exercise alone or are concerned about beginning an exercise routine, consider enrolling in one of these programs.

2. Eat for the Heart.

Instead of eating your heart out, eat for your heart. The heart is the most important muscle in our body, constantly in motion, constantly pumping the lifeblood through our system. It makes sense that it functions best when given the proper nutrients.

Heart disease was rare before the 20th century, so it is wise to look back to see what our ancestors ate and how they lived. Saturated fats and sugar were generally not available to them, while unsaturated fats, whole grains, nuts, and fresh fruits and vegetables were mainstays of their diets. Today, experts in the field of cardiovascular health all agree that a low-fat diet, comprised primarily of the foods our ancestors lived on, provides the foundation for a healthy heart.

Foods that are highly recommended for a healthy heart include:

● **Essential fatty acids.** Essential fatty acids (EFAs) contribute to healthy skin and help strengthen the heart. They are not manufactured 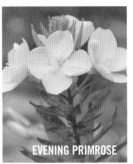 in the body and must be obtained through diet. Evening primrose, borage seeds, black currant seeds, bilberries, elderberries, blueberries, olive oil, most nuts, and fish and fish oils are all rich in EFAs.

EVENING PRIMROSE

- **Fresh fruits and vegetables.** An eight-year study of almost 40,000 men found that those who ate five or more servings of fruit and vegetables each day had a 39 percent lower risk of stroke than those who didn't.

- **Garlic and onions.** It's amazing how many cultures prize the alliums, especially these two fine-smelling members of the family. Alliums, and especially garlic and onions, are rich in compounds that lower cholesterol. Make them a part of your daily diet.

- **High-fiber foods.** Whole grains and fresh vegetables and fruits are great sources of fiber; however, studies have shown that fiber from cereal grains such as oat bran tends to be the most beneficial.

- **Seaweed.** Seaweeds are packed with nutrients, including calcium and phophorus, and are highly recommended for heart health. There are many varieties available in most supermarkets and natural foods stores.

- **Shiitake mushrooms.** A small serving of three or four mushrooms twice a week can lower cholesterol by as much as 12 percent. Join a shiitake mushroom club and have fresh organic shiitakes delivered to your doorstep!

- **Unsaturated oils.** In cooking, primarily use unsaturated oils (such as sunflower seed, safflower, and corn) and monounsaturated oils (such as olive and sesame seed). Olive oil is particularly excellent, because it also offers benefits to the heart.

- **Water.** Fresh, pure water is the best natural diuretic for a healthy heart. Most people feel they are getting enough if they drink one or two glasses a day. But as one recent study showed, simply drinking five or more glasses of water a day can reduce the risk of heart disease by as much as 50 percent! This may be the hardest part of the prescription for a healthy heart, however, as our water sources are less than ideal. If you don't have ready access to springwater, do your heart and body a favor and buy bottled springwater. City and town water supplies often contain substances, such as fluoride, that are harmful to the health of the heart.

- **Whole grains.** Whole grains provide dietary fiber, essential fatty acids, and heart-friendly nutrients.

Foods to avoid include:

- **Excess salt.** Although salt is an essential nutrient for the human body, we need it in only small amounts. Salt occurs naturally in many foods, including seaweeds, vegetables, and some herbs; we can get all the salt we need from these natural sources. Excess salt contributes to hardening of the arteries. Sadly, salt, like sugar, is added to almost all commercially prepared food. Most Americans get much more salt than their bodies need.

- **Excess sugar.** Sugar is found in almost all commercially prepared foods. Do your best to keep your sugar consumption to a minimum.

● **Fried foods.** Deep-fried foods, including onion rings, French fries, potato chips, and many other snack foods lining the shelves of our supermarkets, are highly toxic to the liver and heart.

● **Processed meats.** Avoid commercially prepared lunch meats, hot dogs, sausage, and other forms of processed meat. This food is toxic to the heart muscle. Processed meat should be required to wear a warning sign: "Eat me! I'm bad for you."

USE CAUTION

There are several other herbs that are indicated for the heart, including foxglove, ephedra, and lily of the valley, but they are rich in alkaloids that can be harmful when used inappropriately. I would not recommend using them without the guidance of a qualified health care practitioner. Night-blooming ceres is also widely prescribed for heart conditions; however, this plant is in sore decline due to habitat destruction and overharvesting by zealous wildcrafters. Wild sources of ceres should not be used, and, unfortunately, there is little or no cultivation of this important medicinal plant.

● **Saturated oils.** These are found in almost all baked goods, including breads, crackers, and cookies, and in candy.

● **Soda pop.** Sodas are high in just about everything that causes stress on the heart muscle: salt, caffeine, sugar, and preservatives.

● **Stimulants.** Stress and anxiety are major causes of hypertension, high blood pressure, and rapid heartbeat. Anxiety puts added stress on an often overburdened heart. Strong stimulants will always exacerbate the condition.

It makes sense that in order to reverse the epidemic of heart disease evidenced in this country, we need to make some obvious shifts in the way our nation eats. Do we need any greater evidence that the standard American diet is not adequate to support the functions of a healthy body than a country dying of heartache? Yet it seems we're intent on making the heart's job as difficult as possible. A stroll through a modern supermarket is a heart attack in the making. Something is tragically wrong when the very food we produce contributes to the ill health of the nation.

3. Every Day Use Herbs That Support the Heart.

The heart-healthy herbs in the chart at right can be taken as *tonics* — they nourish, tone, rehabilitate, and strengthen the heart. Use them often in tea, capsule, or tincture form. Consult appendix 1 for dosage guidelines.

HERBAL TONICS FOR THE HEART

Herb	Effect
Cayenne (*Capsicum frutescens* and related species)	One of our most important circulatory tonics; has an especially tonic effect on the heart muscle.
Garlic (*Allium sativum*)	Reduces cholesterol and lowers blood pressure.
Ginkgo (*Ginkgo biloba*)	Improves circulation, lowers blood pressure, dilates peripheral blood vessels, increases peripheral blood flow, and has proved helpful in treating vascular insufficiency.
Hawthorn (*Crataegus oxyacantha* and *C. monogyna*)	The most important cardiac tonic we know of in Western herbology. Can be used beneficially for most heart conditions, is nontoxic, and can be used safely with heart medication.
Linden (*Tilia* spp.)	A relaxing herb used to reduce hypertension and lower blood pressure.
Motherwort (*Leonurus cardiaca*)	Used for all heart conditions caused by stress and anxiety; is especially useful for tachycardia and rapid heartbeat.
Oats (*Avena fatua* and *A. sativa*)	A relaxing, tonic herb that is especially useful for hypertension, rapid heartbeat, and stress and anxiety.
Passionflower (*Passiflora incarnata*)	Highly regarded for its nervine and relaxing properties; a specific medication for hypertension, high blood pressure, and tachycardia.
Prickly ash (*Zanthoxylum americanum*)	Used to treat circulatory problems and acts as a cardiac stimulant; functions much like cayenne, though it is slower in action and doesn't have that "fire."
Siberian ginseng (*Eleutherococcus senticosus*)	An important herb for the heart; has long been recognized as an effective remedy for hypertension, stress, and overwork.
Valerian (*Valeriana officinalis*)	A cardiac relaxant that strengthens and tonifies the heart; used for hypertension and irregular and rapid heartbeat.
Yarrow (*Achillea millefolium*)	Helps lower blood pressure by dilating the peripheral blood vessels; its diaphoretic action also helps relieve pressure on the heart.

HAWTHORN BERRY CONSERVE

This conserve makes a tasty excuse for incorporating hawthorn — a heart tonic extraordinaire — into your diet. I've added chopped oranges, dried cranberries, and chopped walnuts to the conserve; you can make it as fancy or simple as you like.

Dried seedless hawthorn berries

Apple juice

Honey

Ginger (grated or powdered)

Cinnamon

1. Place the hawthorn berries in a pan with just enough apple juice to cover them. Simmer over low heat for 15 minutes. Cover and let sit overnight.

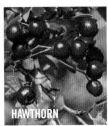
HAWTHORN

2. Sweeten with honey, ginger, and cinnamon to taste. Store in the refrigerator, where the conserve will keep for 2 to 3 weeks.

You can also make a wonderful syrup from hawthorn berries; in fact, it's one of my favorite ways to take advantage of the amazing benefits of the berries. In Europe you can find the syrup in grocery stores as well as pharmacies and herb shops. To make the syrup, simply follow the instructions on page 382. You can add other heart-healthy herbs such as lycium berries and elderberries for a truly delicious heart tonic.

4. Take Daily Supplements That Support a Healthy Heart.

Supplements recommended for a healthy heart are many of the same suggested for maintaining good vision, improving mental acuity, and preventing or slowing the progression of Alzheimer's disease. These include omega-3 fatty acids, spirulina, antioxidants, vitamin E, lecithin, and folic acid. You can find these supplements in vitamin shops and most natural foods stores.

In addition, consider supplementing with coenzyme Q10 (CoQ10). This compound is found in every organ system of the body but is especially concentrated in the heart muscle. It is an important immune-system booster, strengthens the heart and cardiovascular system, and normalizes blood pressure. The amount of CoQ10 in

"When **touched** by the beauty of a spring meadow in bloom or the profound sense of presence felt in a grove of redwood trees, the **heart** figuratively **takes flight** and the spirit is healed. But nature brings physical healing as well, offering nourishment and strength to a troubled heart."

— **David Hoffmann,**
Healthy Heart

our body diminishes as we age, and low levels of CoQ10 have been linked to a number of age-related disorders, including heart disease and even congestive heart failure. The severity of heart failure often correlates to the severity of the deficiency of this important nutrient. CoQ10 is fairly common in our food and can be found in meat (especially organ meats), eggs, fish, and nuts. You can also find CoQ10 supplements in most vitamin shops and natural foods stores. The recommended daily dosage is 50 to 300 mg daily. Unfortunately, CoQ10 is fairly expensive, and supplements are often not of exceptional quality. Check your sources and buy from reliable companies (my favorite is Rainbow Light).

energizing for elders

Low energy is a problem that many elderly people experience. There are countless reasons for lack of energy — lack of sleep, poor digestion, lack of exercise, compromised immune systems, worn-out adrenals, to name just a few — but with an improved diet, a good exercise program, and nights filled with restful sleep, your energy is easily restored and the bloom of life again felt deeply in the heart.

Try this five-step energy program for 4 weeks and you will note a steady return of your inner fire and juice. Try it for 8 weeks and you will find your health restored.

vitamin E for the heart

Vitamin E is a potent antioxidant, strengthens the heart muscle, and improves circulation. When heart problems are prevalent, take only small dosages, not exceeding 50 I.U. daily. Otherwise, 200 to 400 I.U. daily are recommended.

1. Sleep. Get 8 hours of sleep every night. If you don't sleep well, follow the suggestions given in chapter 3 for relieving insomnia (see page 61).

2. Exercise. Every day, undertake at least 30 minutes of some type of low-impact exercise. Yoga is ideal for restoring energy; in addition to the benefits of simple exercise, it offers certain postures that are specific to a depleted and worn system. Short walks to begin and end the day are wonderfully restorative. In fact, for me there is no better way to restore balance and energy than a walk in our wild woodlands.

3. Digestion. Restore your digestive system, following the suggestions given in chapter 4 (see page 93).

4. Adrenals. Restore adrenal function by drinking 2 cups of Pick-Me-Up Tea (see recipe on page 299) daily for 4 to 6 weeks.

5. Green power. To improve and restore energy, every day drink a "green" drink or take capsules of spirulina, chlorella, or blue-green algae. My favorite is Rachel's Green Drink; it is available in most natural foods stores.

ELDER ENERGY BALLS

This formula is adapted for elders and contains less "zoom" than my famous Zoom Balls. All herbs are in powdered form.

> Tahini or other nut butter
> Honey
> 1 part American or Asian ginseng (organically
>   cultivated)
> 1 part astragalus
> 1 part hawthorn berry
> 1 part fo-ti
> 1 part Siberian ginseng
> ¼ part guarana
> Carob or chocolate chips (optional)
> Coconut (optional)
> Lycium berries or raisins (optional)
> Slivered almonds (optional)
> Carob powder

1. Mix equal parts of tahini and honey, or mix to taste (you may prefer less honey and more tahini, for example).

2. Combine the powdered herbs. Add enough of them to the tahini–honey mixture to make a thick batter or paste.

3. Mix in whatever goodies you like, such as carob or chocolate chips, shredded coconut, lycium berries, or slivered almonds.

4. Add enough carob powder to thicken into a dough. Roll into small balls. Store in the refrigerator, where they will keep for 2 to 3 months. But why let them sit so long?

ENERGY SHAKE

This delicious shake is packed with energy-building nutrients. It's easy to prepare and easy to digest. This is my favorite formula, but you can use any combination of fruits and fruit juices, and add various herb powders for an added lift.

> 2 cups pineapple juice (or another fruit juice,
>   Rice Dream, or almond milk)
> 1 tablespoon Rachel's Green Drink
> 1 teaspoon powdered Asian or Siberian ginseng
> 1 teaspoon powdered hawthorn
> ½ cup yogurt
> ¼ to ½ cup blueberries, raspberries, peaches, or
>   whatever fruit is in season
> 1 banana (fresh or frozen)

Combine all ingredients in a blender and process.

QUICK ENERGY RUSH

This recipe is designed for only occasional use, when you need a quick fix of energy, such as when you have a long drive ahead. Guarana contains caffeine, which is contraindicated for exhaustion and depletion. The Alacer Emergen-C provides 2,000 milligrams of vitamin C, plus a wide range of bioflavonoids.

> **2 packages of Alacer Emergen-C (available in natural foods stores)**
> **⅛ teaspoon guarana powder**
> **1 cup water or juice**

Combine the Alacer Emergen-C and guarana in a small container. Shake well. Stir into the water or juice and drink.

PICK-ME-UP TEA

> **2 parts hawthorn berry, leaf, and/or flower**
> **2 parts nettle**
> **1 part ginkgo**
> **1 part licorice (see caution at right)**
> **¼ part cinnamon**
> **¼ part ginger**

Prepare as an infusion, following the instructions on page 380, using 1 ounce of herb mixture per quart of water, and allowing it to steep for 45 minutes or longer. Drink 2 to 3 cups daily.

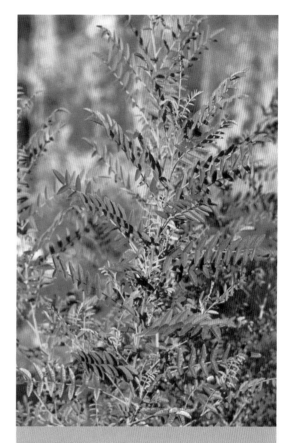

LICORICE CAUTION

Licorice is not recommended for individuals who have high blood pressure due to water retention; individuals who are on heart medication should check with their health care provider before using licorice.

treating varicose veins

Varicose veins occur when capillaries and veins lose their elasticity and become distended and distorted. More than a cosmetic problem, varicose veins can be painful and make walking and sitting uncomfortable, and are a sign that the vascular system needs attention. Older people experience varicose veins most often because of circulatory problems and weakening of the vein walls.

To prevent and lessen the symptoms of varicose veins, do not stand on your feet for long periods of time, especially on cement or other hard surfaces. The blood will pool in the weakened capillaries, causing further distention. Sit, when possible, with your legs elevated slightly above the hips. If you must stand for any length of time, be sure there is a soft cushioned pad under your feet. When you sleep at night, elevate your legs.

Vitamin C and bioflavonoids are essential for healthy capillaries and veins. Eat lots of foods rich in vitamin C, such as rose hips, bilberries, and blueberries. I would also suggest taking a vitamin C supplement. My favorite is Alacer Lite Emergen-C (available at most supermarkets), which is high in bioflavonoids and is quickly absorbed into the system. (But don't take the Alacer supplement in the evening, as it stimulates the system and can keep you up for hours.)

Supplement your diet with herbs that improve circulation. Cayenne, elderberries, ginger, ginkgo, and hawthorn are all good choices.

HEALING LINIMENT FOR VARICOSE VEINS

To help heal varicose veins, apply this liniment every evening. Butcher's broom is specific for varicose veins.

> **2 parts calendula flowers and leaf**
> **2 parts horse chestnut**
> **1 part butcher's broom**
> **1 part witch hazel bark**
> **Witch hazel extract**

1. Place the herbs in a quart jar and cover with 2 to 4 inches of witch hazel extract (the kind that you buy at pharmacies). Place in a warm location and let it steep for 2 weeks.

2. Strain and rebottle. Store in a cool location.

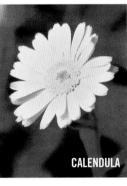

CALENDULA

3. Sit with your legs slightly elevated. Have handy a bowl filled with the liniment and a lightweight cotton hand towel. Soak the towel thoroughly in the liniment and use it to slowly, steadily rub your legs upward toward the heart. Continue for 10 to 12 minutes.

4. Wrap the liniment-soaked towel around each leg. Sit with your legs elevated for 20 minutes.

HEALING TEA
FOR HEALTHY VEINS

This herbal infusion will help prevent or relieve varicose veins.

    2 parts butcher's broom
    2 parts hawthorn
    2 parts rose hips
    1 part white oak bark

Combine all the ingredients and prepare as an infusion, following the instructions on page 380. Drink 2 to 3 cups daily.

VITAMIN C POULTICE

    1 part calendula
    1 part comfrey
    1 part yarrow
    5,000 I.U. vitamin C
    Witch hazel extract

Chop and mix together the calendula, comfrey, and yarrow. Mix in the vitamin C. Add enough witch hazel extract to make a thick paste. Apply directly to the varicose veins or wrap in a muslin cloth and place over the veins. Leave on for 30 to 45 minutes.

preventing and treating ulcers

Many elders suffer from painful gastrointestinal ulcers. Most are the result of stress, poor eating habits, and gastrointestinal disturbances. Remarkably common — one in ten Americans suffers from some form of an ulcer — ulcers offer a sad statement about American health. Once considered an affliction of the elderly and those living an opulent lifestyle, ulcers were most commonly seen in rich, portly, elderly men and women. Nowadays, age and class are no longer determining factors; everyone seems equally affected by the stress and tension of our busy modern lifestyles, and most Americans have unhealthy eating habits and thrive on rich, sugar-laden diets.

Helicobacter pylori, a common stomach bacterium, is thought to be a primary cause of stomach ulcers. When the body's protective intestinal mantle fails, *H. pylori* invades, releasing large amounts of ammonia and carbon dioxide that irritate the stomach lining. But *H. pylori* is not the sole culprit behind ulcers. This bacterium is a natural inhabitant of our intestines and generally causes no problems. When our system is thrown out of balance, however, by poor eating habits and overwhelming stress, the body becomes the perfect medium for excess bacterial growth, and an ulcer results.

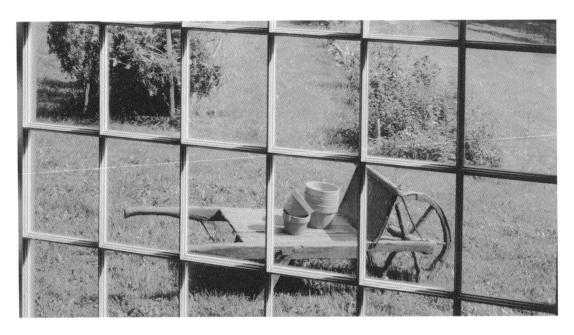

My all-time favorite remedy for ulcers is one my grandmother taught me many years ago. Shortly after my grandfather died, my grandmother developed a painful ulcer. And no wonder! She'd spent her life depending on my grandfather for everything that had to do with the outer world. Grandpa did the shopping, drove her wherever she needed to go, and took care of any business dealings. It wasn't that my grandmother wasn't busy. Quite the contrary! She was as busy as he — but busy raising an armload of children, minding the boardinghouse, cooking up the most sumptuous meals I've ever had, and saving our souls from eternal damnation. Maintaining a home and attending to bills and finances were quite another issue. Having to take over Grandpa's duties after he passed away, in addition to her grief at losing her life partner, created an unbearably stressful situation. She recognized the telltale signs of the ulcer — severe burning stomach pains after eating, nausea, and loss of energy — so she hastened to the store to stock up on green cabbage. She fasted for seven days, eating only an occasional piece of fruit and drinking fresh cabbage juice religiously two or three times daily. In less than seven days, that ulcer was gone, and she never did get one again.

GRANDMA MARY'S CABBAGE JUICE COCKTAIL

Fresh green cabbage

Place cabbage leaves in a juicer and process. As soon as the cabbage is juiced, pour it into a glass and drink it up. Cabbage juice starts to oxidize very quickly, losing most of its valuable properties. Fresh cabbage juice tastes sweet and good, but cabbage juice that has sat for any length of time tastes and smells pungent and very unflavorful, like an old goat in rut.

STRESS-RELIEF TEA

This tea blend soothes both mind and ulcer.

3 parts oats (milky green tops)
1 part licorice root
1 part marsh mallow
1 part purslane or chickweed

Combine all the ingredients. Prepare as an infusion, following the instructions on page 380, using 2 teaspoons of herb mixture per cup of water, and steeping for 30 to 40 minutes. Drink 2 to 3 cups daily.

ULCER-RELIEF TEA

Herbs that are soothing, mucilaginous, and supportive of the immune system are excellent for ulcers. This is a good tea blend that works as well as it tastes.

Uña de gato is a wonderfully healing herb from the rain forest. If you have trouble finding it, however, substitute the more readily available pau-d'arco.

2 parts licorice root
1 part blueberries or huckleberries
1 part marsh mallow root
1 part uña de gato or pau-d'arco
¼ part cinnamon bark

Combine all the ingredients. Prepare as a decoction, following the instructions on page 380, using 2 teaspoons of the herb mixture per cup of water and letting it steep for 20 minutes or longer. Drink 2 to 3 cups a day.

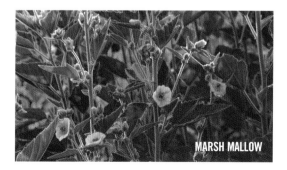

MARSH MALLOW

hearing loss and tinnitus

An estimated one in ten Americans has some form of hearing loss. While most hearing loss is experienced by people over 65, studies show that younger people are experiencing a higher percentage of hearing loss than ever before, primarily due to noise pollution. For example, both my father (in his late 70s) and my partner, Robert (in his mid-40s), have varying degrees of hearing loss. My father's is a result of medication for heart disease, while Robert's is a result of noise pollution at his former job.

Though more than one-third of people over the age of 65 experience hearing loss, it is not necessarily the result of advancing years but, rather, of a change in blood supply to the ear generally due to heart disease, diabetic conditions, and circulatory imbalances. Noise pollution is another major factor. People of all ages are subjected to noise pollution, but the sensitive ears of the elderly (and children) are often most deeply affected. Built into the sensitive hearing mechanism of the ear is a protective device that warns us when noise becomes too loud or irritating — if we but listen to it. When noise becomes assaulting or damaging to the ears, we often hear a distinctive hissing or high-pitched ringing in the ears, or it sounds as if we're hearing underwater. This warning sign is termed temporary threshold shift (TTS), and it is an indication that the fine hairs in the inner ears that transmit sound have been injured by the powerful sound waves. Overnight rest and relief from the assaulting noise are necessary to restore hearing to normal. If we continue to subject our ears to the noise, the damage can become irreversible and permanent threshold shift (PTS) results.

Tinnitus, which occurs in approximately 85 percent of people with impaired hearing, is a particularly distressing form of hearing loss. It is generally thought to be due to nerve damage, noise pollution, or congestion in the ear canals resulting from allergies. Tinnitus is characterized by a constant or recurring ringing or buzzing sound in the ears. Some people hear it constantly, while for others it comes and goes in what seems to be a random pattern. It can be extremely irritating and often debilitating. At this time, allopathic medicine has little to offer to alleviate the symptoms of tinnitus, but there are several natural and herbal therapies that have proved helpful.

Boosting Circulation to Alleviate Tinnitus

Some cases of tinnitus result from poor circulation to the brain. Ginkgo, a potent circulation booster, has proved helpful for many people with this type of tinnitus. I generally prefer to use whole-plant tinctures and extracts and have found these to be effective in most cases. Take ½ to 1 teaspoon of the tincture three times daily or 2 capsules (60 mg) three times daily. However, if the whole-plant tincture doesn't appear to be helping within a 3- to 4-week period, switch to a commercial extract that is standardized to 24 percent flavone glycosides (what some researchers consider the active constituents). Use the recommended dosages on the container as a guide, adjusting them according to the age and health of the patient.

CIRCULATORY TEA FOR EARS AND TINNITUS

This formula makes a tasty and effective circulatory stimulant, helping increase circulation throughout the body, with the benefit of improving some cases of tinnitus and hearing loss.

- 1 part ginkgo
- 1 part hawthorn berries
- ¼ part cinnamon
- ¼ part ginger

Combine all the ingredients and prepare as an infusion, following the instructions on page 380. Drink 3 to 4 cups daily.

This blend can also be made into a syrup, following the instructions on page 382.

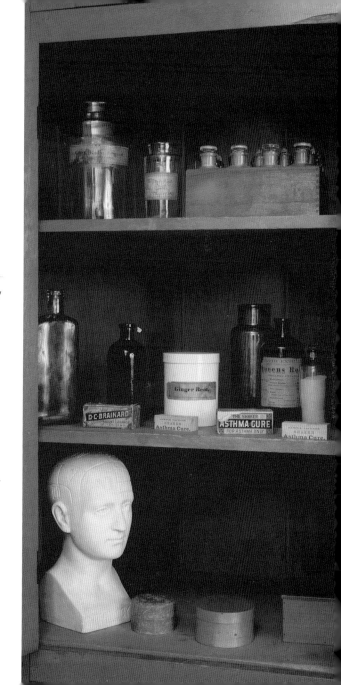

Allergies and Hearing Loss

Allergies and food sensitivities often cause sinus congestion, which can irritate the ear canals and hearing mechanism. Little is known about the effects of allergies and food sensitivities on hearing loss, but it has been proved that eliminating a food that triggers an allergic reaction can radically change the personality, clear long-standing illnesses, and energize, invigorate, and revitalize the mind and the body.

A good example of this was noted in my beautiful Bernese Mountain dog. I purchased Deva from a breeder, and she already showed symptoms of a compromised immune system and allergies by the time she landed in my welcoming lap at 12 weeks of age. Unsuspectingly, I started her on an all-natural diet, as my teacher, Juliette de Bairacli Levy, an avid dog lover and breeder of world-renowned hounds, had instructed me: organic raw meat, cottage cheese, whole grains, and vegetables. It was an awesome diet, but Deva didn't thrive on it. Though an unusually sweet puppy, she became irritable, snappy, and hyperactive. Her ears had a foul odor and were filled with excess wax, and she would often shake her head in an attempt to clear them. She also didn't hear well. Finding the allergens took time, but we were committed and eventually found that she was allergic to beef, lamb, wheat, and dairy.

You should see this dog now. Except for her recent encounter with a porcupine, she is the picture of health and vitality. If she could have shared her experience with us verbally, telling us what she had experienced during her allergy attacks, I'm quite sure she would have complained of ringing in her ears.

I'm convinced that allergic reactions cause tinnitus and hearing loss as often as noise pollution, stress, and poor circulation. Food allergy tests can be costly and are not always accurate, but if you can afford them, they are certainly worthwhile. It is also worth your time to undertake a food elimination diet, removing from your diet one food group at a time, each for 1 to 2 weeks, and examining the results. It can be challenging, but the results are often amazing. Allergies are many and varied, but wheat, dairy, and sugar are the most common triggers.

"Live each season as it passes; breathe the air, drink the drink, taste the fruit, and resign yourself to the influences of each."

— Henry David Thoreau

In addition to eliminating foods that may be causing allergic reactions, you can clear the sinuses by eating horseradish, ginger, and cayenne. My favorite remedy for sinus congestion is horseradish sauce.

HORSERADISH SAUCE FOR SINUS CONGESTION AND TINNITUS

People experiencing sinus congestion or tinnitus should make this sauce themselves. It's part of the therapy — and don't use a food processor, or you won't get the full effect!

Horseradish root

Apple cider vinegar

Honey

1. Using a hand grater, finely grate the horseradish root. Grate until your eyes are watering and your nose begins to water. The effects of horseradish have begun!

2. Mix the grated horseradish with vinegar and honey to taste. Store the sauce in a glass jar with a tight-fitting lid in the refrigerator, where it will keep for 6 months. Eat 1 to 2 teaspoons daily; I like to mix it with grains and vegetables or spread it on crackers. It's very tasty and is a powerful remedy for sinus congestion.

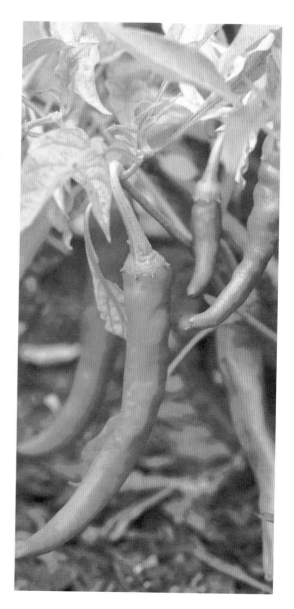

Appendix I
The Herbal Apothecary: An A-to-Z Guide

Though it's always a challenging task to decide which of the many wonderful herbs to include in listings such as this, I've limited my discussion to those herbs that have the longest history of use and that are common ingredients in home remedies. Most of these herbs can be used successfully and safely over a long period of time for a variety of purposes. Warnings are given when appropriate. For a more complete listing of beneficial herbs or for further information on the herbs that I have included, consult any one of the encyclopedic herbal compendiums available today.

Reading will fill your head with the wonderful facts and stories about each plant, but herbalism is more than "head" learning. Plants teach by interacting with us, so the best possible way to learn about each herb is to experience it. After you've read about it, if it seems like an herb that is appropriate for your situation, try it. Your body — tasting, smelling, analyzing the effect of the herb on your being — is the best laboratory you have for determining an herb's effectiveness.

When teaching my students how to use herbs, I insist they first try each one as a tea. In

this way, they learn about each herb's flavor and effects. Next, I ask them to research the herb in several good reference books. Learning the various uses that different herbalists recommend for an herb augments your direct experience with it.

Learning about herbs is, most important, listening carefully: to the wisdom of your body, to the feeling of the herbs as you're using them, and to the book knowledge you gain as you read about them.

do your research

I've always felt it requisite, when studying herbs, to research each one I'm planning to use in at least three herb books. Because herbs are so multifaceted, no one book will give you a complete picture of what an herb is or what it can do. Reading about the herb in several books will paint a more complete picture for you and give you a broader understanding of its depths and possibilities.

aloe vera *(Aloe vera)*

Parts used: Fresh leaves, dried leaf resin, and gel extracted from the fresh leaf

Benefits: A virtual first-aid kit in a plant, aloe may well be one of the most useful houseplants you can grow. The fresh leaves are a soothing emollient agent for skin abrasions, wounds, and burns, including radiation burns. The gel of the inner leaf has a natural pH of around 4.3, making it excellent for skin and hair preparations. Many people have found that aloe, used both internally and externally, is helpful for skin problems such as pimples, acne, and rosacea. Aloe vera also contains aloin, a natural sunscreen that blocks as much as 30 percent of the sun's ultraviolet rays. In addition, there has been some promising research into using aloe as a mild antiviral treatment for people with HIV and AIDS.

Aloe is one of the most famous cleansing herbs, having been used for centuries as a laxative. The outer skin of the fresh leaves must be peeled away before the herb can be used internally, as aloin, a brown gel concentrated near the leaf blade, can be an irritant. Generally, for internal purposes, fresh preserved aloe juice is used.

Suggested uses: Grow this herb and use it! For external use, cut a leaf from the plant at its base. A clear gel will ooze from the fresh wound, but it will quickly heal. Stored in the refrigerator, the leaf will keep for several weeks, always ready when needed. Apply gel squeezed from the leaf,

growing aloe

Though requiring little day-to-day maintenance, aloe is a warm-weather plant; it needs lots of sunshine and, like most succulents, does best in hot, dry locations. The mother plant generously produces many "pups," or small plantlets. These are easily detached and will thrive on their own when repotted in well-drained soil.

or the leaf itself, to burns, skin irritation, and bedsores, and use as an ingredient in cosmetic formulas.

For internal use, find fresh preserved aloe juice — available at most natural foods stores. Follow the manufacturer's recommended dosage.

Caution: Aloe should be used internally with caution, following recommended dosages diligently, as it can cause griping and painful stomach cramps and diarrhea. Nursing mothers will want to avoid using aloe internally; it will pass through the breast milk and affect the nursing child. Pregnant women also should not take aloe internally.

Although aloe is highly recommended for most skin problems, do not use it on staph, impetigo, or other staphlike infections. The sweet gel of the aloe creates a perfect petri dish for staph bacteria to grow in.

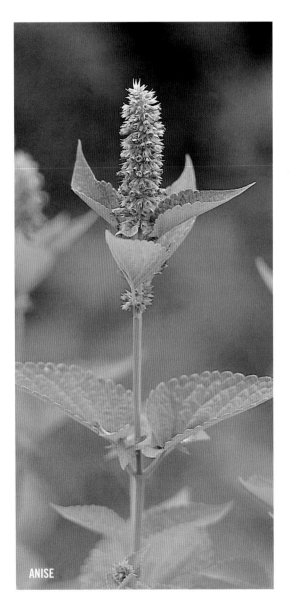

ANISE

anise *(Pimpinella anisum)*

Parts used: Primarily seeds, but leaves are useful

Benefits: Anise is a carminative (gas-expelling), warming digestive aid. It has a tasty licorice-like flavor.

Suggested uses: Use as a tea for colic and other digestive problems. Because it has a sweet flavor, you can blend anise with less tasty herbs to disguise their flavor.

meetin' seeds

Our Puritan forefathers (and mothers!) used to mix carminative seeds such as anise, dill, fennel, and caraway. They would carry the mixture in little containers to the long church services. When the children's tummies growled from hunger or boredom, they would chew on these "meetin' seeds" to calm their stomachs — but I'm not sure it calmed their restless spirits.

artichoke *(Cynara scolymus)*

Parts used: All plant parts are useful, but the large lobed leaves (not the leaves of the flower heads, which we eat) are the most useful medicinally

Benefits: Like its cousin milk thistle and related members of the thistle family, artichoke is rich in cynarin, a chemical that aids and protects the liver. It also contains bitter principles that actively stimulate the liver and the gallbladder. It is especially indicated for slow or sluggish digestion and poor absorption. The entire plant is medicinal, but the leaves are particularly rich in inulin, cynarin, and bitter principles and are the parts most often employed in herbal medicine. I think artichoke is one of our finest bitters; considering that it is easily cultivated in many areas of the country, it is sadly underused. And in its native Mediterranean territory, artichoke is well known as an excellent food for diabetics, because it helps lower blood sugar levels.

Suggested uses: Blend artichoke leaves with other liver tonics, such as dandelion, yellow dock, and burdock, for an effective digestive tonic.

ashwagandha (*Withania somnifera*)

Parts used: Roots

Benefits: An ancient Ayurvedic herb, ashwagandha is often referred to as the "Indian ginseng," and, in fact, it is used in very much the same manner that ginseng is used in Asia. An excellent adaptogenic herb, ashwagandha increases the body's overall ability to adapt to and resist stress. In India, it is used to increase memory and facilitate learning. It is both energizing and soothing. Ashwagandha is primarily classified as a male tonic herb, but women use it as well. It is a classic reproductive tonic and will help restore sexual chi, or energy.

Suggested uses: This herb is specifically indicated for reduced levels of energy, general debilitation, reduced sexual energy, nervous tension, stress, and anxiety. It promotes general well-being and enhances stamina (thus explaining its popularity with athletes).

Said to have the smell of a female horse's urine and the stamina of a stallion, ashwagandha isn't the best-tasting herb you'll ever meet. I recommend blending it with other more flavorful herbs, such as ginger, sarsaparilla, and cinnamon, to make a suitable-tasting tea. Powder the root and mix it with milk for a classic Indian rejuvenating drink, or try blending it with your favorite chai tea blend. You can also use it in tincture or capsule form.

astragalus (*Astragalus membranaceus*)

Parts used: Roots

Benefits: A wonderfully energizing and tonic herb, astragalus is one of the most outstanding herbs for building immune strength and energizing the entire body, particularly the spleen and lungs. It is a superior tonic herb and is used in the treatment of chronic imbalances. It stimulates the rebuilding of the bone marrow reserve that supports and regenerates the body's "protective shield," or immune system. It is used to both prevent and treat long-term infections, including chronic colds, recurring flus, and candida, as well as the Epstein-Barr virus. Astragalus promotes circulatory health and stimulates regular metabolism of dietary sugars. It is often used by people with diabetes.

There have been some promising studies on using astragalus with cancer patients undergoing radiation and/or chemotherapy. Though there doesn't appear to be anything in astragalus that kills cancer cells directly, these studies have indicated that the herb strengthens the immune system's ability to resist infection, thereby contributing to the overall well-being of the patient.

Suggested uses: Use astragalus as a tea to treat long-term illness, to rebuild energy levels, and to support and build deep immune strength. You can also add it to soups; simply place a whole root or two in a pot of soup and simmer several hours. Astragalus can also be served in capsules.

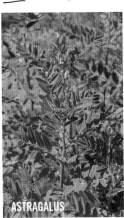
ASTRAGALUS

Astragalus comes in many grades and qualities. The root is sliced and pressed and bears a remarkable resemblance to tongue depressors used by doctors. Look for long, wide, straight roots, generally whitish or cream-colored, with a yellowish core. The root has a sweet flavor that's quite tasty, and children enjoy chewing on the root as if it were a stick of licorice candy.

bilberry *(Vaccinium myrtillus)*

Parts used: Leaves and berries

Benefits: Bilberry is both a preventive and a curative for eye problems. The leaves and especially the berries have a high concentration of antioxidants and bioflavonoids, particularly a complex group known as anthocyanosides, which increase blood flow to the eyes and strengthen the tiny capillaries in and surrounding them.

Both the fruit and the leaves of bilberry reduce excess sugar in the blood and have proved beneficial for diabetics. Bilberry can help regulate hyperglycemia if used over a period of several months. It also is a stimulating tonic for the urinary system and strengthens bladder and kidney function. As an antiseptic and diuretic, bilberry is used for treating urinary infections; it is often combined with cranberry or uva-ursi for this purpose. In addition, bilberry has a good reputation for enhancing circulation, treating varicose veins and hemorrhoids, and rebuilding connective tissue.

Suggested uses: Bilberry can be purchased as a .25 percent standardized extract. Though I would suggest the whole-plant tincture or tea for most purposes, for macular degeneration and diabetic retinopathy, the standardized preparation would be indicated because of its concentration.

Don't leave bilberry jam and bilberry wine out of your medicinal repertoire. These sweet treats are both excellent ways to indulge in this plant's medicine.

blackberry (*Rubus* spp.)

Parts used: Fruit, leaves, and roots

Benefits: Long used by native people as a delicious food, blackberries have also been an important folk medicine. They contain a host of nutrients, including vitamin C, tannins, organic acids, and flavonoid compounds, which may explain their medicinal action. Though the fruits have mild laxative properties, the roots and leaves of the blackberry plant are effective remedies for diarrhea and dysentery. The leaf is milder in action and is particularly good for children with loose bowels. The root is my favorite remedy for "touristo," and I carry blackberry root tincture with me every time I travel in Central and South America, with excellent results.

Suggested uses: Blackberries are excellent in pies, jams, and jellies. They make a delicious and nutritious wine and cough syrup. The leaves are also flavorful; they are often combined with leaves of other *Rubus* species, such as raspberry. Blackberry leaf tea is effective for young children with mild diarrhea and loose bowels. The root contains the most tannins and is a strong remedy for diarrhea and dysentery. It is best when harvested in the early spring or late fall — but it's a bear to dig up, which may account for why there isn't more of this excellent remedy on the market. Use young roots that are easily sliced, not the hard woody rootstalks, which contain less of the medicinal components.

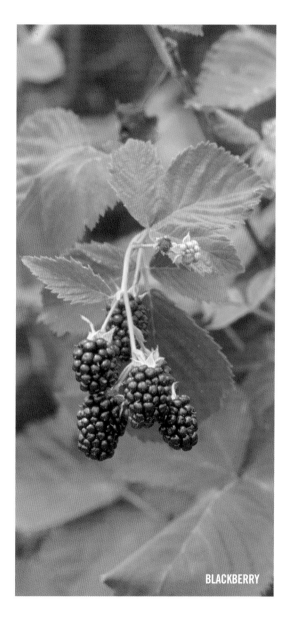

BLACKBERRY

black cohosh *(Cimifuga racemosa)*

Parts used: Rhizomes and roots

Benefits: Black cohosh and blue cohosh are unrelated, but they are often used together; they are not interchangeable, but they are synergistic. Black cohosh has an estrogen-like action. It regulates and normalizes hormone production and is often used in formulas for balancing women's hormonal systems. It is also highly regarded as a nervine and muscle relaxant.

Suggested uses: Black cohosh is used in combination with blue cohosh to stimulate uterine contractions. It is often given during the last week of pregnancy to prepare the uterus for childbirth, and it is especially helpful for moving along overdue pregnancies when the mother or infant is in stress. Because of its estrogen-like qualities, black cohosh has a special affinity for menopausal women and is used in formulas to balance hormone production. It is often taken to bring on delayed menstruation and is helpful for relieving the stress and nervous tension that often accompany the menstrual cycle.

Black cohosh is also recommended for relieving headaches and muscle spasms. Its anti-inflammatory action makes it useful for arthritis and muscular and neurological pain.

Caution: Do not use black cohosh during pregnancy, except in preparation for childbirth, and then only under the supervision of a qualified holistic medical practitioner.

black walnut *(Juglans nigra)*

Parts used: Nuts and their green hulls

Benefits: The stately black walnut tree is greatly prized by furniture makers and other artisans for its rich hardwood. Herbalists treasure the black

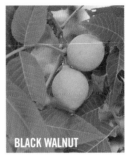

BLACK WALNUT

walnut for the hulls of its unripe nuts, which are used internally to cleanse the blood and intestines and externally to heal the skin.

In North America, preparations containing black walnut hull were popular folk remedies — and are still used today — for curing athlete's foot and other fungal infections; in Europe the butternut, a close relative of black walnut, is used similarly. I have found black walnut to be very effective for all types of fungal infections; I use it in foot powders, liniments, and as a wash for athlete's foot and infectious skin disorders, though it will stain the skin a rather interesting color that will last for several days.

The green hulls of black walnuts are a rich source of juglone, an antifungal and antiparasitic compound. Taken internally as a tincture, black walnut can have a very beneficial effect on gastrointestinal problems, including diarrhea and constipation, caused by intestinal parasites, including giardia, and candida.

The nuts themselves are delicious and nutritious; they are considered to be excellent for those with "wasting" diseases, as they are a rich source of high-quality oils and help stabilize weight loss.

Suggested uses: Use powdered black walnut hull in foot powders, in foot soaks, and as a wash for skin infections. The powdered hull can also be encapsulated for internal use. I generally recommend mixing it with other herbs, such as ginger and fennel for gastrointestinal problems, or chaparral and goldenseal for parasites. Dosages should not exceed 2 dropperfuls of tincture three or four times daily or 2 size-00 capsules three times daily over a period of 3 to 4 weeks. If further treatment is necessary, discontinue the treatment for a week, then repeat the cycle as needed.

As a tincture, black walnut can be applied topically to herpes and cold sores.

Caution: Black walnut is not recommended for long-term use. The hulls are a rather strong remedy, so when using them internally, pay particular attention to dosage and frequency.

Black walnut hulls, whether fresh or dried, will quickly stain the skin if applied topically. I never mind, because they are just so effective for treating athlete's foot and other fungal infections. It seems to me a blackish green foot is better than an itchy, painful one! And the stain lasts for only a few days.

blue cohosh *(Caulophyllum thalictroides)*

Parts used: Roots and rhizomes

Benefits: Formerly known as papoose root and squaw root, blue cohosh was commonly used by Native American women during the latter stages of pregnancy to ensure an easier labor and childbirth. Dr. Shook, an early Physiomedical herb doctor, stated, "This exceedingly valuable herb is well called 'women's best friend' for the reason that it is much more reliable and far less dangerous in expediting delivery in those cases where labor is slow and very painful. This is a very old Indian remedy. They believed it to be the best parturient in nature, and it was the habit of their women to drink the tea several weeks before labor." Blue cohosh was listed in the United States Pharmacopoeia from 1882 until 1905 as a labor inducer and was generally given during the last few weeks of pregnancy. It was also used before pregnancy to prepare the uterus for childbirth.

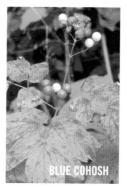

BLUE COHOSH

Suggested uses: Blue cohosh is still widely used among herbalists; it is considered one of the best uterine stimulants and emmenagogue herbs. Caulosaponin, a chemical constituent of blue cohosh, actively stimulates uterine contractions and promotes blood flow to the pelvic region, which can help relieve menstrual cramps.

Caution: A strong medicinal herb with very active properties, blue cohosh should be used responsibly and only under the supervision of an experienced herbalist. Because it is a uterine stimulant, it should not be used during pregnancy. Avoid the berries, which are poisonous.

blue cohosh controversy

Caulosaponin, one of the active constituents of blue cohosh, has been under clinical observation by the scientific community. When researchers isolated the chemical from the mother plant and injected it into animals, it had the effect of narrowing the arteries. From these very limited and, I might add, inhumane studies, researchers have concluded that blue cohosh may contribute to heart damage.

However, caulosaponin is only one constituent of the blue cohosh chemical blueprint. To isolate it, test it on clinically doomed animals, then give a verdict on its toxicity seems horribly ludicrous. This plant has been used safely and effectively for hundreds of years.

borage
(Borago officinalis)

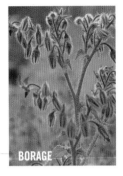

BORAGE

Parts used: Flowers and leaves

Benefits: Traditionally used for relieving anxiety and stress, borage is especially useful when the spirits need lifting. Taken throughout the day, borage will help allay depression.

Suggested uses: This plant loses much of its medicinal qualities when dried, so use it fresh whenever possible. Make a flower essence from borage, or drink a tea made with the flowers and leaves.

buchu *(Barosma betulina)*

Parts used: Leaves

Benefits: A healing herb from South Africa, buchu became an important medicine in North America in 1847, when Henry Helmbold introduced it as a patented medicine. Helmbold's Compound Extract of Buchu quickly became the most popular medicine for kidney and urinary problems and for "diseases arising from imprudence." Helmbold, the self-proclaimed Buchu King, became a millionaire and was, in part, responsible for the demise of *Barosma betulina* in the wild.

The leaves of the buchu plant have a strong, aromatic, almost mintlike taste. They contain high amounts of volatile oils, sulfur compounds, flavonoids, and mucilage and act as a urinary antiseptic, diuretic, and stimulant. Buchu is an excellent herb for treating a variety of kidney and bladder conditions, including cystitis, urethritis, edema (water retention), and kidney stones. It stimulates the flow of urine; clears away mucus, uric acid, and other substances from the kidneys and bladder; and strengthens the tissues of the urinary system. It offers particular relief in cases of pain associated with urinating.

Suggested uses: Buchu's pleasant flavor and water-soluble compounds make it particularly suitable for tea. For chronic urinary problems, drink 2 or 3 cups of tea daily. For acute situations such as cystitis and other urinary infections, every hour drink ¼ cup of a tea made from 1 part buchu mixed with 1 part marsh mallow root and/or corn silk until the infection clears. Buchu leaf tincture is also effective, though teas are generally to be preferred for urinary tract infections. If using the tincture, take 1 to 2 dropperfuls three times daily for chronic problems or ¼ dropperful every hour for acute situations.

Caution: Pregnant women should not take buchu. The herb contains pulegone, a compound also found in pennyroyal that is a strong abortifacient and emmenagogue.

At-risk warning: Buchu is rare in the wild, so be sure to buy only organically cultivated stock. It is widely cultivated in Africa and parts of South America.

burdock *(Arctium lappa)*

Parts used: Primarily roots and seeds, but leaves can be used externally

Benefits: Burdock is truly a superior tonic herb, and it is used as both a preventive and a medicinal plant. Burdock is rich in iron, magnesium, manganese, silicon, and thiamine, as well as a host of other vitamins and minerals. It is simply the best herb for the skin and can be used internally and externally for eczema, psoriasis, acne, and other skin-related imbalances. It is a specific for the liver, and because of its pleasant flavor, it is often formulated with other less tasty "liver herbs."

Cooling and alkalizing, burdock is used for treating stagnant conditions of the blood and is an excellent blood purifier or alterative. It promotes healthy kidney function and expels uric acid from the body, so it is helpful for gout and rheumatism.

Suggested uses: Fresh, young burdock root can be used like carrots in soups, stir-fries, and other dishes. In Japan, burdock is considered a premium vegetable and is often featured in fine restaurants as gobo root. When it's grated, lightly steamed, and sprinkled with toasted sesame seed oil, you'd hardly recognize it as the tenacious backyard weed

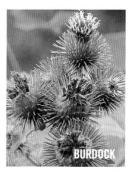
BURDOCK

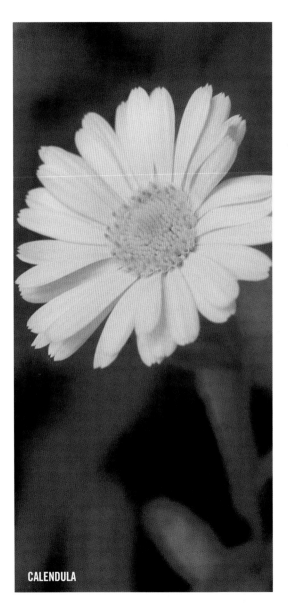

CALENDULA

that it is. Burdock also makes a fine-tasting tea and can be adapted for teenagers with problem skin by serving it with juice or other herb teas; it is useful externally as a wash for treating "hot spots" on animals. The tea can also be served with meals as a digestive aid. Use burdock leaves in salves and as a wash for itchy, irritated skin; the seeds can be used in ointments for the skin. Burdock tinctures well in an 80-proof alcohol solution, but don't be alarmed by the thick white "milk" that may settle in the bottom of your tincture bottle. That is the inulin of the burdock separating from the alcohol.

calendula *(Calendula officinalis)*

Parts used: Flowers

Benefits: This sunny little flower brightens most gardens. It is a powerful vulnerary, healing the body by promoting cell repair, and acts as an antiseptic, keeping infection from occurring in injuries. Calendula is most often used externally for bruises, burns, sores, and skin ulcers. It is also used internally for fevers and for gastrointestinal problems such as ulcers, cramps, indigestion, and diarrhea. And, of course, you see it used in many cosmetics for its skin-soothing effects.

Suggested uses: Use calendula in salves for burns and irritated skin and as an infusion for skin problems, fevers, and gastrointestinal upsets. Brewed in a tea at triple strength, it makes a wonderful hair rinse.

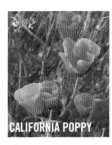

california poppy
(Eschscholzia californica)

Parts used: Seeds, flowers, and leaves

Benefits: This vibrant, golden blossom, California's state flower, is a kissing cousin of the notorious opium poppy; it has similar sedative and narcotic properties but is much milder and nonaddictive. It is quite gentle in its action and is excellent in establishing equilibrium and calming nerve stress and excitability. California poppy is especially recommended for children who have difficulty sleeping and who are overly excitable.

Suggested uses: Juliette de Bairacli Levy, world-renowned herbalist and my mentor, suggests grinding the seeds into a meal and mixing them with honey. She dries these "cakes" in the sun and then feeds them to children experiencing stress and anxiety. Poppy seeds can also be prepared as a tea (1 teaspoon of seeds per cup of water, infused for 20 minutes) or as a tincture.

cascara sagrada *(Rhamnus purshiana)*

Parts used: Aged, cured bark

Benefits: It seems that constipation has always plagued the human race. Cascara sagrada is a large shrub that grows only in the Pacific Northwest. Native Americans introduced it to Spanish explorers, who then popularized it in Europe. Its fame as a laxative quickly spread. The plant's name is Spanish for "sacred bark" — an interesting name for a laxative! The herb relieves constipation by stimulating peristalsis in the large intestine while counteracting harmful bacteria in the digestive tract. Although it is a safe laxative that restores tone to the colon, cascara sagrada is nonetheless very strong and should be used sparingly. It also tonifies the hepatic system and is especially useful for the gallbladder. It may be taken in small doses as a liver tonic and for treating gallstones.

Suggested uses: Although it is one of the safest laxatives, cascara sagrada can cause griping and stomach pain. It is always best to formulate it with other digestive herbs, such as ginger, cinnamon, and fennel, to alleviate any intestinal griping. The aged bark can be prepared as tea, tincture and capsules. Many herbalists suggest that cascara can be used over time as a bowel toner, but long-term use of any laxative, natural or not, can be habit-forming. However, if chronic constipation is an issue, it is better to use cascara to stimulate regular elimination than to have no movement at all. Always incorporate dietary changes when treating chronic constipation.

Caution: Cascara sagrada is not recommended if you have or develop diarrhea, loose stools, or abdominal pain. Consult your physician before using cascara sagrada if you are pregnant, nursing, or taking medication. Above all, be sure that the cascara sagrada bark is aged; the fresh bark is toxic.

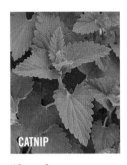
CATNIP

catnip *(Nepeta cataria)*

Parts used: Leaves and flowers

Benefits: Another versatile wonder plant, catnip is safe, effective, and easy to use. It grows easily both in and out of the garden — if you keep your cats away long enough for it to get a head start. While it sends cats into spasms of pleasure, it calms and sedates people, both young and old. An excellent calming herb, catnip can be used for all manner of stress. It is particularly beneficial for lowering fevers and for the pain of teething or toothaches. It is especially valued as a safe, effective relaxant for babies and young children. It is also a restorative digestive aid used for indigestion, diarrhea, and colic. Jethro Kloss, that famous herb doctor, writes in *Back to Eden,* "If every mother had catnip herb on the shelf, it would save her many a sleepless night and her child much suffering."

Suggested uses: Catnip is quite bitter, so it is often formulated with other more pleasant-tasting herbs such as oats and lemon balm. Serve as a tea throughout the day during teething pain. Give a couple of drops of the tincture before meals to serve as a digestive aid. A few drops of the tincture before bedtime will help calm a fussy child. To reduce fevers, both catnip tincture and a catnip enema are effective.

cayenne pepper *(Capsicum annuum)*

Parts used: Fruits

Benefits: There's a growing cult of cayenne aficionados, and it's deserving of all this attention. Cayenne serves as a catalyst to the system, stimulating the body's natural defense system. It has antiseptic properties and is an excellent warming circulatory herb. It is one of the best heart tonics, increasing the pulse and toning the heart muscle. It is a natural coagulant that stops bleeding, and it is an excellent carminative, stimulating the digestive process and helping with congestion and constipation.

Suggested uses: Use cayenne sparingly in formulas (teas, capsules, tinctures, and food preparations) as a catalyst or action herb. The burning feeling it creates is superficial and not harmful.

Caution: Cayenne, though perfectly safe, is hot! Even a pinch of cayenne in a tincture formula can overwhelm, and a grain or more in an herbal pill can send you to the ceiling.

chamomile *(Anthemis nobilis* and *Matricaria recutita)*

Parts used: Primarily the flowers, but the leaves are also useful

Benefits: This small, beautiful, and gentle plant has long been used as a beverage tea but is equally valued for its powerful medicinal properties. Chamomile demonstrates to us that gentle does not mean less effective. It is one of the best all-around children's herbs. It has been used for treating children's colic, nervous stress, infections, and stomach disorders. Remember the story of Peter Rabbit? When little Peter returned from Farmer John's garden — an extremely stressful experience, considering that he barely escaped with his life — his mother whipped him soundly, gave him a cup of chamomile tea, and sent him to bed. Chamomile flowers also have a

scientific proof

Pharmacological and clinical studies confirm what herbalists have long known: The common wayside plant known as chamomile is a very important medication for the nervous system. One of chamomile's major constituents is azulen, a beautiful, azure blue, volatile oil obtained by steam distillation. Azulen contains a whole complex of active principles that serve as anti-inflammatory and antipyretic agents. Its medicinal action is most obvious in three major areas: the nervous system, the immune system, and the digestive system.

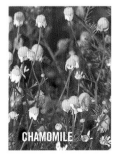

CHAMOMILE

rich supply of essential oil that acts as a powerful anti-inflammatory agent.

Suggested uses: Chamomile tea sweetened with honey can be served throughout the day to calm a stressed or nervous child. A massage oil enhanced with a few drops of chamomile essential oil can be used for similar calming effects and to soothe sore, achy muscles. A few drops of the tincture before mealtime will aid digestion. For a marvelous soothing wash, add chamomile flowers to a baby's bath.

chaparral *(Larrea tridentata)*

Parts used: Leaves, flowering twigs

Benefits: Chaparral stirred up quite a bit of controversy a few years ago. Three cases of liver toxicity suspected to be caused by chaparral were reported, so the United States Food and Drug Administration (FDA) ordered a recall of all products containing chaparral, and a ban was placed on the sale of the herb in both the United States and Great Britain. The year that those three cases were reported, 30,000 tons of chaparral had been sold for medicinal purposes both in the United States and abroad. If the FDA were to use the same standards to judge the toxicity of over-the-counter drugs, there wouldn't be any products on the pharmacy shelves. Though it's possible that these three cases of liver toxicity were due to chaparral, none of the cases was proved, and the FDA eventually dropped both its charges and the ban.

In the meantime, however, although chaparral wasn't available commercially, there was a steady supply of it available "underground." Why? Long used by the native peoples of the American Southwest as a cure-all, chaparral is considered a superior blood cleanser, anti-inflammatory, and, most important, antitumor agent. It is often included in formulas and health programs designed for addressing tumors, fibroids, and cysts. Though its action is different from that of goldenseal, I often use it in place of goldenseal (an endangered plant) for deep-seated colds and flus that aren't responding to other treatments. It promotes sweating and has antibacterial properties. It is also one of the most important antifungal herbs we have and is often combined with black walnut for treating skin infections. Though there have been few scientific studies to document chaparral's effectiveness, the existing evidence warrants further study.

Suggested uses: Chaparral is extremely bitter, and there are few flavors strong enough to mask its rather unpleasant one. Because of this, and also because it is high in resins, which are not water soluble, chaparral is most often administered in tincture form. You can also use it in salves and ointments for athlete's foot and other skin infections.

Caution: Chaparral is a powerful herb and should be used with caution. Follow recommended dosages carefully, and do not use for extended periods of time.

chaste tree *(Vitex agnus-castus)*

Parts used: Berries

Benefits: Chaste tree, also known as vitex, has a stimulating effect on the pituitary gland, which regulates and normalizes hormone production in both men and women. It has an excellent reputation as a tonic for the endocrine gland and is used to normalize the reproductive systems of both men and women. In historical times, monks and priests used vitex to suppress libido; from this tradition came its folk names "monk's pepper" and "chaste berry." (However, by all accounts, it wasn't very successful.) In normalizing and balancing hormone production, vitex will either stimulate or suppress sexual expression as necessary.

Through its effect on the endocrine system, vitex restores and balances our stores of energy. It is the herb of choice for many women to relieve the symptoms of menopause and PMS and to regulate any kind of menstrual dysfunction. Many people use it to enhance their sexual vitality.

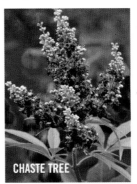

CHASTE TREE

Suggested uses: Use vitex as a reproductive tonic, for balancing hormones, and for relieving the depression and anxiety associated with midlife crisis. Vitex can be prepared as a wine or liqueur or in tincture or capsule form. It has a rather spicy flavor that is not always appropriate for tea. Try it in Longevity Chai (see page 38) or Chai Hombre (see page 244) in place of peppercorns.

chickweed *(Stellaria media)*

Parts used: Aerial parts of the plant

Benefits: This weedy plant can be found growing around the world, especially anywhere moist, cultivated soil can be found. It is highly esteemed for its emollient and demulcent properties and is used to treat skin irritations, eye inflammation, and kidney disorders. It is a mild diuretic and is indicated for water retention. It is an excellent poultice herb and is often found in salve formulas because of its soothing effects on the skin. In addition, it is a treasure trove of nutrients, including calcium, potassium, and iron.

Suggested uses: The fresh tender greens are delicious in salads. They can be juiced or blended with pineapple juice and are often made into salves. A light infusion of chickweed is quite soothing. The plant doesn't dry or store well, so to preserve it for future use, it is best to tincture it fresh.

cinnamon *(Cinnamomum zeylanicum)*

Parts used: Bark and essential oil

Benefits: What a marvelous plant! As well known for its medicinal properties as for its delicious flavor, the cinnamon tree is native to India but is widely cultivated in most tropical regions of the

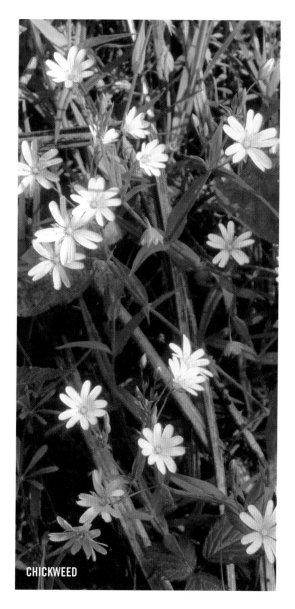

CHICKWEED

world. Though cinnamon is considered to be simply a spice by most Westerners, herbalists have been using it for centuries as a warming digestive aid. It is a wonderful mild stimulant and can be combined with ginger to treat circulatory and digestive problems. The plant is rich in volatile oil, tannins, mucilage, and coumarins. It has antiviral and antiseptic activities, making it useful for fighting infections. Because of its wonderful flavor, it's often used in herbal formulas to mask the taste of less flavorful medicinal plants. There are few blends that aren't enhanced by cinnamon's warm, spicy flavor.

Suggested uses: To make a warming tea, infuse ½ to 1 teaspoon of cinnamon bark in 1 cup of boiling water for 15 to 20 minutes. Cinnamon is most often combined with other herbs to enhance its effectiveness — for example, with ginger for circulatory problems, with chamomile for poor digestion, and with yarrow and peppermint for colds and flus. Use the powdered bark in cooking; it is a flavorful addition to many main courses and desserts. The powdered bark can also be encapsulated. Add cinnamon essential oil to salve recipes and use them topically as analgesics and as warming, stimulating balms.

Note: Cassia, a related species native to China and Japan, with similar constituents, is often used in place of cinnamon. I love them both, but I find cinnamon to be more subtle and perhaps a bit more active medicinally, while cassia has a stronger flavor and scent.

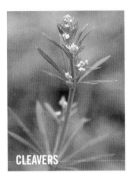

CLEAVERS

cleavers
(Galium aparine)

Parts used: Aerial parts of plant

Benefits: Another common garden weed, cleavers is often found growing near chickweed; the two are often combined in formulas. Both are mild, safe diuretics and both tone and soothe irritations of the kidneys and urinary tract. In addition, cleavers is an excellent lymphatic cleanser and is often used as a safe, effective remedy for swollen glands, tonsillitis, and some tumors.

Suggested uses: The fresh tender greens are delicious in salads. They can be juiced or blended with pineapple juice and are often made into salves. Cleavers doesn't dry or store well, so to preserve it for future use, it is best to tincture it fresh.

coltsfoot *(Tussilago farfara)*

Parts used: Leaves

Benefits: Coltsfoot was so popular in medieval times that it was chosen as the emblem to identify the local apothecary. The plant's genus name, *Tussilago*, means "cough dispeller," and, indeed, coltsfoot has long been cherished as a remedy for coughs, colds, and bronchial congestion. It is an antiasthmatic and expectorant, helping dilate the bronchioles and expel mucus.

Suggested uses: Coltsfoot makes an excellent tea; it is best combined with other lung herbs such as comfrey, elecampane, mullein, and nettle.

Caution: There are some safety concerns about coltsfoot because it has been found to contain PLAs (pyrrolizidine alkaloids, substances that have been linked to fatal liver disease). However, studies have been inadequate and inconclusive. Since coltsfoot has been used safely and effectively for hundreds of years, I continue to use it.

comfrey *(Symphytum officinale)*

Parts used: Leaves and roots

Benefits: Rich in allantoin and mucilage, comfrey is highly valued for its soothing qualities and is a common ingredient in poultices, salves, and ointments. It facilitates and activates the healing of damaged tissue. It is one of the best herbs for treating torn ligaments, strains, bruises, and any injury to the bones or joints.

Suggested uses: Comfrey root and the leaf have similar properties; the root is stronger, but the leaf is more palatable. Use them both in salves and ointments. When served as a tea, comfrey will soothe inflammation in the tissues. The root is decocted, the leaf infused. Comfrey can also be administered via capsules.

Caution: Comfrey was widely used by herbalists in the 1960s and '70s, but studies a few years ago found traces of PLAs in the plant. However, the studies were never conclusive. I'm so absolutely convinced that comfrey is safe that I continue to use it personally, though I don't recommend it to others. You must make the choice for yourself.

corn silk *(Zea mays)*

Part used: The golden, not brown, silk of corn

Benefits: Corn silk, the flower pistils from maize, has long been used as a urinary tonic. It has antiseptic, diuretic, and demulcent actions on the urinary system. It stimulates and cleans urinary passages while soothing inflammation. It is among the most effective herbs for treating bedwetting and incontinence.

Suggested uses: To help strengthen the urinary system, drink corn silk tea during the day, ceasing 3 to 4 hours before bedtime. Take corn silk tincture just before bedtime to help prevent bed-wetting.

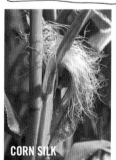
CORN SILK

Note: Corn silk will not often cure bed-wetting on its own. For maximum effectiveness, it should be used in conjunction with other therapeutic treatments, such as counseling and kegel exercises. I also recommend testing for allergies, as they can play a role in the development of this dysfunction.

Be sure that the corn silk you use is from an organic source; most corn available in supermarkets has been heavily treated with pesticides.

crampbark *(Viburnum opulus)*

Parts used: Bark, young stems

Benefits: An incredible uterine nervine, crampbark is remarkably effective for relaxing the uterine muscles. It is one of my favorite remedies for menstrual cramps, and I've also found it to be invaluable in cases of threatened miscarriage due to nerve stress and uterine tension. Dr. Christopher, among the most famous of herb doctors, claimed that crampbark is "possibly the best female regulator-relaxant that we have for the uterus and ovaries, and it is especially useful for painful and difficult menstruation and for nervous afflictions during pregnancy that threaten abortion."

Suggested uses: Like valerian, crampbark is rich in valerianic acid and is sedating and relaxing; however, its actions are specific to the reproductive system. It is also rich in tannins and is often recommended as a tonic and remedial herb for women — especially menopausal women — who bleed excessively during their menstrual cycle.

damiana *(Turnera aphrodisiaca)*

Parts used: Leaves

Benefits: Though damiana has a strong reputation as an herb of passion and romance, I include it in my list of favorite longevity herbs because it is completely restorative; it restores exhausted nerves, exhausted dreams, and exhausted spirit. It will help restore sexual vitality; its species name, *aphrodisiaca,* is a sure giveaway. Damiana has long been known to strengthen the reproductive systems of both men and women.

Its nervine and toning properties make damiana a good general herb for the nervous system, as well, and as a relaxant and antidepressant. It is also a favorite herb to use for dream work. It stimulates and promotes one's ability to remember dreams and often will promote colorful, though not always positive, dreamlike states.

Suggested uses: Use in cases of diminished sexual vitality, impotence, infertility, nervous exhaustion, anxiety and depression associated with sexual factors, and muscle and nerve exhaustion, as well as for dream therapy. Damiana is most often administered in tincture or capsule form. It is also very effective as tea but should be blended with other, more tasty herbs, such as oats and lemon balm, because of its bitter flavor. The most delicious way to take it is the famous Damiana Chocolate Love Liqueur (see the recipe on page 245).

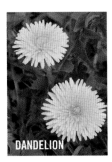

DANDELION

dandelion

(Taraxacum officinale)

Parts used: Leaves, roots, and flowers

Benefits: Dandelion is, I'm convinced, one of the great tonic herbs of all times. The entire plant is restorative and rejuvenating. The root is a prized digestive bitter. It is particularly stimulating to the liver, inducing the flow of bile and cleaning the hepatic system. Dandelion root is also considered one of the safest and most effective diuretics. It tones the kidneys and aids in proper water elimination while maintaining appropriate potassium levels. The jagged leaves are high in vitamins and minerals, including calcium, magnesium, iron, and vitamins A and C, and the flowers make a delicious wine.

Suggested uses: Dandelion is both a food and a medicine. The young, tender roots can be added to stir-fries, soups, and casseroles. They are bitter, so don't add more than a few. They can also be decocted and served as a tonic tea. The leaves, also bitter, are either infused for tea, steamed, or added raw to salads. Marinated in oil and vinegar, they are almost tamed of their bitterness. My favorite way to eat the leaves is to steam them, then marinate them overnight in Italian dressing and honey. Oh, my — this is good!

dill *(Anethum graveolens)*

Parts used: Primarily the seeds, but leaves are also useful

Benefits: Dill is a good digestive aid, and it has an even greater reputation for expelling gas.

Suggested uses: Use dill as a culinary herb. You can also grind and encapsulate the seeds or brew them in teas for their colic- and gas-relieving properties.

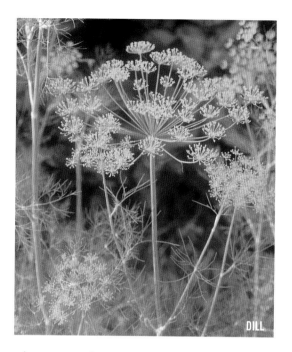

DILL

dong quai *(Angelica sinensis)*

Part used: Root

Benefits: Dong quai is one of the most useful female tonic herbs. It has often been called the "the female ginseng," though women and men can use either herb successfully. Used over time, dong quai is excellent for strengthening and balancing the uterus. It is nourishing to the blood and has a mild stimulating and cleansing action on the liver. Though it has no specific hormonal action, through its positive action on the liver and endocrine system it exerts a regulating and normalizing influence on hormonal production.

Suggested uses: Dong quai is recommended for almost every gynecological imbalance because of its strengthening and building qualities. Use for menstrual irregularities, for dysmenorrhea, and for delayed or absent menses.

Caution: Dong quai may stimulate menstrual bleeding and is not recommended during menstruation or for the duration of pregnancy. If you take dong quai over an extended period, discontinue its use one week before the onset of menses, resuming after menstruation has ceased.

echinacea *(Echinacea angustifolia, E. purpurea, and E. pallida)*

Parts used: Roots, leaves, and flowers

Benefits: This immune-system booster is one of the most important herbs of our times. Echinacea was listed in the United States Pharmacopeia until 1950, but it had fallen out of favor in this country until it was rediscovered in the mid-1970s by a group of errant herbalists. Though incredibly effective, it is not known to have any side effects or residual buildup in the body. Echinacea works by increasing macrophage T-cell activity, thereby boosting the body's first line of defense against colds, flus, and many other illnesses. It is used as a preventive as well as a curative. Though potent and strong, it is 100 percent safe for children, the elderly, and everyone in between. Contrary to what many believe, not only the root of the plant but also

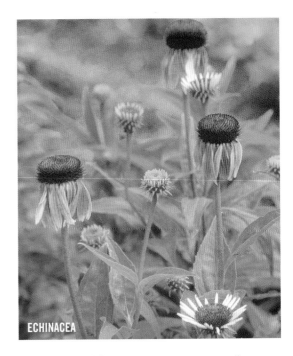

ECHINACEA

the leaves and flowers are very potent and enhance immune functions.

Suggested uses: Most of the compounds in echinacea are water soluble, so it makes a fine tea. The roots are prepared as a decoction; the aerial part of the plant is infused. The entire plant can also be used to make a tincture. Echinacea is active in dried form and can be powdered and encapsulated, or the powder added directly to food or drinks. My favorite way to use it is to nibble on the young buds and leaves fresh from the garden throughout the growing season. Fresh echinacea produces a tingling, numbing sensation on the tongue.

Take echinacea in frequent small doses in tea or tincture form to boost immunity at the first sign of a cold or flu or to treat a bronchial infection. Echinacea tea is also useful as a spray for sore throats. For sore gums and mouth inflammation, make a mouthwash from the root, with peppermint or spearmint essential oil added for flavor.

Note: Echinacea's effectiveness will decrease if it is used continuously. It is best to use it in cycles, generally 5 days on, 2 days off, repeated until the infection or illness has corrected itself.

At-risk warning: Because of the huge demand for echinacea, it is being poached mercilessly from its wild habitats. *E. pallida* and *E. angustifolia* are primarily harvested from the wild and are rapidly becoming scarce in their entire native range. Therefore, I recommend using only organically cultivated echinacea. *E. purpurea*, in particular, not only is easy to propagate in a variety of habitats but also is an exceptionally handsome plant, gracing any garden setting.

elder *(Sambucus nigra)*

Parts used: Berries and flowers

Benefits: Elder flower syrup is Europe's most esteemed formula for colds, flus, and upper respiratory infections. Both the flowers and the berries are powerful diaphoretics; by inducing sweating, they reduce fevers. Elder also has immune-enhancing properties and is especially effective when combined with echinacea.

Suggested uses: There are several varieties of elder; use the variety that produces blue berries. Elderberries make some of the best syrups and wines you'll ever taste. The flowers are often used in teas to treat fever and are the main ingredient in elder flower water, a traditional cosmetic wash. Elder flowers are also edible; every summer, I collect the large, flat clusters and make a few elder flower fritters as a treat. They are delicious served with elderberry jam, itself another magnificent method for enjoying this plant's good medicine.

the popularity contest

Echinacea is the most researched plant in the modern world. Though it is native to the North American continent and was used by the native peoples here for hundreds, if not thousands, of years, most of the recent research on echinacea has been conducted in Germany. Commonly known as purple coneflower, echinacea is one of the greatest medicinal plants and probably the single most popular plant in the marketplace. Though there are nine species of echinacea native to North America (several are endangered), only three are commonly sold in natural foods stores.

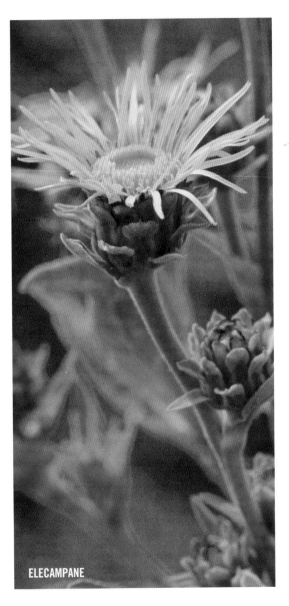

ELECAMPANE

elecampane *(Inula helenium)*

Parts used: Roots

Benefits: A giant, sunny, sunflower-like plant, elecampane is beautiful in any garden, and it's easy to grow. As an expectorant and stimulating tonic, it is often recommended for coughs, bronchitis, asthma, chronic lung ailments, and even tuberculosis. Elecampane is one of my favorite herbs for treating wet, mucus-type bronchial infections.

Suggested uses: Elecampane root can be decocted for tea; it tastes somewhat acrid and bitter, so first-time users may prefer to take it as a tincture. Combine it with echinacea to combat deep-seated bronchial infections.

eucalyptus *(Eucalyptus globulus)*

Parts used: Leaves and essential oil

Benefits: Eucalyptus is a strikingly beautiful tree native to Australia, where it has a long history of medicinal use. It was a favorite remedy of the Australian aborigines, who used it to treat colds, fevers, and coughs, and was highly prized for its aromatic oil. Eucalyptus is used in much the same manner today.

Eucalyptus is an ingredient in Vicks VapoRub and other over-the-counter medications for coughs and colds, and many of us have strong memories of eucalyptus-scented days when we were home sick in bed as children. It can also be found in throat lozenges and cough remedies.

Eucalyptus is excellent for treating respiratory colds and coughs. The essential oil is among its most important medicinal constituents and is a strong, broad-based antibiotic, antibacterial agent. The tree is also rich in tannin, resin, and flavonoid compounds.

Suggested uses: Add the essential oil to a hot bath or use as a steam inhalant for colds and respiratory infections; this is an excellent remedy for sinus infections. Added to a salve base, the essential oil makes an effective chest rub for respiratory infections. The oil can also be applied topically as a disinfectant and antibiotic cleanser. Infuse the leaves and use the tea as a gargle for sore throats; you can also combine the leaves in a tea with coltsfoot and peppermint for relieving a cold.

fennel *(Foeniculum vulgare)*

Parts used: Primarily the seeds, but the leaves and flowers are useful as well

Benefits: A well-known carminative and digestive aid, fennel was used by early Greek physicians to increase and enrich milk flow in nursing mothers. It is also an antacid, which both neutralizes excess acids in the stomach and intestines and clears uric acid from the joints. More generally, it stimulates digestion, regulates appetite, and relieves flatulence.

Suggested uses: Fennel tea not only is tasty but can help relieve colic, improve digestion, and

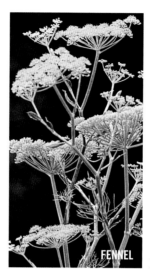

FENNEL

expel gas from the system. Nursing mothers can drink 2 to 4 cups daily to increase and enrich their flow of milk. Use a wash of warm fennel tea for conjunctivitis and other eye inflammations. Because of its delightful licorice-like taste, fennel is a useful flavoring agent for less tasty herbs.

fenugreek *(Trigonella foenum-graecum)*

Parts used: Seeds

Benefits: One of the earliest medicines mentioned in the recorded annals of herbalism, fenugreek seeds are rich in oil and mucilage and can be used to soothe irritated membranes in the throat and stomach. They are exceptionally nourishing and are used to treat debilitating and wasting disorders. The seeds also help regulate blood sugar levels.

Suggested uses: Because of its bitter flavor, fenugreek will definitely have to be formulated with other herbs to make it palatable. Combine fenugreek seeds with other, more pleasant-tasting herbs to create a tea for sore, irritated throats and digestive tracts. Nursing mothers can take fenugreek tea to help enrich the flow of their milk.

the feverfew migraine fix

I prefer to blend feverfew with lavender and other nervine herbs for an effective remedy for migraine relief. Pour 1 quart of boiling water over 1 ounce of feverfew flowers and leaves; add other desired herbs. Let steep for 20 minutes, covered tightly. Strain and drink ¼ cup every 30 minutes until the headache is gone.

When using a tincture of feverfew, dilute ¼ teaspoon in ½ cup of warm water or lemon balm tea every hour until the headache is cleared.

feverfew *(Tanacetum parthenium)*

Parts used: Leaves and flowers

Benefits: Recent pharmacological studies have proved this plant's remarkable value in alleviating migraine headaches, common headaches, inflammation, and stress-related tension. In 1772, an American herbalist wrote, "In the worst headache, this herb exceeds whatever else is known." Parthenolide, feverfew's active ingredient, controls chemicals in the body responsible for producing allergic reactions. It also inhibits the production of prostaglandins that are implicated in inflammation, swelling, and PMS.

Suggested uses: Though feverfew will help alleviate the pain of an active migraine, it is far more effective when taken over a period of 1 to 3 months as a preventive. Its action is similar to that of aspirin, with a stronger but slower effect. Some people find that eating a fresh leaf or two a day directly from the garden helps prevent migraines. Parthenolide is highly sensitive to heat and will be easily destroyed if feverfew is exposed to high heat in the drying or preparation process. If the product you are using is not effective, try another brand.

Caution: Feverfew can be taken over a long period of time by most people with no side effects; however, it does require some cautionary measures. Since one of feverfew's medicinal actions is to promote menstruation, it may stimulate the menstrual cycle unnecessarily or promote cramping and painful menstruation. It also is not recommended for pregnant women or for people taking anticoagulant drugs.

fo-ti *(Polygonum multiflorum)*

Parts used: Roots

Benefits: Of all the classic Chinese tonic and longevity herbs, fo-ti, also known as ho shou wu, is the most renowned and one of my personal favorites. It is said to restore vitality and purportedly will restore original color to hair that has gone gray, though I've yet to see this. This is one of the herbs that have been used for hundreds of years by millions of people to increase vitality and inner strength. It was one of master herbalist Li Ch'ing Yuen's favorite herbs; he is said to have consumed it daily, combined with ginseng, lycium berries, and other famous tonic herbs.

As with many of the longevity herbs, fo-ti has a solid reputation for enhancing sexual energy, increasing sperm count in men, and strengthening fertility cycles in women. It is specific for cleansing the liver and strengthens kidney chi, or energy. Though a great tonic and energizer, it is relaxing and is useful during times of stress and anxiety. Modern studies have shown fo-ti to contain resveratrol and lecithin, two compounds that have a beneficial effect on cholesterol levels and enhance circulatory function.

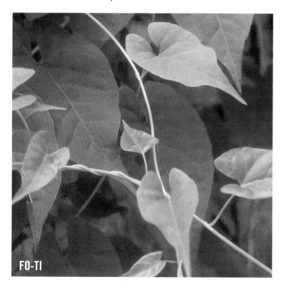
FO-TI

Suggested uses: Fo-ti is best when consumed on a regular basis. It is excellent when combined with astragalus, burdock root, ginseng, and lycium berries. It can be used in tea or as capsules. I powder fo-ti and companion herbs, such as ginseng, licorice, cinnamon, and cardamom, and mix them into a paste with honey. I eat the mixture daily on toast, on crackers, or sometimes right from the spoon. Quite tasty!

garlic *(Allium sativum)*

Parts used: Bulbs

Benefits: Garlic is one of the oldest remedies known to humans. Its sulfur and volatile oils make it a potent internal and external antiseptic. It stimulates the body's immune system and is a well-known vermifuge, used for expelling intestinal worms in humans and animals. It is very effective for maintaining healthy blood cholesterol levels and lowering high blood pressure. And if all that healing power weren't enough, garlic is just plain tasty.

Suggested uses: The best way to take advantage of garlic's potent healing powers is to add it to your meals. According to the latest studies, and contrary to popular opinion, garlic's active ingredients may diminish a bit with cooking, but they are still present, so go ahead and add it to your stir-fries, sauces, soups, and other dishes. I like to tincture garlic, pickle it (with tamari and vinegar), and make herbal oils with it.

gentian *(Gentiana lutea)*

Parts used: Roots

Benefits: Gentian may well be the most highly regarded digestive bitter tonic in Europe. It has been used for centuries in bitters formulas, including the famed Angostura bitters. Gentian root promotes the secretion of bile, saliva, and gastric juices and has a tonifying effect on the gastrointestinal system. It is often recommended to stimulate the appetite and improve digestion. In addition, gentian is a good source of iron.

Suggested uses: Combine gentian with other digestive and warming herbs, such as cardamom, cinnamon, fennel, and ginger, to make a bitter digestive tonic. For maximum effect, take digestive bitters 30 minutes before meals.

Caution: Gentian is not recommended for people with ulcers or stomach inflammation or irritation.

At-risk warning: Gentian is on the United Plant Savers "at risk" list and is considered an endangered plant by many global conservation groups. Never buy any products that contain wildcrafted gentian. If a product's label doesn't say ORGANICALLY CULTIVATED GENTIAN, leave it on the shelf.

ginger *(Zingiber officinale)*

Parts used: Roots

Benefits: Ginger is prized both for its delicious flavor and for its remarkable healing powers. It is one of the classic herbs of traditional Chinese medicine. It is highly regarded as a primary herb for the reproductive, respiratory, and digestive systems. It is one of the main ingredients in reproductive tonics for men and women and helps improve poor circulation to the pelvis; it is my favorite remedy for cramps. It is a safe and often effective herb for morning sickness and motion sickness — without unpleasant side effects. Ginger is also a good diaphoretic that opens up the pores and promotes sweat. It improves digestion and helps the body efficiently move out waste.

Suggested uses: Ginger is excellent in stir-fries and Asian-inspired dishes. Grated ginger with lemon and honey makes a delicious tea. Ginger is rich in volatile oils, and as a tea, even though it's a root, it is best infused. Try making ginger syrup; it is simply delicious. A particularly pleasant way to enjoy your "medicine" is to suck on candied ginger. For cramps and stomach tension, apply hot poultices of ginger over the pelvis.

ginkgo *(Ginkgo biloba)*

Parts used: Leaves and fruit

Benefits: Though the fruits and seeds of the venerable ginkgo tree are considered to have medicinal value, it is the fan-shaped leaves that are most often used. Historical evidence from China suggesting that the leaf can be used to improve brain function is supported by more than 40 years of clinical research in Europe. Ginkgo leaf is one of the best herbs for enhancing memory, vitality, and circulation. I suggest it as a regular tonic herb for everybody over 45. The active ingredients of ginkgo leaf improve circulation and vasodilatation. Though this action is evidenced throughout the body, it is most noted in the cerebral region. It is a promising remedy for age-related declines in brain function such as Alzheimer's, strokes, and short- or long-term memory loss. Ginkgo is also an antioxidant and is useful against free radicals, substances that damage cellular health and accelerate aging.

While most of the literature written about ginkgo focuses on its great memory-enhancing qualities, some of its other outstanding features are often overlooked. Ginkgo is one of the best herbs for the circulatory system; it serves as a cardiac tonic by increasing the strength of the arterial walls. It also reduces inflammation in the blood vessels and helps prevent platelet aggregation and blood clotting that can lead to blocked arteries. It is one of the best herbs available for promoting blood flow and oxygenation throughout the body. It is also an excellent herb for treating vertigo and is an effective remedy for tinnitus, or ringing in the ear. It has proved to be an excellent treatment for arterial erectile dysfunction.

Suggested uses: Some studies suggest that ginkgo doesn't break down in water, but I have found it wonderfully effective as a tea. And since herbalists throughout the ages have used it primarily in a

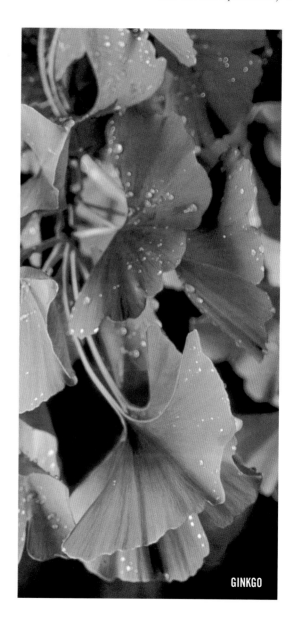

GINKGO

water base, I'm unsure how those studies arrived at that conclusion. As a tea for improving memory, ginkgo blends well with sage, rosemary, and gotu kola. For a circulatory tea, blend ginkgo with hawthorn and lemon balm. For stress and anxiety, especially when it's mental worry, blend ginkgo with oats and nettle.

You'll often find standardized ginkgo products on the market, and I would recommend these, as well as tea and whole-plant tincture. Ginkgo works as a nutrient, not a drug, so it must be used with consistency, and in adequate amounts, for several weeks or months before any benefit is noticed.

a prehistoric plant

Ginkgo is the sole remaining survivor of the oldest known tree genus, *Ginkgoaceae*, which dates back more than 200 million years. In fact, there are fossil remains of ginkgo that date to the dinosaur era. This is certainly a plant that can teach us about aging gracefully. An excellent brain food and memory enhancer, perhaps ginkgo works in part because it holds the memories of an entire species — indeed, an entire age — in the cellular makeup of its being.

ginseng, american
(Panax quinquefolius)

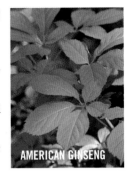

AMERICAN GINSENG

Parts used: Roots

Benefits: This is one of my favorite woodland plants, though it's difficult to find in its native habitat these days. Connoisseurs of ginseng consider American ginseng the best variety in the world, and Asian practitioners often prefer it. Though used similarly to Asian ginseng, it differs in chemical makeup and energetics. While Asian ginseng is warming and builds energy and heat in the body, *quinquefolius* is more neutral in its effects and tends to cool and soothe the system, making it a better choice for many American men. It has the same tonic, adaptogenic effects as the Asian variety and has a long history as a restorative and building herb.

American ginseng is a balancing tonic for the entire body. It helps restore energy if used over a period of time. Use it to treat general debilitation, to augment mental clarity, and as an excellent adaptogenic herb to tone the entire system. It can also be used to treat anemia and other blood weaknesses and is good for exhaustion and for sexual inadequacy, especially when due to exhaustion or stress.

Suggested uses: Roots should be at least five or six years old, and the older, the better. Prepare the

the versatility of ginseng

In Shen Nung's materia medica from A.D. 196, ginseng was described as "a tonic to the five viscera: quieting the spirits, establishing the soul, allaying fear, expelling evil effluvia, brightening the eyes, opening the heart, benefiting the understanding, and, if taken for some time, invigorating the body and prolonging life."

However, in the early 1980s an American study cited ginseng as the cause of digestive disorders, hypertension, and general malaise. Called GAS (Ginseng Abuse Syndrome), this "discovered" condition baffled longtime users of ginseng. Shortly after the report was released, it was found that the studies had been badly flawed. Much of the herb material being tested was, in fact, not ginseng at all but a type of *Rumex* found growing in the prairies of the United States.

same as described for Asian varieties, below. It has a wonderful bittersweet flavor and can be chewed.

At-risk warning: Wild American ginseng is considered at risk in most of its native habitat. It is important to verify where your roots are coming from. Use only organically cultivated or woods-grown ginseng (ginseng that has been planted and tended in woodland settings). It's futile to try to become healthier using herbs that may themselves be suffering as a result of overharvesting and habitat destruction.

ginseng, asian *(Panax ginseng)*

Parts used: Roots

Benefits: Considered the king of all tonics, ginseng boasts one of the best reputations in the herbal kingdom. Its genus name, *Panax,* is Greek for "cure-all," and the herb has long been renowned as a male tonic. Often the older roots grow in the shape of men. Much of what is touted about ginseng — its incredible potency and healing powers — is true, if you use good-quality, mature roots. There are many varieties of *Panax* ginseng on the market (Asian, Korean, and Chinese); all of them are superior adaptogenic agents that help the body resist a wide spectrum of illnesses.

Asian ginseng is often sold as either "white" or "red" ginseng. Red ginseng is really white ginseng that has been slowly steamed, cured, and dried. The steaming process affects the ginsenosides, active ingredients of ginseng, and makes red ginseng more stimulating than its white counterpart. Red ginseng is frequently given to people who have low energy.

When used over a period of time, ginseng revitalizes and restores energy and is especially good for building sexual vitality. Though it is most often associated with the male reproductive system, I've found ginseng to be equally good for women, especially women who need the "yang" (masculine) or grounding energy it's famous for. Ginseng rejuvenates the entire nervous system, regenerates frayed or overtaxed nerves, and discourages mood swings and depression. It rebuilds and restores energy if used consistently over a 3- to 4-month period.

Suggested uses: Ginseng roots should be at least 5 to 6 years old; the older, the better. They have a fine, bittersweet, robust flavor. Many people enjoy simpy chewing on the fresh "sing root." Sliced and soaked in honey, it makes a tasty treat. A classic preparation is a strong decoction of a high-quality mature root. It blends well with many other tonic nervine herbs, such as astragalus, burdock, dandelion, fo-ti, ginger, and nettle, to make a delicious concoction that can be used directly in tea or spread on crackers (see Longevity Tonic, page 38). I especially enjoy it served with ginger and cinnamon in a chai blend (see Longevity Chai, page 38). Ginseng extracts and capsules are readily available, but because of its good flavor and ease of preparation, I suggest using ginseng in powder form, cooking the roots in soups, and making tea with this granddaddy of all herbs.

Caution: Though ginseng is an excellent restorative tonic, it can sometimes produce too much heat or congestion in the body, especially in those who tend toward hypertension. I have found ginseng to be counterproductive in Type A personalities.

Much of the Asian ginseng imported into this country and those Asian roots grown here are heavily sprayed with toxic substances. In one recent undercover operation, the U.S.D.A. found more than 36 illegal toxic substances in roots harvested in Wisconsin. If the roots look large, overly plump, and whitish, be suspicious of their quality. Buy only woods-grown or organically cultivated ginseng.

which ginseng should i use?

I prefer using Siberian (eleuthero) rather than *Panax* varieties of ginseng, both because I find that it works as well and because, unlike Asian and American varieties, it grows readily and in great abundance. Though not much eleuthero is cultivated in the United States, I've seen healthy specimens growing in parks and arboretums in the Northeast, suggesting that there are possibilities for commercial cultivation.

ginseng, siberian
(Eleutherococcus senticosus)

Parts used: Roots and bark

Benefits: Siberian ginseng, also called eleuthero, has almost the same properties as its cousin, *Panax* ginseng. It's a superior adaptogenic herb with an impressive range of health benefits. It has a long history of stimulating male virility and is commonly employed as a tonic for the reproductive systems of men.

Siberian ginseng helps produce a state of nonspecific resistance against an underlying imbalance, regardless of the specific nature of the stressor. This is one of our best herbs for increasing endurance and stamina and for building and enhancing our resistance to stress factors, whether emotional, physical, or psychological.

Suggested uses: The flavor of eleuthero is rather inconspicuous and blends well with other tonic and adaptogenic herbs in tea. I also frequently use the powder in foods and candies. The roots are an important ingredient in wines and elixirs. For best results, use it over a period of time, several weeks to a few months.

goldenseal *(Hydrastis canadensis)*

Parts used: Roots and leaves

Benefits: This is possibly one of the most useful and valuable plants of North America. Particularly effective at healing mucous membranes, goldenseal is used in cleansing washes

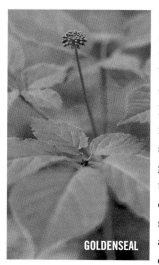

GOLDENSEAL

for the eye, as a douche for infections (careful; it can be too drying for the vagina if not formulated correctly), in mouthwashes for sore mouths and gums, and in the topical treatment of eczema and psoriasis. It is a natural antibiotic and is often combined with echinacea to help fight infections and ward off colds and flus. Goldenseal also is strongly bitter and is often used as a bitter tonic and as a digestive aid.

Suggested uses: To make a bitter tea, infuse (instead of decocting) the root. The tea can be used as a mouthwash for gum infections and as a wash for cuts. The root is often powdered and used in poultices for infections, abscesses, and wounds.

Caution: If used continually over long periods, goldenseal becomes an irritant to the mucous membranes, causing inflammation and irritation. Do not take for longer than 3 weeks at a time.

At-risk warning: Use only organically cultivated varieties of this endangered plant. If you have woodlands, grow your own goldenseal.

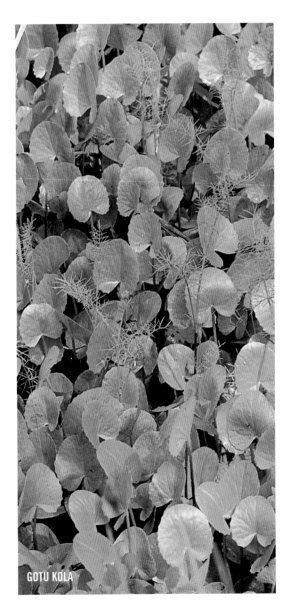

GOTU KOLA

gotu kola *(Centella asiatica)*

Parts used: Leaves

Benefits: This beautiful violet-like plant is native to tropical and subtropical regions of the world. It grows easily in the warmer areas of the United States or can be grown in greenhouses for a daily fresh supply of the tasty little leaves.

Gotu kola is one of my favorite herbs for nourishing the brain; I use it frequently combined with ginkgo. It is especially recommended for memory loss. Considered one of the best nerve tonics, it has been used successfully in treatment programs for epilepsy, schizophrenic behavior, and Alzheimer's disease. It is superb in formulas for nervous stress and debility. It gently but firmly increases mental alertness and vitality by feeding and nourishing the brain. Gotu kola also improves the body's nonspecific response to disease and stress.

Suggested uses: I prefer to use gotu kola as a tincture to strengthen memory function. It must be used consistently for at least 4 to 6 weeks before a difference is noticed. What should you expect? Well, you won't wake up one morning feeling like Einstein. Rather, you may experience a subtle but noticeable increase in memory and a pleasant feeling of being more mentally alert.

Fresh gotu kola is quite tasty and can be served raw as a salad green or infused as a tea.

Caution: Most of the gotu kola available commercially is of very poor quality. I recommend that, if possible, you grow this important herb or purchase only organically grown gotu kola from reliable sources.

hawthorn *(Crataegus oxyacantha* and *C. monogyna)*

Parts used: Leaves, flowers, berries, and tips of branches

Benefits: Hawthorn may well be the herb supreme for the heart, and a healthy heart is essential to a long and productive life. The flowers, berries, tips of branches, and leaves nourish, strengthen, and tone the heart muscle and its blood vessels. As a tonic for the heart, it has the amazing ability to either gently stimulate or depress the heart's activity as needed.

Hawthorn dilates arteries and veins, allowing blood to flow more freely and releasing cardiovascular constrictions and blockages. It lowers blood pressure and also helps maintain healthy cholesterol levels. Hawthorn is outstanding both for preventing heart problems and for treating heart disease, edema, angina, and heart arrhythmia. It is another of those herbs, along with ginkgo and saw palmetto, that I suggest regularly for men over 45. Because of its strong concentrations of bioflavonoids, hawthorn is an effective antioxidant and is used to fight free radicals in the system.

Though it is little is mentioned in literature, hawthorn is also a wonderful remedy for "broken hearts" and for depression and anxiety. It is a spe-

The **hawthorn tree** has been planted in or near most herb gardens throughout Europe and has been revered and surrounded by legend for centuries. When my grandmother came to this country, she planted hawthorns in the yard of each home she lived in. Many of those old hawthorns planted by her strong, worn hands still bloom.

cific medicine for those who have a difficult time expressing their feelings or who suppress their emotions. Hawthorn helps the heart flower, open, and be healed.

Suggested uses: Hawthorn is a tonic herb and should be used over a period of time to be effective. Use in the form of tea, tincture, capsules, syrup, and jam or jelly. The general dose would be 3 to 4 cups of tea a day, 1 teaspoon of the tincture three times daily, or 2 capsules three times daily. However, hawthorn tastes so good that I generally recommend more culinary-style preparations, such as jam, jelly, and liqueur, which taste exquisite and retain all of the herb's nourishing benefits. Hawthorn berry jam, in particular, is delicious and readily available in grocery stores, as well as pharmacies. Spread it on crackers and consume to your heart's delight.

Hawthorn berries also make a delicious tea and are often combined with lemon balm and oats for hypertension. Another treatment for high blood pressure is a tea made of hawthorn leaves, berries, or flowers combined with yarrow and motherwort. Hawthorn berries, leaves, and flowers are also excellent combined with ginkgo leaves as a vascular tonic.

Caution: I have found hawthorn perfectly safe to use in combination with heart medication, but if you decide to do so, first consult with your health care practitioner.

hibiscus *(Hibiscus sabdariffa)*

Parts used: Flowers

Benefits: High in vitamin C and bioflavonoids, hibiscus has slightly astringent properties. It is useful for treating mild colds, flus, bruising, and swelling.

Suggested uses: This is the plant that made Celestial Seasonings famous. The large tropical hibiscus flowers make a beautiful ruby red tea. The flavor is somewhat tart, with a sweet aftertaste.

hops *(Humulus lupulus)*

Parts used: Strobiles (the leaf bracts surrounding the tiny flowers) and pollen

Benefits: Where I grew up, in the beautiful hills of northern California, the surrounding area was

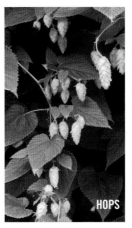

HOPS

planted in hops. It is a beautiful plant whose gold-dusted strobiles blossom in the late summer and hang from a golden green vine. It is these strobiles that contain the inconspicuous green flowers and the golden pollen grains that are the medicinal parts of the plant. Rich in lupulin, volatile oils, resins, and bitters, hops is a potent medicinal herb highly valued for its relaxing effect on the nervous system. It is my favorite remedy for insomnia. It is especially useful for hypertension and eases tension and anxiety in men, as well as decreasing excessive sexual desire. Hops is one of the most potent bitters and is excellent as a digestive bitter. It's especially useful for indigestion due to nervous energy and anxiety.

Suggested uses: Hops is extremely bitter. Nothing really disguises the taste well, so hops is generally tinctured or encapsulated. It is also a fine medicine when made into beer, serving as both a sedative and a digestive bitter. Be sure the beer is of high quality, or grow the hops and make your own brew.

To treat insomnia, I prefer to mix tinctures of hops and valerian. Take a dose a couple of hours before bedtime. Keep the tincture bottle by the bedside. If you wake up in the middle of the night, take several more large dropperfuls diluted in a bit of warm water.

To aid in balancing excessive sexual drive, take ½ teaspoon of hops tincture diluted in warm water three or four times a day.

You can make your own digestive bitters by combining hops with other bitter herbs, such as mugwort, motherwort, artichocke leaf, dandelion root, and yellow dock; prepare as a tincture, following the instructions on page 384. Take ½ teaspoon of the tincture before meals.

Caution: Because it has such strong sedative properties, hops is not recommended in large dosages for those suffering from depression.

kava-kava *(Piper methysticum)*

Parts used: Roots

Benefits: Kava has the unique ability to relax the body while awakening the mind. It produces a sense of relaxation and at the same time heightens awareness and makes you feel brighter. It helps reduce tension, anxiety, and stress. Its analgesic properties help alleviate pain.

Suggested uses: Kava is available as tincture, extract, and capsules. The tincture is a quick, effective, and handy form to use. It is helpful in times of stress when you need a quick relaxant, something that helps put the world in perspective. Capsules are effective for long-term stress and anxiety.

the kava cool

Native to Polynesia, Melanesia, and Micronesia, kava has been highly revered for hundreds of years in its native cultures. It played an important part in every ceremony and was served at most social functions, celebrations, inaugurations, and meetings. I have seen ads for it in newspapers, have heard people talking about it in drugstores, and have been to more than one party where the beverage of choice has been kava. It truly is a remarkable herb, and it's no wonder that it has gained such popularity here. The traditional saying is, "There can be no hate in the heart when one has kava."

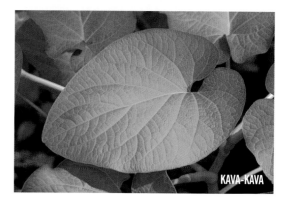

KAVA-KAVA

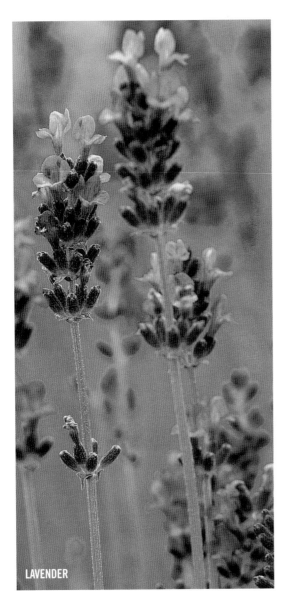

LAVENDER

The unique flavor may take some getting used to. Don't be alarmed the first time you try it; it will numb the tongue and create tingling sensations throughout the mouth. These sensations are temporary and are caused by kava's active chemical compounds, called kavalactones.

I generally prefer kava as a tea or a punch. Prepare a strong tea; add cinnamon, ginger, and cardamom for flavor. Let the tea sit several hours or overnight, then strain. Add pineapple juice and coconut milk for flavor and serve chilled. I've served this kava punch at many large herbal functions. It definitely seems to elevate the spirits and brighten the mood.

Caution: Kava-kava can be overused and abused. Though an herb of celebration, it was not meant to be drunk to the point of intoxication. Too much kava can make you nauseated and induce sleepiness, impair physical coordination, and even lead to unconsciousness. There have been several cases of people arrested for driving "under the influence" who were actually not drunk but had overindulged in kava. Be respectful of the power of this herb. Used judiciously, it is a wonderful relaxant and stress reliever.

lavender (*Lavandula* spp.)

Parts used: Flowers

Benefits: Native to the Mediterranean, beautiful, fragrant, and hardy, lavender blesses us with a range of uses. It is a strong nervine and a mild antidepressant, and it offers great relief for headache sufferers. Combined with feverfew, it helps alleviate migraines. It is one of the best herbs to add to the bath for alleviating tension, stress, and insomnia. The essential oil is excellent for soothing insect bites, bee stings, and burns (mix with honey).

Suggested uses: Add small amounts of lavender to tea (use just a pinch, as its flavor can be over-powering). It makes a tasty glycerin- or alcohol-based tincture. Add lavender essential oil to bathwater to soothe the nerves. For headaches, apply 2 or 3 drops to the temples and nape of the neck. Apply lavender tea topically for insect bites or as a wash for cuts.

first aid in a bottle

Lavender essential oil has been called "a first-aid kit in a bottle" and can be used effectively for a number of situations. Once I was working in the garden with Lila, a student. She knelt on a bee, and the unsuspecting creature stung her quite ferociously. But Lila pulled a bottle of lavender oil from her pocket and applied a few dabs to the wound. The area hardly swelled, and she reported very little pain.

lemon balm
(Melissa officinalis)

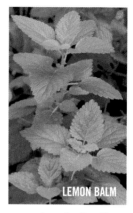
LEMON BALM

Parts used: Leaves and flowers

Benefits: Calming, antiviral, and anti-septic, this beautiful and fragrant member of the mint family is one of nature's best nervine herbs. Lemon balm's leaves and flowers contain volatile oils, tannins, and bitters that have a definite relaxing, antispasmodic effect on the stomach and nervous system. It is excellent for stomach distress and general exhaustion and can be used as a mild sedative and for insomnia. Applied topically, lemon balm has been found to be helpful for herpes. It is often made into a cream for this purpose, though I find that the tincture works as well, and the essential oil is the treatment of choice in European countries.

Suggested uses: Fresh lemon balm is most effective for medicinal preparations. It makes a delicious tea and can be served with lemon and honey throughout the day to alleviate stress and anxiety. For a delicious nervine tonic, blend equal amounts of lemon balm, oats, and chamomile. Lemon balm also makes one of the tastiest tinctures. Tinctured in a glycerin base, it makes a lovely remedy for children.

licorice *(Glycyrrhiza glabra)*

Parts used: Roots

Benefits: Sweet-tasting licorice root is an outstanding tonic for the endocrine system and is specific for the reproductive system. It is particularly effective for relieving adrenal exhaustion, which is so prevalent in those who suffer from depression. In fact, what is often classified as a midlife crisis may be closely or directly associated with adrenal exhaustion. Licorice supports the adrenals and will revitalize them if used over a period of weeks or months. It has constituents that are similar in function to the natural steroids in the human body.

Licorice is also highly regarded as a remedy for the respiratory system, and it is used as a soothing demulcent and anti-inflammatory remedy for respiratory problems.

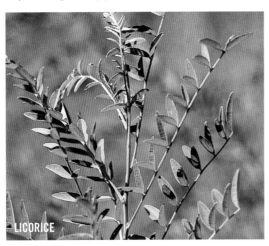

LICORICE

The effective yet delicious qualities of this herb help make it one of the most important herbal remedies for children. It is used for treating a multitude of ailments, including bronchial congestion, sore throat, coughs, and inflammation of the digestive tract (such as ulcers or nonspecific sores).

Suggested uses: Because of its extremely sweet flavor, licorice is best used with other herbs. It is an excellent harmonizer — when used in multiherb formulas, it alleviates unpleasant symptoms caused by the action of harsher herbs without interfering with their beneficial qualities. It has a rich mucilaginous consistency and adds a soothing quality to any syrup or tea it's mixed with. I use licorice powder to flavor other herbal powders and then roll them into tasty little pills and balls. Children enjoy chewing on licorice sticks.

For adrenal exhaustion, lethargy, and fatigue, drink 2 to 3 cups of tea made from licorice blended with astragalus, sarsaparilla, burdock root, and dandelion or with wild yam, sarsaparilla, burdock root, and sassafras. Licorice is often made into cough syrups for sore throats, mixed with pleurisy root and elecampane for deep-seated bronchial inflammation, and combined with marsh mallow root for digestive inflammation and ulcers.

Caution: There have been studies indicating licorice's ability to induce water retention and thus raise blood pressure levels, but most of the studies were done on licorice extracts, licorice

chinese licorice

Chinese licorice *(Glycyrrhiza uralensis),* a close relative of *Glycyrrhiza glabra,* is one of the most important herbs in Chinese herbal medicine. It is known as the "Grandfather of Chinese Herbs" and the "Great Adjunct" because it is used in so many formulas to blend and harmonize with other herbs. It is a superior longevity herb and is used to restore and revitalize the entire system. When used over a prolonged period of time, Chinese licorice is said to promote long life and produce radiant well-being.

candy, and allopathic medication — not on the whole plant or crude preparations made from licorice root. However, licorice is not recommended for individuals who have high blood pressure due to water retention. And those who are on heart medication should check with their health care provider before using licorice. Though most children don't suffer from these ailments, licorice should not be given to children who have hypertension or kidney/bladder problems, or those youngsters on steroid therapy.

Although there are many warnings against using it, it must be remembered that licorice is one of the most widely prescribed herbs in the world; there are very few reported cases of toxicity due to its use. It is generally safe for children and the elderly, which usually means it's safe for everyone in between. And licorice is particularly beneficial for weakened individuals who suffer from debilitating and wasting diseases.

lobelia *(Lobelia inflata)*

Parts used: Aerial parts of the plant, especially the seeds and leaves

Benefits: This may be one of the more maligned but useful medicinal plants we have for serious respiratory problems. Lobeline, one of lobelia's major active ingredients, has been demonstrated to stimulate the respiratory center in the brain, producing deeper and stronger breathing. It is a powerful antispasmodic herb, meaning that it relaxes the chest and opens constricted bronchial passages, and is a superb expectorant, as well as an excellent remedy for spastic or "dry" coughing and wheezing. Lobelia is among our best remedies for asthma and bronchitis. In addition, applied externally, lobelia soothes inflammations and reduces the pain of boils and rheumatism.

Lobelia was highly regarded by the early Eclectics and herbalists for its relaxing effect on the muscles, and Cascade Anderson Geller notes in *Planting the Future,* a book written by United Plant Savers, that she "knows of a number of children who have been aided in their birth process when their mothers were given a modest oral dose of lobelia extract to relax the uterus."

Lobelia has a diverse reputation and, because of its variable effects, has always caused quite a stir among herbalists. There's just one thing that everyone seems to agree on: This is one powerful herb. It is best formulated with other herbs and taken with moderate amounts of water. Otherwise, as one of its common names, pukeweed, implies, the herb will likely induce vomiting.

Suggested uses: It is always important when you're using an herb for the first time to start with small dosages, but it is especially important with lobelia. This herb has greatly varying effects on people, depending on their sensitivity to its constituents. Begin with small dosages, use the herb in formulation (with other herbs), and dilute in tea or water. Even following recommended dosages given on tincture and capsule bottles may give you unpredictable results. Three drops to ½ dropperful of tincture is a standard adult dosage.

Caution: Lobelia is not recommended during pregnancy.

At-risk warning: Because of its limited native range and its increasing popularity, lobelia is on the United Plant Savers "to watch" list. Very limited harvesting from the wild is acceptable when no alternatives are available. Whenever possible, however, use lobelia that has been organically cultivated.

lycium *(Lycium chinense)*

Parts used: Berries

Benefits: Lycium berry is one of my favorite tonic herbs. It is delicious and colorful and is said to brighten the spirits. In China, it has gained a solid reputation as a longevity herb; it was among those herbs frequently used by long-lived sages. Li Ch'ing Yuen, for example, who lived to be more than 200 years old (and proof of his age has been given by scientific study!), was reported to greatly enjoy the delicious lycium berries, which were an essential ingredient in his famed "long-life soup."

Lycium berries are a specific tonic for the liver. They are also a circulatory aid and are used as a blood tonic.

Suggested uses: A famed Chinese longevity tonic formula is the combination of equal proportions of schisandra berries and lycium berries. Making a tea from this mixture and drinking 2 to 3 cups daily over a couple of weeks is said to brighten the spirit and promote cheerfulness.

Lycii berries are quite tasty on their own; they can be eaten plain as a snack, added to breakfast cereal, and used in baking. I often substitute them for raisins in my baking; I enjoy their effects and prefer their flavor. They also add a nice touch of sweetness to tea.

For a delicious tonic beverage, soak lycium berries in fruit juice or wine. This is one of my favorite ways to "take my medicine."

marsh mallow *(Althaea officinalis)*

Parts used: Primarily the roots, but the leaves and flowers are useful

Benefits: A soothing mucilaginous herb, marsh mallow can be used much like slippery elm. However, marsh mallow is much more readily available and is easy to grow in most garden settings. It makes a good substitute for slippery elm, which is on the United Plant Savers "at risk" list, in topical applications.

Suggested uses: Serve marsh mallow as a tea for treating sore throats, diarrhea, constipation, and bronchial inflammation. Mix it into a paste with water and apply topically to soothe irritated skin. Marsh mallow can also be used in the bath as a soothing wash; combine it with oatmeal for maximum effect.

marsh mallow at the campfire?

Who would believe that the mucilaginous root of this common herb was the original marshmallow, the sticky, sugary concoction that kids love to skewer on a stick and roast over an open fire? Our pioneer parents cooked the root with honey or sugar, formed it into soft balls, and gave it to their children to suck on to soothe a sore throat.

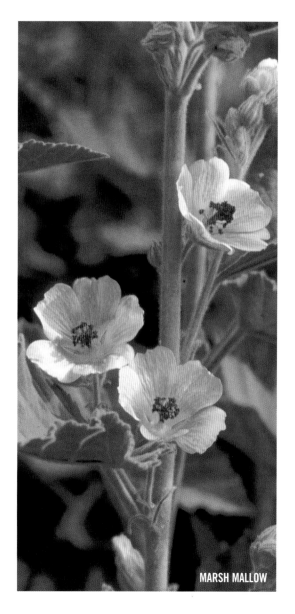

MARSH MALLOW

milk thistle *(Silybum marianum)*

Parts used: Seeds; wild-food enthusiasts enjoy the leaves as food

Benefits: Milk thistle seed is a powerful antioxidant. It helps fight the damaging effects of free radicals, ameliorating the effects of many age-related diseases. It stimulates liver function and rebuilds liver cells that have been damaged by illness, rich food, hepatitis, or alcohol consumption. The seeds are rich in a substance called silymarin, which stimulates the liver cells to regenerate through a process known as protein synthesis. Milk thistle seed has remarkable abilities to protect the liver against damaging chemicals. It is the only known substance to provide any relief from poisoning by death cap mushroom, the most virulent liver toxin known. Milk thistle seed is also helpful for the gallbladder and the kidneys.

Suggested uses: Though an amazingly powerful herb, milk thistle seed is nontoxic and can be used effectively as both a therapeutic agent and a preventive tonic herb. I've found that the most effective method to extract the active ingredients from the hard seeds of the milk thistle is to grind them in a coffee mill or smash them with a hammer. The resulting powder is tasty and can be made into a tea, added to cereal and soups, or encapsulated.

When tincturing milk thistle seed, grind the seed with some of the alcohol in a blender. This will better enable all of the healing properties of the seed to be rendered into the alcohol and start the tincturing process more quickly.

motherwort *(Leonurus cardiaca)*

Parts used: Leaves

Benefits: Motherwort is best known for its beneficial properties for women, especially for menopausal women, but it's equally beneficial as a heart tonic. Its botanical name, *Leonurus,* means "lionhearted." Motherwort is a superb tonic for nourishing and strengthening the heart muscle and its blood vessels. It is a remedy for most heart disease, neuralgia, and an overrapid heartbeat. It is valued for many women's health issues, including delayed menstruation, uterine cramps associated with scanty menses, water retention, and hot flashes and mood swings during menopause.

Suggested uses: Prepare as an infusion, flavored with tastier herbs, or as a tincture.

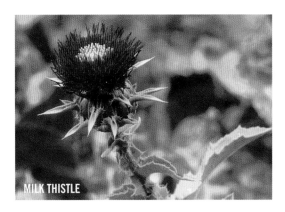

MILK THISTLE

learning from history

"My opinion is that [milk thistle] is the best remedy that grows against all melancholy diseases," John Gerard wrote in the sixth century. At that time, melancholy referred to diseases of the liver. In the 17th century, famed herbalist and astrologer Nicholas Culpeper decreed milk thistle good for "removing obstructions of the liver and gallbladder." German scientists, taking a lead from these and other early uses of the plant, began researching milk thistle in the 1970s and discovered that it contained one of the most valuable chemicals for damaged liver tissue.

muira puama *(Ptychopetalum olacoides* and *Liriosma ovata)*

Parts used: Bark

Benefits: Native to Brazil, muira puama is used as an aphrodisiac throughout South America and in Europe, and it is slowly being "discovered" in North America. It is a favorite remedy for men who are unable to attain or maintain an erection.

Muira puama may well be one of the best-kept herbal secrets; it offers tremendous benefit for those suffering from impotence and depressed sexual activity. The herb is often referred to as "potency wood" and has a long-standing reputation as a powerful aphrodisiac and nervine. Its mode of action is unknown at this time, but it seems to have no side effects. It is also used to treat dysentery, diarrhea, and other diseases for which a strong astringent is indicated.

Suggested uses: Muira puama is often combined with ashwagandha, Siberian ginseng, and circulatory herbs such as ginkgo and hawthorn to help build reproductive health and vitality. It is an excellent reproductive tonic that can be prepared as a tea, as a tincture, or in capsule form. For tea, drink 1 cup three or four times daily. For a tincture, take ½ to 1 teaspoon twice daily for several weeks. (It can be taken in more frequent doses just before lovemaking.) The general dosage recommendation for capsules is 2 capsules taken three times daily.

Caution: Muira puama is considered a tonic herb, and it doesn't seem to have any harmful side effects when used in therapeutic dosages. However, there is very little known about this herb, so be mindful as you use it. If you notice any undesirable side effects, discontinue use immediately.

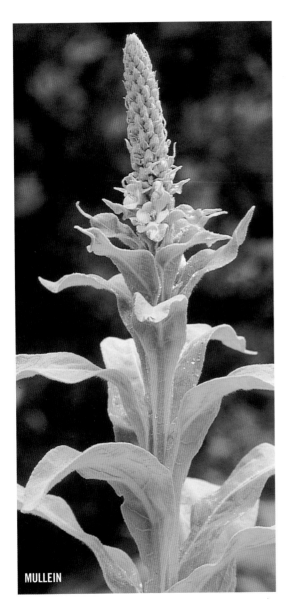

MULLEIN

mullein *(Verbascum thapsus)*

Parts used: Leaves, flowers, and roots

Benefits: Mullein is one of my favorite wayside weeds. It is a stately plant, sending its flowering stalk sometimes several feet into the sky. That stalk is full of beautiful, fragrant yellow flowers that make absolutely the best oil for ear infections. Mullein used to be called torch plant, because its long, flowering stalks were dried, dipped in fat or oil, and lit as a slow-burning torch.

The leaves are used most often, especially in cough formulas and for respiratory infections, bronchial infections, asthma, and glandular imbalances.

Suggested uses: Prepare the flowers as an infused oil for treating ear infections (see the recipe on page 82). The leaves can be prepared as a tincture or an infusion for bronchial congestion, colds, and coughs. For glandular problems, combine mullein with echinacea and cleavers.

myrrh *(Commiphora myrrha)*

Parts used: Dried resin

Benefits: Myrrh has been used as an aromatic healing plant for thousands of years. According to Christian legend, it was one of the gifts given by the wise men of the East to the baby Jesus.

An excellent herbal antiseptic with high concentrations of volatile oils, myrrh is often used, in combination with goldenseal, for treating the flu, colds, and lung congestion. It helps increase macrophage activity, thereby raising the potency of our protective shield (surface immune system). Myrrh's thick consistency helps coat the mouth and throat, making it particularly effective for sore throats and infections of the mouth, gums, sinuses, and upper respiratory system.

Suggested uses: Because it is a thick resin, myrrh is not water soluble, so it must be either used in dried powdered form or prepared as a tincture. Dilute the tincture and use it as a wash for sore throats, gingivitis, and other infections of the mouth. The powder can be used as a poultice or encapsulated and taken internally to treat mouth ulcers, gingivitis, pyorrhea, pharyngitis, sinusitis, and laryngitis. A myrrh poultice is also effective for treating boils, abrasions, and wounds.

nettle *(Urtica dioica)*

Parts used: Leaves, seeds, roots, and young tops

Benefits: This is the stinging nettle that farmers despise, hikers hate, and children learn to avoid. But herbalists around the world fall at the feet of this green goddess/green man herb. I am convinced that it is one of the superior tonic herbs and is as important as many of the famous Chinese "long life" herbs. It is a vitamin factory, rich in iron, calcium, potassium, silicon, magnesium, manganese, zinc, and chromium, as well as a host of other vitamins and minerals. One of my favorite all-around remedies, it makes a great hair and scalp tonic. It activates the metabolism by

nettles through the seasons

The tips of the nettle plant in early spring and summer are superior, though I've eaten them throughout the season. If you have a stand of nettles nearby, it is good practice to trim them constantly throughout the season so they will keep producing those tasty tops until fall.

strengthening and toning the entire system. It is useful for growing pains in young children, when their bones and joints ache (just like older folks'!). An excellent reproductive tonic for men and women, nettle is used for alleviating the symptoms of PMS and menopause. It's a superb herb for the genitourinary system and will strengthen weak kidneys, essential for vitality and energy. It is indicated for liver problems and is excellent for allergies and hay fever. All this and it tastes good, too!

Suggested uses: For any liver disorder, take nettle in tea, tincture, or capsule form. To tone the nervous system, combine nettle in a tea with lemon balm, oats, and chamomile. For reducing the symptoms of allergies and hay fever, take freeze-dried nettle capsules. For urinary health and for treating edema, drink several cups of nettle tea combined with dandelion greens. To combat reduced energy and sexual dysfunction, combine nettle in a tea with green milky oat tops and raspberry leaf. To decrease prostate enlargement, combine in a tincture with saw palmetto.

Fresh young nettle leaves have a rich green flavor. They can be used to replace spinach in any recipe, but they must always be well steamed; they'll sting if undercooked! I often serve this herb on toast or in omelettes, soups, and spinach-nettle pies. Try the tops in place of spinach in spanikopita or with feta cheese and olive oil. The roots can also be steamed and eaten, though most people ignore them in favor of the tender tops.

Ryan Drum, herbalist and wildcrafter extraordinaire, considers nettle seeds, which can be collected in the fall, among the best and most nourishing of herbal stimulants.

oats (*Avena sativa* [cultivated] and *A. fatua* [wild])

Parts used: Green milky tops, seeds, and stalks

Benefits: Oats are among the best of the nerve tonic herbs and are a superior cardiac tonic. Those who are overworked, stressed, or anxious, or who have irritated and inflamed nerve endings due to burns or hemorrhoids, should make oats a regular part of their diet. Oats provide energy by increasing overall health and vitality. They are frequently used for nervous system disorders, depression and anxiety, low sexual vitality, irritability, and urinary incontinence. The plant's mucilaginous properties make it particularly helpful for damage to the

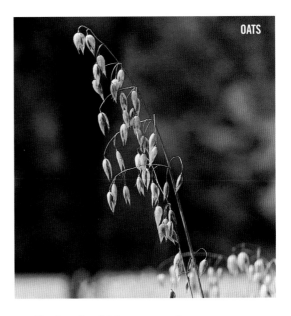

OATS

myelin sheath, which covers and protects nerve fibers. Oats help soothe irritation from nicotine and other chemical withdrawals. They are one of the principal herbal aids used for convalescing after a long illness; oatmeal is often included as a healing agent in diets for people who are weak and debilitated and can't hold in food.

Oat tops are exceptionally rich in silica, calcium, and chromium and are one of the highest terrestrial sources of magnesium. The stalks of oats, though not as rich in minerals as the milky green tops, are also medicinal.

Suggested uses: Though oat stalks are rich in silica and calcium, it is the fruit, or seed, that is primarily used. The fruit contains several active alkaloids, including trigonelline and gramine (found also in barley and passionflower), as well as starch and B vitamins. I recommend using the stalks and fruits together. They are at their best harvested when green-gold and not fully ripe. Much of what is commercially available is the yellow stalks. Though this may be good for mulching the garden, it is not as good for medicinal tea. Look for the green-gold milky tops and stalks.

We're used to thinking of oats in the classic form of oatmeal. But to herbalists, oatmeal is for breakfast, while the delicious oat tops are for tea. Both the milky green tops and the stalks make a delicious, nutritive tea — one of the best, I think. Make it strong and mix it with fruit juice.

Combine oats with lemon balm and passionflower for a good nervine, with valerian for a good sleep aid, or with digestive bitters for any liver or digestive upset. And, finally, oats (both the meal and the unripened milky tops) make one of the most soothing herbal baths for nervous stress and irritated, itchy skin. Add several drops of lavender oil for an especially relaxing experience.

oregon grape *(Mahonia aquifolium)*

Parts used: Roots

Benefits: The roots of this beautiful hollylike plant are gaining fame — not to its demise, I hope — because they contain berberine, a compound similar to that found in goldenseal, and there's some indication that Oregon grape root can be used in place of goldenseal, an endangered herb. Oregon grape root has exceptional anti-inflammatory, antiseptic, and antiviral properties. It is excellent for fighting systemic infection, as well as for topical cleansing, making it especially useful for treating skin conditions such as acne, eczema, and psoriasis.

Suggested uses: Decoct the root and use it as a topical wash for infections, or take it internally for infections, for poor digestion, and as a tonic for the liver.

At-risk warning: Be cautious of harvesting Oregon grape from the wild. Though often prolific where it is found growing, Oregon grape is a slow-growing perennial with a limited range. In the near future, we may determine that this herb should be gathered only from cultivated sources and that wild stands should be left to grow.

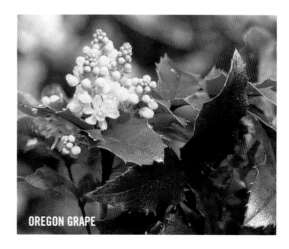

OREGON GRAPE

passionflower *(Passiflora incarnata)*

Part used: Leaves and flowers

Benefits: Contrary to what its name implies, passionflower is a calming, relaxing herb. It has a long history of use in its native range in South America, where it is used to treat epilepsy, anxiety, insomnia, and panic attacks. An effective but gentle herb, passionflower can be used for hyperactive children as well as adults. Passionflower has some analgesic effects and is somewhat effective as a pain reliever for toothache, headache, and menstrual pain. It has strong antispasmodic actions, which make it useful for cramps and spastic or convulsive muscles. This plant is well known for its sleep-inducing properties and is often combined with valerian for this purpose. It is one of the best herbs for stress, anxiety, and depression and can be effectively combined with St.-John's-wort.

Suggested uses: Brew the leaves and flowers as an infusion and drink throughout the day. Use the tincture at bedtime to promote deep, restful sleep.

peppermint *(Mentha × piperita)*

Parts used: Leaves and flowers

Benefits: Peppermint has often been called "a blast of pure green energy." It's not that there aren't stronger stimulants, but few make you feel as renewed and refreshed as peppermint does. Peppermint is most commonly used as a digestive aid. It is also effective for easing nausea and stomach cramps and for freshening the breath.

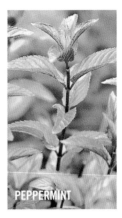

PEPPERMINT

Suggested uses: Peppermint can be made into a tea or tincture (which should be diluted). It is a common ingredient in toothpaste and tooth powders. Because of its pleasant and familiar flavor, it is often used to flavor less tasty herbs. I think it is most refreshing when just grazed from the garden.

pipsissewa *(Chimaphila umbellata)*

Parts used: Leaves

Benefits: Pipsissewa comes from a Cree word meaning "to break into small pieces"; the herb breaks kidney stones into small pieces so they can be passed. Also known as prince's pine, pipsissewa is generally helpful for the urinary system and acts as both a diuretic and a urinary antiseptic, much like uva-ursi but with a gentler, milder action. It also helps prevent or treats various degrees of prostatic irritation and the frequently accompanying cystitis (bladder inflammation). It acts by cleaning, toning, and soothing the irritation, restoring the organs to normalcy. As a poultice, pipsissewa was used by native people to heal blisters, sores, and swellings and to relieve painful joints.

Suggested uses: Pipsissewa is generally made into a tea for urinary problems, though the capsules or tincture can also be used.

At-risk warning: Pipsissewa is a small woodland plant with limited range in North America, and it is on the United Plant Savers "at risk" list. Habitat destruction and overharvesting by the herbal industry have taken a toll on this beautiful plant, and at this time, there is no large-scale cultivation of pipsissewa. Do not collect pipsissewa from the wild, and purchase only supplies that are clearly labeled ORGANICALLY CULTIVATED.

plantain *(Plantago major* and *P. lanceolata)*

Parts used: Seeds, roots, and leaves

Benefits: Plantain is a common weed across almost all of North America and is a highly nutritional food. It is one of the best poultice herbs and is often referred to as the "green bandage." It's among my favorite herbs for treating blood poisoning, used externally on the infected area and internally as a tea. Plantain seeds are rich in mucilage and are often used in laxative blends for their soothing bulk action; in fact, psyllium seeds used in Metamucil are produced from a *Plantago* species. This herb is also very effective for treating liver sluggishness and inflammation of the digestive tract.

Suggested uses: Though it is often considered a bitter, plantain is quite mild in flavor and makes a nice infusion. It can also be powdered and added to food or used as an herbal first-aid powder for infections. Or make a poultice with the fresh leaves to soothe irritation and infection.

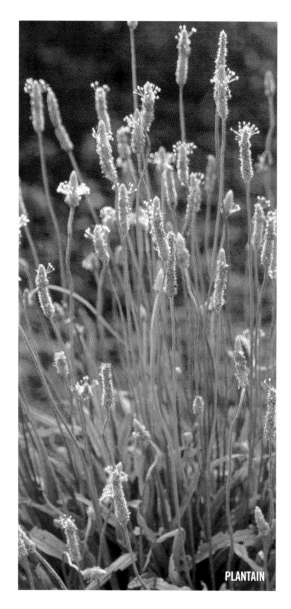

PLANTAIN

pumpkin *(Cucurbita pepo)*

Parts used: Seeds

Benefits: Because of their high zinc content, pumpkin seeds have a good reputation for being a non-irritating treatment for benign enlargement of the prostate gland. A cytotoxic compound also makes them valuable in the treatment of cancer-induced prostate enlargement. The seeds are also rich in phytosterols, anti-inflammatory agents that make them particularly beneficial in conjunction with pygeum and saw palmetto for the prostate.

Suggested uses: Keep a bowl handy and munch on pumpkin seeds throughout the day. They are excellent in trail mix and can be sprinkled on salads or in soups and casseroles. Eat as much as ¼ cup daily to maintain prostate health and as a zinc supplement. Any pumpkin seeds will do, but those of *Cucurbita pepo* are most commonly sold commercially.

pygeum *(Pygeum africanum)*

Parts used: Bark

History: Used in Africa for centuries for male health, prostate enlargement, and impotence and infertility, pygeum was introduced into the Western herbal medical field in only the late 1800s. Little information on this amazing herb is found in early literature.

Pygeum is one of the most popular herbs in Europe for the treatment of benign prostatic hyperplasia (BPH), because it promises to reverse the condition, not just control the symptoms. Pygeum also reduces cholesterol levels that have been found to contribute to BPH. It is used to treat enlarged prostate, inflammation, edema, infertility and impotence, and sterility when due to insufficient prostate secretions.

Suggested uses: Combine pygeum with saw palmetto or pumpkin seeds to treat prostate enlargement, inflammation, and edema. Pygeum's mode of action is different from, though complementary to, that of saw palmetto, so this combination is helpful for many men with congested prostate glands or BPH.

Traditionally, pygeum bark was powdered and mixed with warm milk. Sometimes other spices were used to flavor this drink. In North America today, pygeum is available primarily in capsules and extracts, seldom in raw bulk form.

At-risk warning: Pygeum is threatened in its native range due to habitat destruction and overharvesting; only commercially farmed pygeum should be bought.

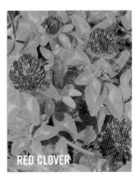
RED CLOVER

red clover *(Trifolium pratense)*

Parts used: Flowering tops and leaves

Benefits: One of the best detoxification herbs and respiratory tonics, red clover is especially useful for easing chronic chest complaints such as coughs, colds, and bronchitis. Red clover is rich in minerals, most notably calcium, nitrogen, and iron. It is used for all skin conditions, as it is an excellent detoxifier or blood purifier. It is commonly used in antitumor formulas.

Suggested uses: Red clover makes a delicious tea. Blend it with other herbs, such as mullein, for persistent respiratory problems. In addition, you can use the tea for building blood and improving the skin. The tea or tincture can be used when there are growths on the body such as cysts, tumors, and fibroids.

Caution: Hemophiliacs or people with "thin" blood should not use red clover regularly, as the herb can exacerbate the condition.

red raspberry *(Rubus idaeus)*

Parts used: Leaves, roots, and berries

Benefits: Raspberry is a highly nourishing reproductive tonic, providing nutrients that tone and strengthen the entire genitourinary system. One of the richest sources of iron, raspberry is used to replenish iron-poor blood and is often combined with nettle for anemia and related low energy levels. It is also a rich source of niacin and among the richest sources of manganese, a trace mineral used by the body to produce healthy connective tissue, such as bone matrix and cartilage, and an important factor in energy metabolism.

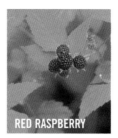

RED RASPBERRY

As a tea or tincture, raspberry leaf is invaluable for treating diarrhea and dysentery. It helps reduce excessive menstruation and is one of the superior tonics for pregnancy and childbirth. Because of its astringent properties, it is a good mouthwash for sore or infected gums. Use as a nutritive tonic when energy is low, when recovering from illness, and at times when an endocrine tonic is needed.

Suggested uses: The leaf is quite tasty and is generally prepared as an infusion. Drink several cups of the tea daily to experience its toning effects. Raspberry leaf can also be blended with other reproductive tonic herbs and made into a tincture to be used daily. The berries, too, are medicinal and delicious. Use them to make divinely flavored cordials for toasting the gods.

rose hips *(Rosa canina* and related species)

Parts used: Primarily the seeds, but also the leaves and flowers

Benefits: Rose hips contain more vitamin C than almost any other herb, many times the amount found in citrus fruit when measured gram by gram. Vitamin C is a noted antioxidant with disease-fighting abilities. The leaves are astringent and toning. The flowers are used in love potions and flower essences.

Suggested uses: Make fresh rose hips into a vitamin-rich syrup or jam. Rose hips also make a delicious, mild-flavored tea, perfect on a cold New England night, sipped by a roaring fire.

rose hips jam

Dried seedless rose hips make a delicious and easy-to-prepare jam. Simply cover them with fresh apple juice and let them soak overnight. The next day, the jam is ready to eat. Cinnamon and other spices can add more flavor, but the jam is quite good as is.

rosemary *(Rosmarinus officinalis)*

Parts used: Leaves

Benefits: We've only begun to uncover the many uses of rosemary. It has long been renowned as a memory aid. It has a tonic effect on the nervous system and is good for circulation. It strengthens the heart and reduces high blood pressure. It has been used for hundreds of years as a cosmetic herb for its beneficial effects on the hair and skin.

Suggested uses: Blended with other herbs in the famous Queen of Hungary's Water (see the recipe on page 130), rosemary makes a bracing astringent cosmetic preparation. It also makes a pleasant tea when infused with other herbs and is often blended with ginkgo and gotu kola in tincture and tea form as a memory aid.

sage *(Salvia officinalis)*

Parts used: Leaves

Benefits: Warming and strengthening, sage is an excellent herb for rebuilding vitality and strength during long-term illness. Its name, *Salvia*, derives from the Latin *salvus*, "safe," and *salvere*, "to be well." It clears congestion and soothes sore throats, tonsillitis, and laryngitis.

Suggested uses: An infusion of sage is pleasant and warming. An infusion is also useful as a gargle for sore throat and infections in the mouth. Perhaps because of its grounding nature, sage is helpful for menopausal women, specifically for hot flashes. Of course, sage is excellent as a culinary herb and enhances the flavor of many foods.

st.-john's-wort *(Hypericum perforatum)*

Parts used: Leaves and flowers (approximately 70 percent flower to 30 percent leaf)

Benefits: St.-John's-wort has become a popular herb for depression and anxiety. A classic remedy for nerve damage and depression, St.-John's-wort has been used for centuries and is held in high esteem by herbalists throughout western Europe and the Mediterranean. It is primarily valued as a treatment for damage to the nerve endings such as in burns, neuralgia, wounds, and trauma to the skin. It is also highly effective for relieving the symptoms of stress, anxiety, depression, seasonal affective disorder, chronic fatigue, and personality disorders. It lifts the spirits and puts a bit of sunshine into the day. Early speculation targeted the plant as an MAO inhibitor, but this information has been scientifically rejected. The action of the plant is not, in fact, fully understood, nor has the chemical constituent responsible for its antidepressant activities been identified. Look to the whole wonder of this plant.

Suggested uses: Definitely make St.-John's-wort oil (see the recipe on page 98); it is one of the finest medicinal oils and is used for bruises, sprains, burns, and injuries of all kinds. It's a joy to behold and a joy to prepare.

St.-John's-wort combines well with other herbs and is often mixed with hops and valerian for insomnia, with lavender and lemon balm for depression, and with chamomile for children going through emotional upheaval. I often combine it with passionflower for anxiety. St.-John's-wort is effective for depression, but it is best used in conjunction with other supportive therapies, such as counseling, massage therapy, and foods that nurture the nervous system (see chapter 3).

Caution: Though some people claim St.-John's-wort causes sensitivity to the sun, many people use the herb in sunscreen to protect them from sunburn.

There has been concern that St.-John's-wort works similarly to Prozac as an MAO inhibitor, but studies have proved this theory to be false. Therefore, the restrictions imposed on MAO-inhibiting antidepressants do not apply to St.-John's-wort.

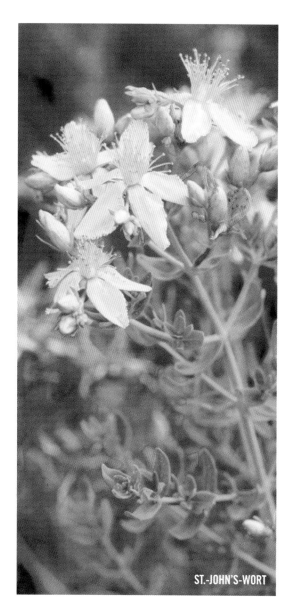

ST.-JOHN'S-WORT

People often ask whether it's appropriate to take St.-John's-wort in combination with prescription or over-the-counter antidepressants, with the hope of being able to decrease or eliminate those drugs altogether. Of course, it depends on the individual situation, but generally, if a person is not suicidal and doesn't have chronic clinical depression, I have found that St.-John's-wort serves very well as a transitional herb. Because prescription antidepressants block the nerve responses and St.-John's-wort serves as a nerve tonic, building and strengthening aid to the nervous system, they don't interfere with each other and create greater possibilities for healing when used together. It is important, however, that you work closely with an experienced holistic practitioner if you intend to use these medications simultaneously.

sarsaparilla *(Smilax officinalis)*

Parts used: Roots and rhizomes

Benefits: Native to Central and South America, sarsaparilla was taken to Europe in the fifteenth century as a cure for syphilis. Sarsaparilla is a wonderful aromatic root tonic that is effective as a cleanser or "blood purifier" for the genitourinary system, liver, and gallbladder. Because of its cleansing action, it is often used in formulas to treat skin conditions. The roots are rich in steroidal saponins that provide the building blocks necessary for the body to produce steroidal hormones. It is very rich in trace minerals, primarily selenium and zinc. Psoriasis and other skin conditions, arthritis and rheumatism, hormonal imbalances, low energy, poor elimination, and sluggish liver can all be treated with this versatile herb.

herbs are not miracle drugs

After a feature on a national television series that detailed the story of a woman — who is, incidentally, the daughter of one of my students — who had great success in using St.-John's-wort to ease depression, sales of products made from this herb shot up an unprecedented 1,000 percent in one year. Stores across the country found it impossible to keep St.-John's-wort products in stock.

Unfortunately, people with little knowledge of how to use herbs attempted to use St.-John's-wort in the same manner as antidepressant drugs, and they did not have the results they had hoped for. Though wonderfully effective and uplifting, St.-John's-wort is not a miracle drug; it alone will not cure depression. It must be used in conjunction with lifestyle changes.

Suggested uses: I usually prepare sarsaparilla as a tea because of its rich, wonderful vanilla-like flavor. It adds that classic root beer taste to teas and is wonderful to blend with sassafras, birch bark, dandelion root, and echinacea for a super immune formula that's delicious. Add a pinch of stevia for sweetness.

sassafras
(Sassafras albidum)

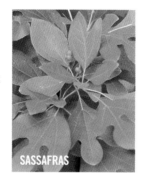
SASSAFRAS

Parts used: Bark and root bark (the root bark is the most potent part of the plant, but you have to dig up the plant — thus killing it — to get to the root)

Benefits: This has long been one of my favorite herbs for flavoring teas, especially teas made from roots and barks. It was traditionally the main ingredient in old-fashioned "root beers," tonic drinks that were made from roots and barks for seasonal cleansing.

Sassafras is cleansing to the entire system and stimulating for congestion in the liver and gallbladder. It has a grounding (yang) action and is often associated with the male system. A powerful astringent, it can be used externally for insect bites and internally for diarrhea and dysentery. I find it to be one of the best herbs for enhancing the flavor and healing properties of male tonic drinks, which can be used to address hormonal imbalances, liver congestion, diarrhea, skin disorders, and disruptions in the genitourinary system.

Suggested uses: Sassafras is water soluble and is quite delicious as tea. It can also be made into tasty elixirs and tonic brews.

Caution: Sassafras is not mentioned often or used in teas anymore, not because it isn't effective or safe, but because it's currently illegal to sell it for internal use. In the 1970s safrole, a highly toxic chemical constituent found in sassafrass, was isolated, extracted with chemical solvents (it, unlike other constituents, is not water soluble), and tested on laboratory rats. It was found, not surprisingly, that in large amounts it produced carcinogenic cells in the rats. No human case of cancer from sassafras has ever been reported. The soft drink industry, which up to that time had been using pure sassafras extracts for flavoring root beer, was forced to substitute synthetic chemicals. (Is that better for us?)

Interestingly, the population of the southeastern United States, where sassafras tea is a traditional folk remedy, has the lowest rate of throat cancer in the country. I continue to use it because I know it's a valuable, safe, and effective herb, though regulations prevent me from using it in my commercial formulas, and (for ethical reasons) I don't recommend it to my clients unless they request it.

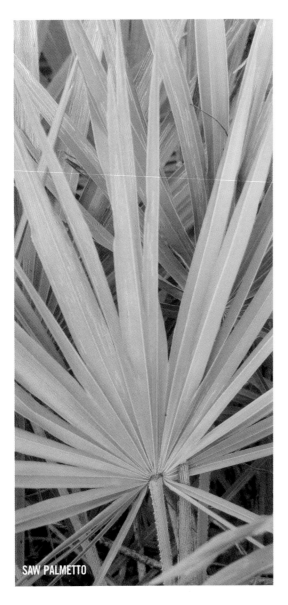

SAW PALMETTO

saw palmetto *(Serenoa repens)*

Parts used: Berries

Benefits: Though long used by the native people of the subtropical coast of North America, saw palmetto has risen rapidly in popularity in recent years. It is simply the best remedy for inflammation of the prostate gland. It is tonic in action and serves as an effective diuretic and relaxant. It is strengthening to those individuals who are continuously nervous and stressed and who lack energy and vitality. Its fatty fruit is one of the few Western herbs that are anabolic; it encourages weight gain and bulk by strengthening and building body tissue. It is used by women to firm sagging breast tissue. As a tonic herb, it can be taken on a regular basis to strengthen the urinary and endocrine systems and to prevent future problems with the prostate gland. Why wait?

Nicknamed the "plant catheter," saw palmetto has the ability to strengthen the neck of the bladder and to reduce enlarged prostate glands. It reduces many of the problems associated with an enlarged prostate gland: dribbling urine; slow, painful urination; the need to urinate several times during the night; and incomplete urination, which can lead to low-grade cystitis.

Suggested uses: Saw palmetto has a fatty, pungent flavor that is hard to swallow and hard to disguise. It is difficult to conceive of the taste of this herb until you've tried it. I don't know of many people who enjoy its flavor in tea. It's usually available in tincture form. It can be used in capsules as well, but they should be fresh and of good quality, because the fats in saw palmetto quickly turn rancid.

schisandra *(Schisandra chinensis)*

Part used: Berries

Benefits: Schisandra is an adaptogenic herb, raising the body's ability to resist all kinds of stress and disease. It is often associated with the sexual organs, as it's known to increase the staying power of men and to revitalize women's sexual experience. People have used schisandra for hundreds of years to increase endurance and stamina.

Though most schisandra comes from China, it is possible to grow this herb in North America. It is a lovely vinelike plant.

Suggested uses: Schisandra berries have a unique flavor; people either love them or not. They can be soaked in fruit juice or wine for a tonic drink

or cooked in honey until soft and jamlike. In tea they add a sour, lemonlike flavor that is not at all unpleasant. For a more concentrated preparation, schisandra tinctures well in 80-proof alcohol.

Combine schisandra berries with vitex to make a superior reproductive tonic, energizing and warming to the entire genital area. Or combine them with ginseng to increase stamina and endurance; this mix is often used by athletes and hikers.

senna *(Cassia angustifolia)*

Parts used: Leaves and pods

Benefits: Senna is probably the most common laxative in the world. Though primarily known for its laxative properties, senna is also used in Ayurvedic medicine for liver, skin, and respiratory problems. The leaves contain anthraquinone derivatives, which stimulate contractions in the lower gastrointestinal tract. It should not be used over long periods of time, as it will weaken the

the five-flavored plant

Called wu wei tsu, or "the five-flavored plant," in Chinese medicine, schisandra has five distinct flavors: sweet, salty, sour, pungent, and bitter. As you chew the berry, each flavor follows the preceding one until the palate is engulfed in the entire taste sensation. It is said that each flavor activates and

balances a different organ system; because of this, schisandra is known as a superior tonic herb. It has enjoyed a great reputation in China and was used at one time primarily by wealthy upper-middle-class women as a preserver of youth and beauty and as a powerful sexual tonic.

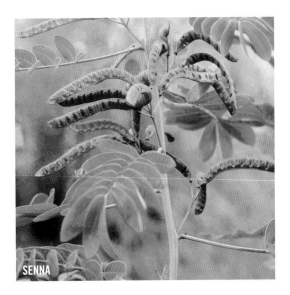

SENNA

bowels and create a dependency, but it is very useful for acute cases of constipation. Senna is most often formulated with other herbs to balance its strong actions and to lessen griping and stomach pain.

Suggested uses: Senna can be taken as a tincture, capsule, or tea as a short-term laxative. Always start with the smallest recommended dosage and increase it as needed. Senna needs up to 8 hours to work, so don't take more, thinking the remedy isn't working. You may be unpleasantly surprised.

Caution: Senna is not recommended if you have or develop diarrhea, loose stools, or abdominal pain. Consult your physician before using it if you are pregnant, nursing, or taking medication or if you develop persistent diarrhea.

skullcap *(Scutellaria lateriflora)*

Parts used: Leaves

Benefits: Skullcap is one of the most versatile of the nervines and is indicated for all nervous system disorders, especially headaches, nerve tremors, stress, menstrual tension, insomnia, and nervous exhaustion.

Suggested uses: This is a strong, effective herb, and there is no danger of overdose or cumulative buildup if it is used over a long period of time. Quite the contrary; to receive the full benefit of skullcap, you should use it over an extended period and in adequate dosages. Skullcap can be prepared in tea, tincture, or capsule form. The suggested adult dose is 2 to 3 cups of tea daily or ¼ teaspoon of tincture diluted in ½ cup of warm water three times daily.

slippery elm *(Ulmus fulva* and *U. rubra)*

Parts used: Inner bark

Benefits: A soothing mucilaginous herb, slippery elm is one of the most beloved of medicinal herbs. This plant is used for soothing any and all inflammations, internal or external. It is particularly valuable for burns, sore throats, and digestive problems, including diarrhea and constipation. A highly nourishing food, it was at one time sold as a medicinal flour and used in cooking.

Suggested uses: This sweet herb combines well with others such as licorice, fennel, and cinnamon. It makes a wonderful tea. My favorite cough medicine is 1 tablespoon of slippery elm, 1 teaspoon of cinnamon, 1 cup of warm water, and 1 tablespoon of honey processed together in a blender.

At-risk warning: Many elm trees have been destroyed by Dutch elm disease. Use slippery elm sparingly, and buy only farm-grown bark or that ethically harvested from limbs of fallen trees. If you intend to use it externally, whenever possible substitute marsh mallow, which has similar mucilaginous properties, for slippery elm.

slippery elm lozenges

The discomfort of burns in the mouth can be quickly eased with slippery elm lozenges. To make the lozenges, mix 1 tablespoon of finely ground slippery elm powder with 1 teaspoon of honey and just enough water to make a paste. Roll into a ball, adding more herb, if needed, to thicken. If the burn is serious, a tiny drop of peppermint oil can be added. Suck on the lozenge, using as many as needed until the pain is gone.

spearmint *(Mentha spicata)*

Parts used: Leaves and flowers

Benefits: Cooling, refreshing, and uplifting, spearmint is, with the possible exception of peppermint, the most popular of all mints.

Suggested uses: Use spearmint to "sweeten" the stomach and breath after sickness, especially vomiting. Add a drop of the essential oil to water or make a cup of fresh tea and rinse the mouth out several times. This herb can be added to uplifting, refreshing tea blends. Spearmint is a nice addition to honey and other foods for a quick pick-me-up. Of course, spearmint is the herb of choice in the dental industry.

stevia *(Stevia rebaudiana)*

Parts used: Leaves

Benefits: Called the sweet herb, stevia is sweeter than sugar but much better for you. It has no calories and doesn't promote tooth decay. It is indicated for pancreatic imbalances and high blood sugar levels and is a type of sugar that diabetics can tolerate. In fact, stevia has been used to help treat diabetes. Though it has been tested extensively in other countries, it was banned in the United States on the pretext that its safety was unknown. Now that several of the large sugar companies have secured an interest in stevia production, the herb suddenly has been legalized in the United States.

Suggested uses: Because of its intense sweetness, stevia is used primarily to enhance the flavor of other herbs. However, it really is exceptionally sweet. If you add even a pinch too much to a cup of tea or a recipe, you'll ruin the flavor. So start with a tiny pinch and taste-test before adding more.

usnea *(Usnea barbata)*

Parts used: Lichens

Benefits: It is odd that an herb so abundant and so useful was not used by modern American herbalists until just a few years ago. This lichen grows primarily on aging trees and is often called "old man's beard"; since several lichens are called by this name, be sure the one you are using is usnea. Usnea's bitter principle, usnic acid, helps soothe the stomach while enhancing digestion. Usnea also has antibiotic properties, making it useful for treating urinary and bladder infections, cystitis, and fungal infections. It is an excellent immune enhancer and is frequently combined with echinacea.

Suggested uses: I often add a small amount of usnea to soup. It is easily powdered and can be mixed with foods or encapsulated; however, its taste leaves something to be desired. Therefore, it is often tinctured, and it seems most effective in an alcohol solvent.

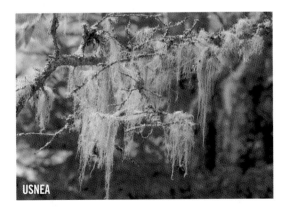

USNEA

uva-ursi *(Arctostaphylos uva-ursi)*

Parts used: Leaves and berries

Benefits: Uva-ursi is a small, wiry shrub that hugs the earth as it grows. Its leatherlike leaves are harvested and used to make a tea for treating kidney and bladder infections. It is an effective diuretic, astringent, and urinary antiseptic that cleans and heals urinary passages. It is an excellent remedy for cystitis, urethritis, kidney stones, leukorrhea, and bed-wetting.

Suggested uses: For treating inflammation and infection of the urinary system, uva-ursi is most effective as an infusion. However, a decoction will bring out a richer concentration of tannins and the plant's astringent properties. Uva-ursi is often infused as a strong tea and mixed with cranberry juice for treating bladder and kidney infections.

valerian *(Valeriana officinalis)*

Parts used: Roots

Benefits: Valerian has been highly regarded as an herbal medicine for centuries. Hildegard von Bingen, a famous 12th-century German abbess and herbalist, valued it as a sedative. In the 1500s, the great herbalist Gerard claimed that valerian was one of the most popular remedies of his time. Today, in spite of its distinct and somewhat offensive odor, valerian continues to be one of the most popular medicinal herbs in the world.

There is no finer herb than valerian for those who suffer from stress, insomnia, and nervous system disorders; it is powerful, safe, very effective, and nonaddictive. Its name is derived from the Latin *valere,* "to be well" or "to be strong." In Europe, where it has been used for centuries, valerian can be found in hundreds of over-the-counter drugs and is relied on primarily as a medicine for stress and tension. It is effective for insomnia, pain, restlessness, headaches, digestive problems due to nerves, and muscle spasms. Depending on the individual, the smell is either relished or deemed offensive. I rather love the odor, which reminds people of violets, rich sweet earth, or dirty underwear, depending on the age of the root.

Valerian is effective both as a long-term nerve tonic and as a remedy for acute problems such as headaches and pain. It has powerful tonic effects on the heart and is often recommended in combination with hawthorn berries for high blood pressure and irregular heartbeat.

Suggested uses: Because the root is rich in volatile oils, it should be infused rather than decocted. Valerian is often tinctured or encapsulated rather than taken as tea because of its odor, though its taste is quite pleasant. Herbalists are in disagreement about whether the fresh or dried herb works better. Without a doubt, it's better tasting when fresh. Cats love it, often better than catnip.

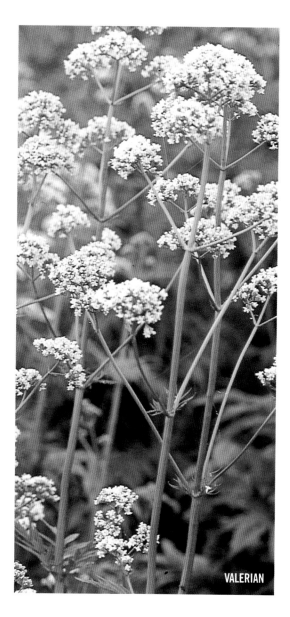

VALERIAN

Caution: Valerian is generally considered a safe, nontoxic herb. It is used as a relaxant, but it can have the opposite effect on people who are particularly sensitive to it. If you become further agitated and restless after taking valerian, discontinue use and consider yourself in that rare 5 percent of the population that cannot tolerate this herb.

dosing valerian properly

Most prescription sedatives carry labels that caution you about their potential addictive qualities and advise you to stay with the prescribed dosage. Valerian, on the other hand, is a nonaddictive, non–habit-forming sedative, and it will not make you sleepy or groggy unless really large amounts are consumed. So don't be afraid to take adequate amounts of valerian. Begin with a low dosage and increase it until you feel its relaxing effects. You'll know you've taken too much if you have a "rubberlike" feeling in the muscles — as if they were too relaxed — or a feeling of heaviness. If that's the case, cut back the dosage so that you feel relaxed but alert.

white oak *(Quercus alba)*

Parts used: Bark

Benefits: The white oak is a huge, stately tree whose bark is a powerful astringent and disinfectant. The bark's high tannin content makes it useful taken internally for treating diarrhea and hemorrhoids; as an astringent antiseptic wash for wounds, poison oak, and poison ivy; and as a gargle for sore throats and mouth infections. It is a good remedy for leukorrhea and varicose veins.

Suggested uses: Decoct the bark for use internally and to make an antiseptic liniment for external use. White oak bark also tinctures well.

wild cherry *(Prunus serotina)*

Parts used: Inner bark

Benefits: This expectorant herb is one of the best for calming coughs. It is one of the few herbs still included in the United States Pharmacopeia's annual drug reference and it is still found in some commercial cough remedies. It also improves digestion and promotes healthy bowel function.

In order not to harm the beautiful trees, I generally collect bark from fallen limbs after a storm.

Suggested uses: Wild cherry can be used in teas, syrups, and tinctures.

wild yam *(Dioscorea villosa)*

Parts used: Rhizomes and roots

Benefits: Wild yam is a primary source of material for steroid production and also serves as a

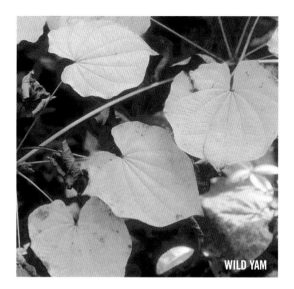

WILD YAM

Suggested uses: Wild yam can be made into teas, tinctures, and capsules. It is bitter and not often prepared by itself as a tea, though it is tolerable when blended with other herbs. I like to mix powdered wild yam with other tonic herbs, add cardamom and cinnamon powder to taste, and mix it into a paste with honey and rose water.

At-risk warning: Native populations of wild yam are under siege, and some varieties are highlighted on the United Plant Savers "at risk" list. Use only cultivated varieties of wild yam.

hormone precursor, thereby aiding the proper function of the reproductive system of both sexes. I have used it successfully to treat all aspects of menstrual dysfunction and to help people increase fertility. Oddly, one sometimes finds wild yam listed as a natural birth-control agent, though it is more often used to promote fertility.

The roots and rhizomes contain bitter compounds that help tone the liver and increase bile flow. Wild yam is one of my favorite herbs for liver congestion and inflammation. It's especially indicated for those who store excess heat (yang) in their bodies or who have high blood pressure. Wild yam is also a nervine and antispasmodic and is excellent for soothing muscle cramps, colic, and uterine pain.

witch hazel *(Hamamelis virginiana)*

Parts used: Bark

Benefits: A pretty North American shrub, witch hazel was a time-honored traditional remedy of native peoples. It is a potent pain reliever and astringent and has antioxidant properties. When taken internally or applied externally, witch hazel is thought to act on the venous system to stop bleeding and inflammation. It is particularly effective for treating intestinal bleeding, bruises, hemorrhoids, varicose veins, dermatitis, sunburn, and diarrhea. It is also indicated for bleeding of the nose and lungs.

Suggested uses: Take witch hazel internally as a tincture and use it externally as a liniment or an astringent, disinfectant wash. It also makes a good cleanser for "troubled" skin. Decocted as tea, it can be taken internally as an astringent for diarrhea and intestinal bleeding.

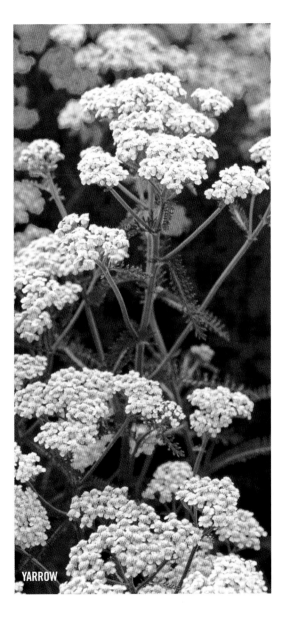

YARROW

yarrow *(Achillea millefolium)*

Parts used: Leaves and flowers

Benefits: A beautiful roadside weed, yarrow is best recognized by its creamy flowers, which bloom throughout the summer months. It is an excellent diaphoretic, often used in teas to promote sweating, thereby helping reduce fevers. Yarrow is a classic first-aid herb and can be used to stop bleeding both internally and externally. It is effective for both menstrual and stomach cramps and is often used in formulas for stomach flus. It also has beneficial effects for the heart and lungs.

Suggested uses: Yarrow makes a bitter infusion, so blend it with tastier herbs as a digestive aid and diaphoretic. The dried, powdered leaf is useful in a first-aid kit; it can be applied to cuts and wounds to disinfect and stop bleeding. A pinch of the powder can be placed in the nose to stop a nosebleed.

yellow dock *(Rumex crispus)*

Parts used: Roots

Benefits: This abundant wild weed of fields, gardens, and roadsides is possibly one of the best herbs for the entire digestive system, including the liver. The large taproot is rich in anthraquinone, which has a laxative action. It contains biochelated iron, which can be readily absorbed. It is one of the best herbs for anemia and fatigue and is useful for women with PMS and men and women with hormonal imbalances.

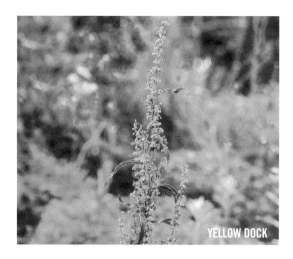

YELLOW DOCK

Suggested uses: Yellow dock makes a somewhat bitter-tasting decoction, so it is best formulated with more flavorful herbs. It can be taken in tincture form for the digestive system, including the liver and gallbladder. It can be added to formulas for its laxative properties. I've also used the root in making iron-rich syrups.

yohimbe *(Pausinystalia yohimbe* and *Corynanthe yohimbe)*

Parts used: Shavings of the inner bark

Benefits: I include this herb in the apothecary with some trepidation. Yohimbe is an exciting herb, but it's very potent, potentially harmful, and has a long list of side effects if used improperly. Even in moderate doses, it can be overstimulating. See the cautions at right.

Yohimbe has a long history of use in its native Africa, where it is used primarily as a potent aphrodisiac and stimulant. It acts both as a central nervous system stimulant and as a mild hallucinogen. It also stimulates blood flow to the erectile tissue. Yohimbine hydrochloride, a product sold by pharmaceutical companies, is a prescription drug used for treating erectile dysfunction. It can also be used — with caution (see below) — to increase libido.

Suggested uses: The traditional way to prepare yohimbe is to bring 2 cups of water to a boil. Add 1 ounce of yohimbe bark to the boiling water and boil for no more than 4 minutes. Reduce heat to low, simmer slowly for an additional 20 minutes, then strain. Sip slowly about 1 hour before you want the desired effect to occur. For a stronger, more effective drink, add 1,000 mg of ascorbic acid (vitamin C) to the brew. The vitamin C reacts with the alkaloids to form yohimbine and yohimbiline ascorbates, more soluble and more active forms of yohimbe.

Caution: Yohimbe is a monamine oxidase (MAO) inhibitor; do not use it in combination with sedatives, tranquilizers, antihistamines, narcotics, or large quantities of alcohol. People with kidney disorders, cardiovascular disorders, diabetes, or abnormal blood pressure or blood sugar should not use yohimbe. Do not use it for long-term treatment.

Appendix II
The Art of Making Herbal Remedies

It took some years to develop the recipes and techniques in this book, and it is with pleasure that I pass them along to you. When I began working with herbs in the late 1960s, what little explanation there was on how to prepare them was difficult to find. When I could find instruction, the steps were often complicated, and sometimes the herbs mentioned were not even available. Through a wonderful, creative trial-and-error process, learning from the old masters and their books, and sharing with and learning from my friends, the instructions for these preparations began to take shape. *This* is the information I wish I had possessed when I first began to study herbs so many years ago.

The most common medicinal herb preparations are tinctures, capsules, and teas. But don't limit yourself to these three. Herbs can be prepared and administered in numerous ways, many of which don't necessarily seem like "medicine." Syrups and elixirs are an incredibly effective way to extract the medicinal properties of herbs, and they're delicious. Add powdered herbs to salads, shakes, hot cereal, stir-fries, soups, and other dishes, or mix the powders into a paste with honey and spices for a delectable daily tonic. Some herbs, such as hawthorn and elder, can be prepared as tasty jams and jellies — not a bad way to take your medicine. Warm baths are one of the most relaxing and enjoyable ways to use herbs. When you soak in a warm herbal bath, the pores of the skin, the largest organ of elimination and assimilation, are wide open and receptive. It's like soaking in a giant cup of tea; your entire body reaps the benefits.

buying versus making

If making your own herbal products is not your cup of tea, you can go to any natural foods store and purchase ready-made products. Though the choices in ready-made products are increasing every day, I encourage you to at least try your hand at herbal medicine making. Allow yourself the pleasure of discovering how simple, easy, and effective it is to make herbal medicines.

buying and storing herbs

In these times, when wild lands are being developed at an alarming pace and cultivation of medicinal herbs has not yet caught up with the rate of their use, it is critical that each of us takes responsibility for where our herbs are coming from and who is growing and harvesting them. You must insist on high-quality organically grown herbs. Though they may cost a bit more, they are far better for our medicines and, ultimately, our planet. Make every effort not to use herbs that are endangered or at risk, whether from the United States or elsewhere. To learn more about endangered medicinal plants, contact United Plant Savers (see Resources).

I have traveled in various parts of the world, and I am astounded by the differences in the quality of herbs in different regions. When I began working with herbs, the quality of herb supplies in the United States was very poor; but in the past 25 years, there has been such an emphasis placed on using high-quality herbs that we now lead the world in quality standards. North American herbalists are hoping we will have the same influence worldwide on preservation as we have had on quality. If we wish to preserve this system of healing for our children as it has been passed down to us from our ancestors, preservation of medicinal plant species is imperative. You are supporting not only your own health but the health of the planet when you buy organically grown herbs.

Buying High-Quality Herbs

The single most important factor when purchasing herbs for making remedies is recognizing and obtaining the best quality available. Buy your herbs from reputable companies, those that have a conscience and are concerned about both the quality of the products they sell and the environment. Ask where their herbs come from. Are they organically grown? Are they wildcrafted? If so, were they collected ethically, with respect for the environment?

Whenever possible, use your herbs fresh. However, for a variety of reasons, it is not always feasible to obtain fresh herbs. Dried herbs, if harvested and dried properly, will generally retain all of their medicinal properties. How do you tell if a dried herb is of good quality? It should look, smell, and taste almost exactly as it does when it's fresh, and it should be effective in your herbal remedies.

> **"My idea of a good herbalist** is not someone who knows the uses of forty different herbs, but someone who knows how to use one herb in forty different ways."
>
> **— Svevo Brooks**

Color

A dried herb should be almost the same color as it is when fresh. Dried quantities of green-leaved plants such as peppermint or spearmint should be vividly green. Blossoms should be bright and colorful. Calendula flowers, for example, should be bright orange or yellow. Roots, though generally very subtly hued to begin with, should remain true to their original color. Goldenseal root should be a golden green, echinacea root a silvery brown, yellow dock root a yellowish brown. You may not always know what the correct color of a plant should be, but look for liveliness, vibrancy, and deep, strong colors. You will soon develop a knack for judging herb supplies by their appearance.

Smell

Herbs have distinctive odors that serve as effective means of determining quality. They should smell strongly, not necessarily "good." The scent of valerian, for instance, has been likened to that of dirty socks; good-quality valerian should smell like really dirty socks. Good-quality peppermint will make your nose tingle and your eyes water. Some herbs, such as alfalfa, just smell "green," but in that green odor is a freshness and unmistakable vitality.

Taste

Herbs should have a distinctive fresh flavor. Judge taste on potency rather than flavor. You will quickly learn that not all medicinal herbs taste good by any stretch of the imagination! Do they taste fresh? Strong? Vital? Distinctive? Do they arouse a distinctive response from your taste buds?

Growing Your Own Medicinal Herbs

The best way to ensure that you're getting quality herbs is to grow your own. Many of the plants that you use for medicine can be grown as part of your

fresh versus dried

There is nothing quite as good as the taste of fresh picked herbs. However, many herbs are not available fresh year-round, and some of our favorites are not grown in North America but are dried and imported. When fresh herbs are unavailable, high-quality dried herbs will do just fine.

Fresh herb blends must be used immediately, of course, while dried mixtures can be stored for several months or longer. You can mix fresh and dried herbs for immediate use. For instance, you can mix fresh peppermint with dried ginger root and cinnamon bark to make a stimulating, refreshing tea.

vegetable and flower garden. Incorporate them into your landscape and use them as they grow and thrive. Though many herbs have specific habitats and limited range — which is one reason they are threatened — we are finding that many of them are far more adaptable than was previously thought. For an excellent book on the subject, read *Growing 101 Herbs That Heal,* by Tammi Hartung.

Storing Herbs

Herbs retain their properties best if stored in airtight glass jars, away from direct light, in a cool storage area. For convenience, you can store them in many other containers — boxes, tins, plastic bags — but most herbalists find that those durable glass bottles work best for storage.

Each herb has its own "shelf life," or duration of time in which it remains viable. Following one set rule for assigning "expiration dates" for herbs could mean you would throw out perfectly fine peppermint while using poor-quality chickweed. Instead, use the standards of quality — look, taste, and smell — outlined above to determine if your herbs have retained their quality.

the kitchen "lab"

A kitchen, with all of its marvelous tools, will supply you with most of the utensils you need for preparing herbal products. One of the few rules that most herbalists agree on is never to use aluminum pans for preparing herbs. Aluminum is a proved toxic substance, and the toxicity is easily released by heat into our food. Use glass, stainless steel, ceramic, cast iron, or enamel cooking equipment.

Some items I've found especially useful are:

- Canning jars for storing herbs and making tinctures
- Cheesecloth or fine muslin for straining herbs
- Coffee grinder reserved for grinding herbs, not coffee (else your herbs will taste like coffee and your coffee like herbs)
- Grater reserved for grating beeswax
- Large, double-meshed, stainless-steel strainer
- Measuring cups (though, heaven forbid, I hardly use them)
- Stainless-steel pots with tight-fitting lids

It is wise to assemble all the ingredients and utensils you need ahead of time. There have been times when I haven't followed this little bit of advice and found that I was out of a necessary ingredient in the middle of a project. This can be either a big or a little inconvenience, but it's always annoying.

As with any culinary recipe, you can substitute ingredients and experiment with medicinal and beauty formulas to create a more personalized product, but be sure you understand what particular ingredients in the formula are "doing," so that you can know what properties you are removing and what properties you may need to put back in. Ask yourself the basic questions: Is this a tonic herb, or does it have a specific action on a particular system? Does this ingredient help thicken the product? Does it add moisture?

In these recipes, there is always lots of room for creativity. I am one of those people who get frustrated with exact proportions. Coffee mugs are most often my measuring cups, and spoons from my silverware drawer serve as measuring spoons. When adding essential oils, I lose count somewhere after the fourth or fifth drop and proceed forward by scent and common sense alone. Nothing is exact in my world, and, needless to say, things don't always turn out exactly the same. But I've learned to follow my intuition, and generally it leads me in its own creative process. Using my common sense rather than exact measurements has often produced exquisite results.

the simpler's method of measurement

Long before the term *herbalist* was coined, people who worked closely with the earth, plants, and the seasons were called simplers. Not at all a derogatory term, *simpler* referred to someone who was observant and relied on intuition and an inner knowing for making preparations. Over the centuries, science developed weights and measures and clinical studies to comprehend, measure, and explain this art of healing. A tablespoon or two of this clinical knowledge is appropriate to the study of herbs and adds a touch of professionalism to the art. More than that, I'm afraid, could be toxic to the creative unfolding of herbal healing.

While many people are converting to the metric system, I've reverted to the simpler's method of measuring, which is extremely simple and very versatile. In the simpler's method, measurements are given as "parts": 3 parts chamomile, 1 part lemon balm, 2 parts oats. A part is a unit of measurement that can be interpreted to mean cup, ounce, pound, tablespoon, teaspoon — any amount at all, so long as you use that unit consistently throughout the recipe. If you were using tablespoons in the recipe just given, for example,

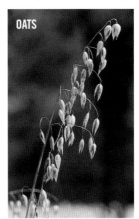

OATS

you would include 3 tablespoons of chamomile, 1 tablespoon of lemon balm, and 2 tablespoons of oats. Or, if you want to make medicine in bulk, use cups instead of tablespoons; just keep the relative proportions of the herbs consistent.

determining dosage

Even in conventional allopathic medicine, determination of dosage is far more arbitrary than we're led to believe. Herbalists are usually quicker to admit that determining dosage involves some skill and experience, a healthy touch of "inner knowing," careful observation, and a bit of guesswork.

To determine the proper dosage of an herbal preparation, you must consider the herbs used to make it: What are their primary actions? Do they have any toxic side effects? Are they tonic in nature or are they used to treat a specific health problem or organ system? Consider the constitution of the person: Is she or he relatively healthy? Robust or sensitive? Weak or debilitated? And, finally, consider the nature of the imbalance or illness you want to address: Is it chronic or acute? Excess or deficient in nature?

These clinical factors will help you determine a reasonable dosage, but ultimately you must trust the wisdom of your own body (or that of the person being treated). Listen to what it tells you. Watch how it responds. The body itself offers the best guidelines for what — and how much — it needs.

For those who are just beginning their herbal studies, the guidelines at right will be helpful in getting started. Remember always to use the smallest dosage that will get the job done, working up only as necessary.

adult dosages

CHRONIC PROBLEMS are long-term imbalances such as hay fever, arthritis, back pain, insomnia, and long-standing bronchial problems. Chronic problems can, however, flare up with acute symptoms. Follow these guidelines for treating chronic problems.

> TEA: 3 to 4 cups daily for several weeks
> EXTRACTS/TINCTURES*: ½ to 1 teaspoon three times daily
> CAPSULES/TABLETS: 2 capsules three times daily

ACUTE PROBLEMS are sudden, reaching a crisis and needing quick attention. Examples of acute problems include toothaches, migraines, bleeding, burns, and sudden onset of cold or flu. Follow these guidelines for treating acute health problems.

> TEA: ¼ to ½ cup served throughout the day, up to 3 to 4 cups
> EXTRACTS/TINCTURES*: ¼ to ½ teaspoon every 30 to 60 minutes until symptoms subside
> CAPSULES/TABLETS: 1 capsule every hour until symptoms subside

*Includes syrups and elixirs

HOW MUCH IS A DROP?

Have you ever been frustrated by a recipe that provides one type of measurement only? Here are some basic conversions to keep in mind:

Teaspoons	Dropperfuls	Milliliters
¼	1 (35 drops)	1
½	2.5 (88 drops)	2.5
1	5 (175 drops)	5

herbal teas

Herbal teas remain my favorite way of using herbs medicinally. The mere act of making tea and drinking it involves you in the healing process and, I suspect, awakens an innate ability for self-healing in the body. Though medicinal teas are generally not as potent or as active as tinctures and other concentrated herbal remedies, they are the most effective medicines for chronic, long-term imbalances.

The making of herbal tea is a fine art, but it is also blessedly simple. If you've never cooked a thing in your life, trust me, you can make a good cup of medicinal tea. All you really need is a quart jar with a tight-fitting lid, the selected herbs, and water that has reached the boiling point.

Herbal teas can be drunk hot, at room temperature, or iced. They can be made into ice cubes with fresh fruit and flowers and used to flavor festive holiday punches. They're delicious blended with fruit juice and frozen as pops for children.

Once brewed, an herbal tea should be stored in the refrigerator. Left at room temperature for several hours, it will go "flat," get tiny bubbles in it, and begin to sour. Stored in the refrigerator, an herbal tea is good for 3 to 4 days.

I seldom direct people to make medicinal teas by the cupful. It is impractical and time consuming. Instead, make a quart of tea each morning or in the evening after work. The herb-to-water ratio varies, depending on the quality of herbs used, whether they are fresh or dried (use twice as much fresh herb in a recipe), and how strong you wish the finished tea to be, though I generally use 1 to 3 tablespoons of herb(s) for each cup of water, or 4 to 8 tablespoons of herb per quart of water, depending on the herb.

For a medicinal tea to be effective, it must be administered in small amounts several times daily. For chronic problems, serve the tea three or four times daily. For acute ailments such as colds, fevers, and headaches, take several small sips every 30 minutes until the symptoms subside. Use the dosage chart on page 379 as a guideline for amounts.

Infusions

Infusions are made from the more delicate parts of the plant, including the leaves, flowers, and aromatic parts. These fragile plant parts must be steeped, rather than simmered, because they give up their medicinal properties more easily than do the tougher roots and barks.

To make an infusion, simply boil 1 quart of water per ounce of herb (or 1 cup of water to 1 tablespoon of herb). Pour water over the herb(s) and let steep for 30 to 60 minutes. The proportion of water to herb and the required time to infuse varies greatly, depending on the herb. Start out with the above proportions and then experiment. The more herb you use and the longer you let it steep, the stronger the brew. Let your taste buds and your senses guide you.

Decoctions

Decoctions are made from the more tenacious parts of the plant, such as the roots, bark, and seeds. It's a little harder to extract the constituents from these parts, so a slow simmer (or an overnight infusion) is often required.

To make a decoction, place the herbs in a small saucepan and cover with cold water. Heat slowly and simmer, covered, for 20 to 45 minutes. The longer you simmer the herbs, the stronger the tea will be.

Solar and Lunar Infusions

Have you ever considered using the light of the moon or the sun for extracting the healing properties of the herbs? It's one of my favorite methods for making herbal tea. Sometimes after I've prepared a tea on my kitchen stove, I'll place it in the moonlight or sunlight to pick up some of the rays of these giant luminaries. We are children of the sky as well as the earth; using the energies of the stars and moon and sun in our healing work adds a special touch.

To make solar tea, place the herbs and the water in a glass jar with a tight-fitting lid. Set it directly in the hot sunlight for several hours.

To make lunar tea, place the herbs and the water in an open container (unless there are lots of night-flying bugs around!) and position it directly in the path of the moonlight. Lunar tea is subtle and magical; it is whispered that fairies love to drink it.

If you wish to have a particularly potent tea, prepare it first as an infusion or a decoction as directed above, then allow the sun or the moon to work its magic.

using a coffee press

A French coffee press is great for making medicinal teas, but don't use the same one for coffee and herbs; the flavors will mingle. Cover the spout of the press with a towel to prevent the steam from escaping; it will carry away many of the vital medicinal properties.

syrups

Syrups are the yummiest of all herbal preparations. They are delicious, concentrated extracts of the herbs cooked into a sweet medicine with the addition of honey and/or fruit juice. Maple syrup and vegetable glycerin may be substituted for honey.

Although there is more than one method for making an herbal syrup, I have been using this technique for many years, and it makes excellent syrups, time after time.

Step 1. Use 2 ounces of herb mixture to 1 quart of water. Over low heat, simmer the liquid down to 1 pint. This will give you a very concentrated tea.

Step 2. Strain the herbs from the liquid. Pour the liquid back into the pot.

Step 3. To each pint of liquid, add 1 cup of honey (or other sweetener, such as maple syrup, vegetable glycerin, or brown sugar). Most recipes call for 2 cups of sweetener (a 1:1 ratio of sweetener to liquid). I find this far too sweet for my taste, but the added sugar helped preserve the syrup in the days when refrigeration wasn't common.

Step 4. Warm the honey and the liquid together only enough to mix well. Most recipes instruct you to cook the honey and the tea together for 20 to 30 minutes over high heat to thicken further. It certainly does make thicker syrup, but I'd rather not cook the living enzymes out of the honey.

Step 5. When the syrup is thoroughly mixed, you may wish to add a fruit concentrate to flavor, or a couple of drops of essential oil, such as peppermint or spearmint, or a small amount of brandy to help preserve the syrup and to aid as a relaxant in cough formulas.

Step 6. Remove from the heat, bottle, and label. Syrups will last for several weeks, even months, if refrigerated.

herbal candy

Far more delightful than tinctures or pills are these delicious medicinal "candies." You can mix just about any herbal formula this way. By carefully measuring the amount of herbs and the number of balls you make, you can calculate fairly accurately an appropriate daily dosage.

Step 1. Grind raisins, dates, apricots, and walnuts in a food processor or grinder. Alternatively, you can mix nut butter (such as peanut, almond, or cashew) with honey (or maple syrup, rice syrup, or maple cream) in equal portions.

Step 2. Stir in shredded coconut and carob powder.

Step 3. Add powdered herbs. Mix well.

Step 4. Roll the mixture into balls. Roll again in powdered carob or coconut. Store in the refrigerator, where they will keep for several weeks.

infused oils

Herbal oils are easy to make, and they can be used on their own or as a base for salves and ointments. By using different combinations of herbs and oils, you can make either strong medicinal oils or sweet-scented massage oils. Though any good-quality vegetable oil will do, the oil of choice for medicine is olive; there is no finer oil for this purpose.

Stored in a cool, dark location, herbal oils will last for several months, sometimes years.

Making Solar-infused Oils

Place the herbs and the oil in a glass jar; cover tightly. Place the jar in a warm, sunny spot and let steep for 2 weeks. Strain the oil through cheesecloth or muslin. When the oil has been poured off, put the herbs in the cheesecloth or muslin and wring thoroughly, squeezing every last drop of the precious oil from the plant material. Then add a fresh batch of herbs to the oil and infuse for 2 more weeks. Strain again. This will give you a very potent medicinal oil.

when good oils go bad

If your herbal oil grows mold, there is either too much water content in the herb or moisture in the jar. Use dry herbs or wilt the herbs before using. Be absolutely certain the container is completely dry. Check the lid for moisture; it is often the culprit.

Using the Double Boiler Method

Although it doesn't provide the magical benefits of sunlight, this is a quick and simple method that makes beautiful oil.

Place the herbs and the oil in a double boiler and bring to a low simmer. Slowly heat for 30 to 60 minutes, checking frequently to be sure the oil is not overheating. The lower the heat, the longer the infusion, the better the oil.

Strain the oil through cheesecloth or muslin. When the oil has been poured off, put the herbs in the cheesecloth or muslin and wring thoroughly, squeezing every last drop of the precious oil from the plant material.

salves and ointments

Once you've made herbal oil, you're a step away from a salve. Salves and ointments (basically different terms for the same product) are made of beeswax, herbs, and vegetable (or animal) oil. The oil is used as a solvent for the medicinal properties of the herb and provides a healing, emollient base. The beeswax also adds a soothing, protective quality and provides the firmness necessary to form the salve. Some people recommend adding natural preservatives to the

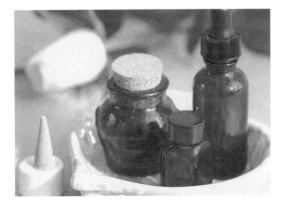

mixture, such as vitamin E or tincture of benzoin, but I've never found it necessary or any more effective.

Step 1. Prepare an infused oil following the instructions above. Strain.

Step 2. To each cup of herbal oil, add ¼ cup of beeswax. Heat until the beeswax is completely melted. To check for consistency, place 1 tablespoon of the mixture in the freezer for just a minute or two. If it's too soft, add more beeswax; if too hard, add more oil.

Step 3. Remove from heat immediately and pour into small glass jars or tins. Store any extra salve in a cool, dark place. Stored properly, salves will last for months, even years.

tinctures

Tinctures are concentrated liquid extracts of herbs. They are very potent and are taken by the dropperful, most often diluted in warm water or juice. Because they are so concentrated, they should be administered carefully and sparingly, following the dosage guidelines on page 379.

Most tinctures are made with alcohol as the primary solvent or extractant. Though the amount of alcohol is very small, many people choose not to use alcohol-based tinctures, for a variety of sound reasons. Effective tinctures can be made with vegetable glycerin or apple cider vinegar as the solvent. Though they may not be as strong as alcohol-based preparations, they do work and are preferred for children and people who are sensitive to alcohol.

If you use alcohol as your tincture solvent, it should be 80 to 100 proof, such as vodka, gin, or brandy. Half of the proof number is the percentage of alcohol in the spirits: 80 proof brandy is 40 percent alcohol; 100 proof vodka is 50 percent alcohol.

There are several methods used to make tinctures, but the traditional or simpler's method is the one I prefer. Herbs, the menstruum (alcohol, vinegar, or glycerin base), and a jar with a tight-fitting lid are all that you need. This extremely simple system produces a beautiful tincture every time.

Step 1. Chop your herbs finely. I recommend using fresh herbs whenever possible. High-quality dried herbs will work well also, but one of the advantages of tincturing is the ability to preserve the fresh attributes of the plant. Place the herbs in a clean, dry jar.

Step 2. Pour in enough of the menstruum to cover the herbs, and continue pouring until the liquid rises 2 or 3 inches above the herbs. The herbs need to be completely submersed. Cover with a tight-fitting lid.

Note: If you are using vegetable glycerin, dilute it with an equal amount of water before pouring it over the herbs. If you are using vinegar, warm it first.

removing alcohol from tinctures

Some of the alcohol in tinctures can be removed by placing the tincture in boiling water for 1 to 2 minutes. This method removes only about 50 percent of the alcohol; some alcohol always remains.

Step 3. Place the jar in a warm location and let the herbs and liquid soak (macerate) for 4 to 6 weeks — the longer, the better.

Step 4. Shake the bottle daily during the maceration period. This not only prevents the herbs from packing down on the bottom of the jar, but also is an invitation for some of the old magic to come back into medicine making. During the shaking process, you can sing to your tincture jars, stir them in the moonlight or the sunlight, wave feathers over them — whatever your imagination and intuition inspires.

Step 5. Strain the herbs from the menstruum using a large stainless-steel strainer lined with cheesecloth or muslin. Reserve the liquid, which is now a potent tincture, and compost the herbs. Rebottle and label. Store out of the reach of children in a cool, dark location, where the tincture will keep almost indefinitely.

herbal liniments

An herbal liniment is made in exactly the same way as a tincture; however, a liniment, which uses rubbing alcohol or witch hazel as its solvent, is for external purposes. Liniments are made either for disinfectant purposes or to soothe sore, inflamed muscles. Be sure to label liniment bottles FOR EXTERNAL USE ONLY.

herb powders

Powdered herbs are simple, effective medicines. They are an excellent way to administer bitter herbs to children, because the flavor usually can be masked. It is also easy to regulate the dosage of the herbs being used. Sprinkle herb powders on food and drinks for a tasty and nutritious treat. Mix them into honey to form a paste. Try blending them in blender drinks. Powders can also be combined with dried fruits, honey, and carob powder to make candy balls, a favorite herbal remedy for young and old alike. I especially like herbal powders added to soups and sprinkled in stir-fries.

Fine herb powders are available commercially, but you can also powder most dried herbs at home in an electric coffee grinder. However, for taste purposes, use separate grinders for your herbs and your coffee. Powdered herbs do not have as long a shelf life as whole herbs, so powder only about ¼ to ½ cup at a time, and store them

in airtight glass containers in a dark, cool area or in the refrigerator. Herbal powders can be mixed and matched as needed.

herbal capsules and pills

Herbal capsules and pills are simple to make and quick and easy to take. There are many ready-made herbal capsules available commercially, but until recently, I seldom recommended them, because they were generally of such poor quality. The herbs they contained were often "purified" by being heated to excesses of 200°F, losing many of their vital constituents in the process. The capsules themselves were made of gelatin, which is difficult to digest and leaves a gummy residue, not to mention that it's also a by-product of the slaughter industry.

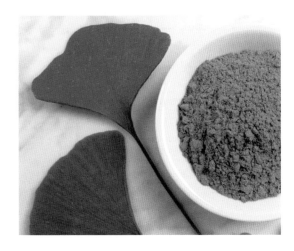

But there has been a transformation in the capsule industry. Veggie caps have recently become widely available. Plant based, these capsules dissolve quickly and are completely digestible. New cryogenic grinders powder the herbs at subzero temperatures, allowing the plant mixture to retain all of its valuable constituents. The powdered plants smell and taste fresh and are of very good quality. When buying capsules, buy from those companies that have gone to the extra trouble to ensure the quality of the product.

You can easily make your own herbal capsules by placing powdered herbs in size 00 capsules (available at health food stores and pharmacies) and then joining the two sides. This process is time consuming. The primary advantages of making your own herbal capsules are that you can customize your herb blend formula and be assured of the quality of the product you're using.

You can formulate recipes for herbal pills — without capsules — that are easy to make, taste good, and work effectively. Just follow the simple steps below.

Step 1. Place the powdered herbs in a bowl and moisten with enough water and honey or maple syrup to make a sticky paste.

Step 2. Add a tiny drop of essential oil, such as peppermint or wintergreen, and mix well.

Step 3. Thicken with carob powder, adding just enough to form a smooth paste. Knead until smooth, like the texture of bread dough.

Step 4. Roll the dough into small balls the size of pills. You can roll again in carob powder for a finished look.

Step 5. Place on a cookie sheet and dry in a very low oven or in the sun. These pills, once dried, will store indefinitely.

Note: I often store pill dough, undried and unrolled, in the refrigerator in a glass jar with a tight-fitting lid, and roll out pills as I need them. It's very unprofessional, I know, but it saves time and is just as effective.

herbal baths

Herbal baths are deeply relaxing. They help take the edge off the day, calm and quiet the mind, encourage deep sleep, and sometimes are just the comfort one needs in a rough and busy world. And aside from your bed, your bathtub may be the most sensuously arousing place in your home, perhaps yet undiscovered.

Several prominent healers administer most of their herbal formulas via the bath. Depending on the herbs you use and the temperature of the water, you can create a bath that is relaxing, stimulating, uplifting, soothing, decongesting, or otherwise curative. Herbal baths open up the pores of the skin, our largest organ of elimination and assimilation.

Herbal bathing used to be far more popular than it is today. But as with so many other things in our busy lives, efficiency has won out over quietude, and the quick "in and out" of showers has replaced the slow, peaceful nature of bathing. Perhaps this is simply because modern bathtubs tend to be so small and shallow. A hot herbal bath is definitely not relaxing if half of you is sticking out of the tub, freezing! You might consider investing in an old-style claw foot tub — it's well worth it.

The temperature of the water will affect the healing quality of the bath. Cool to tepid water is excellent for lowering a fever or normalizing the system. A warm bath is relaxing and soothing to the nervous system. Cold water is stimulating and contracting and will firm and strengthen the entire system if you're brave enough to endure it.

To make an herbal bath, use 3 to 4 ounces of herb per tub. Use the herbs to make an extra-strong herbal tea; strain and add the tea to the bathwater. Alternatively, bundle the mixed herbs in a large cotton scarf or clean nylon stocking and tie it directly onto the nozzle of the tub. Run hot water through the herbal bundle until the tub is half filled, then toss the bundle in the tub and adjust the temperature with cold water. Soak in the bath for 20 to 30 minutes to enjoy the full benefits of the herbs.

Hand baths and footbaths are also wonderful ways to take advantage of the healing power of herbs. All of the nerves in the body pass through the feet and the hands, making them a map of our inner being. Simply choose an appropriate-sized container and adjust the proportion of herbs to water accordingly.

essential oils and the bath

Pure essential oils can enhance the bathing experience enormously. Lavender oil is divine in the bath, creating a lasting relaxing feeling. When I travel, which I often do, lavender oil accompanies me like a steady friend. After a long day of traveling, it is a welcome addition to the bathwater and always, always, brings a sense of calm.

However, be extremely cautious when adding essential oils to the bathwater. I hate to admit it, but my first marriage ended because of a peppermint oil bath! My dear ex-husband, very ill and feverish, stepped into a therapeutic bath to which I had inadvertently added peppermint instead of eucalyptus oil. The poor innocent let out a squeal that I remember to this day. I always like to remind him that he was, after all, well the next day, but he insists that he just never again dared to let me know when he was not feeling well.

resources

Thankfully, herbs and herbal products are now widely available. I generally suggest purchasing herbal products from local sources, as it helps support bioregional herbalism and community-based herbalists. However, here are some of my favorite sources for high-quality herbs and herbal products.

MAIL-ORDER HERBS
Frontier Herbs
P.O. Box 299
Norway, IA 52318
800-669-3275; fax: 800-717-4372
Web site: www.frontiercoop.com
A giant list of supplies and herbs. Frontier is a wholesale supplier but offers price breaks for individuals.

Healing Spirits
9198 Route 415
Avoca, NY 14809
607-566-2701
One of the best sources in the Northeast of ethically wildcrafted and organically grown herbs.

Jean's Greens
119 Sulphur Springs Road
Newport, NY 13416
315-845-6500; fax: 315-845-6501
Web site: www.jeansgreens.com
Fresh and dried organic and wildcrafted herbs.

Mountain Rose Herbs
85472 Dilley Lane
Eugene, OR 97405
800-879-3337; fax: 510-217-4012
Web site: www.mountainrose
  herbs.com
A small herbal emporium.

Trinity Herbs
P.O. Box 1001
Graton, CA 95444
707-824-2040
A small wholesale company that sells bulk herbs in quantities of one pound or more.

Wild Weeds
233 Red Rock Lane
Fieldbrook, CA 95519
800-553-9453
Web site: www.wildweeds.com
Organically grown herbs and cosmetic ingredients; catalog available.

Zack Woods Herb Farm
278 Meade Road
Hyde Park, VT 05655
802-888-7278
Owned and operated by Rosemary's daughter Melanie and her husband, Jeff, Zack Woods supplies some of the finest organic dried herbs available.

MAIL-ORDER HERBAL PRODUCTS
Avena Botanicals
219 Mill Street
Rockport, ME 04856
207-594-0694
Web site: www.avenaherbs.com
A range of organic herbal products.

Empowered Herbals
3481 Myers Lane
St. James City, FL 33956
Supplier of my favorite "green drink" made from spirulina.

Equinox Botanicals
33446 McCumber Road
Rutland, OH 45775
740-742-2548
This small country business has been producing handmade, high-quality products for more than 20 years.

Herb Pharm
Box 116
Williams, OR 97544
800-348-4372; fax: 800-545-7392
Web site: www.herb-pharm.com
A comprehensive line of high-quality tinctures.

Herbalist and Alchemist
51 South Wandling Avenue
Washington, NJ 07882
800-611-8235; fax: 908-689-9071
Web site: www.herbalist-
  alchemist.com
A full line of Western and Chinese herbs and formulations.

Liberty Natural Products
8120 S.E. Stark Street
Portland, OR 97215
800-289-8427; fax: 503-256-1182
Web site: www.libertynatural.com
Offers a variety of herbal extracts,
essential oils, and natural products.

Sage Mountain Herb Products
P.O. Box 6091
Holliston, MA 01746
(508) 429-5265
Founded by Rosemary's daughters,
Melanie and Jennifer, and purchased
by a former apprentice. Features
Rosemary's favorite formulas.

Simpler's Botanical Company
P.O. Box 2534
Sebastopol, CA 95473
800-652-7646
Web site: www.simplers.com
Herbal products from the California
School of Herbal Studies. Offers qual-
ity herbal extracts, essential oils, and
aromatherapy products.

Woodland Essence
392 Tea Cup Street
Cold Brook, NY 13324
315-845-1515
Web site: www.woodland
  essence.com
An incredible array of flower essences.

EDUCATIONAL RESOURCES
American Herb Association
P.O. Box 1673
Nevada City, CA 95959
530-265-9552; fax: 520-274-3140
Web site: www.jps.net/ahaherb
Complete listings of schools, programs,
seminars, and correspondence courses
offered throughout the United States.

American Herbalists Guild
1931 Gaddis Road
Canton, GA 30115
770-751-6021; fax: 770-751-7472
Web site: www.american
  herbalist.com
The only national organization for pro-
fessional, peer-reviewed herbal practi-
tioners. Offers a directory of members.

**The California School
of Herbal Studies**
P.O. Box 39
Forestville, CA 95436
707-887-7457
Web site: www.cshs.com
One of the oldest herb schools in the
United States, founded by Rosemary
Gladstar in 1978.

Herb Research Foundation
1007 Pearl Street, Suite 200
Boulder, CO 80302
303-449-2265; fax: 303-449-7849
Web site: www.herbs.org
A clearinghouse for herb information.
Offers an excellent newsletter.

**Rocky Mountain Center for
Botanical Studies**
2639 Spruce Street
Boulder, CO 80302
303-442-6861; fax: 303-442-6294
Web site: www.herbschool.com
Offers excellent programs for beginners,
as well as advanced clinical training
programs.

**Sage Mountain Retreat Center and
Botanical Sanctuary**
P.O. Box 420
East Barre, VT 05649
Apprentice programs and classes with
Rosemary Gladstar and other well-
known herbalists.

**The Science and Art of Herbalism:
A Home Study Course by
Rosemary Gladstar**
P.O. Box 420
East Barre, VT 05649
The Science and Art of Herbalism was
written in an inspiring and joyful man-
ner for students wishing a systematic, in-
depth study of herbs. The course
emphasizes the foundations of herbalism,
wildcrafting, earth awareness, and herbal
preparation and formulation. The heart
of the course is the development of a deep
personal relationship with the plant
world.

index

Page numbers in *italics* indicate recipes; those in **bold** indicate photographs.

photograph credits

United Plant Savers

United Plant Savers (UpS), a nonprofit organization formed by Rosemary Gladstar and other herbalists in 1994, is dedicated to the conservation and cultivation of endangered native medicinal plants. Indiscriminate harvesting, deforestation, and urbanization have devastated many of the areas where herbs grow in the wild, and North American medicinal plants are being exported in huge quantities to countries whose native plants have already been depleted. The creators of UpS believe that though it's exciting to see the ever-growing demand for herbs, this demand can negatively impact many plant populations.

The mission of UpS is to protect native medicinal plants of the United States and Canada and their native habitat while ensuring an abundant, renewable supply of these plants for generations to come. The creators and members recognize that environmentally responsible cultivation, land stewardship, habitat protection, and sustainable wild harvesting are critical to the sustainability of herbal medicine.

As part of their work, members of UpS have compiled an "at risk" and a "to watch" list of herbs that are endangered in their natural environment. Plants on the "to watch" list have been proposed for inclusion on the "at risk" list but warrant further research. In some cases, these plants are abundant in one bioregion and rare in others.

For more information about United Plant Savers, or to become a member, write to UpS, P.O. Box 98, East Barre, VT 05649.

"AT RISK" LIST

American ginseng (*Panax quinquefolius*)
Black cohosh (*Cimicifuga racemosa*)
Bloodroot (*Sanguinaria canadensis*)
Blue cohosh (*Caulophyllum thalictroides*)
Echinacea (*Echinacea* spp.)
Eyebright (*Euphrasia* spp.)
Goldenseal (*Hydrastis canadensis*)
Helonias root (*Chamaelirium luteum*)
Kava-kava (*Piper methysticum*)
Lady's slipper orchid (*Cypripedium* spp.)
Lomatium (*Lomatium dissectum*)
Osha (*Ligusticum* spp.; esp. *L. porteri*)
Peyote (*Lophophora williamsii*)
Slippery elm (*Ulmus rubra*)
Sundew (*Drosera* spp.)
Trillium (*Trillium* spp.)
True unicorn (*Aletris farinosa*)
Venus fly trap (*Dionaea muscipula*)
Virginia snakeroot (*Aristolochia serpentaria*)
Wild yam (*Dioscorea* spp.; esp. *D. villosa*)

"TO WATCH" LIST

Arnica (*Arnica* spp.)
Butterfly weed/pleurisy root (*Asclepias tuberosa*)
Calamus (*Acorus calamus*)
Cascara sagrada (*Rhamnus purshiana*)
Chaparro (*Castela emoryi*)
Elephant tree (*Bursera microphylla*)
Gentian (*Gentiana* spp.)
Goldthread (*Coptis* spp.)
Lobelia (*Lobelia* spp.)
Maidenhair fern (*Adiantum pendatum*)
Mayapple (*Podophyllum peltatum*)
Oregon grape (*Mahonia* spp.)
Partridge berry (*Mitchella repens*)
Pink root (*Spigelia marilandica*)
Pipsissewa (*Chimaphila umbellata*)
Spikenard (*Aralia racemosa, A.californica*)
Stillingia (*Stillingia sylvatica*)
Stone root (*Collinsonia canadensis*)
Stream orchid (*Epipactis gigantea*)
Turkey corn (*Dicentra canadensis*)
White sage (*Salvia apiana*)
Wild indigo (*Baptisia tinctoria*)
Yerba mansa (*Anemopsis californica*)
Yerba santa (*Eriodictyon californica*)